GENE THERAPEUTICS
Methods and Applications of
Direct Gene Transfer

GENE THERAPEUTICS
Methods and Applications of Direct Gene Transfer

Jon A. Wolff
Editor

Foreword by James F. Crow

92 Illustrations with some color art

Birkhäuser
Boston • Basel • Berlin

Jon A. Wolff
University of Wisconsin Medical School
Departments of Pediatrics, Medical Genetics, and Neurology
Waisman Center, Room 607
1500 Highland Avenue
Madison, WI 53705-2208
USA

Library of Congress Cataloging-in-Publication Data

Gene therapeutics: methods and applications of direct gene transfer / Jon A. Wolff, editor; foreword
by James F. Crow.
    p. cm.
    Includes bibliographical references and index.
    ISBN 0-8176-3650-1 (h: acid-free). — ISBN 3-7643-3650-1 (h: acid-free)
    1. Gene therapy. I. Wolff, Jon A. (Jon Asher), 1956– .
    [DNLM: 1. Gene Therapy—methods. 2. Transfection—methods. QW 51 G3256 1993]
    RB155.8.G46 1993
    616.042—dc20
    DNLM/DLC   93-42919
    for Library of Congress   CIP

Printed on acid-free paper.   *Birkhäuser*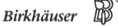

ISBN 0-8176-3650-1
ISBN 3-7643-3650-1

Camera-ready copy prepared by the editor and formatted using Aldus PageMaker®
Printed and bound by Quinn-Woodbine, Inc., Woodbine, New Jersey
Printed in the United States of America

9 8 7 6 5 4 3 2

To my wife Katalin,
for her understanding and inspiration.

Contents

III APPLICATIONS

Foreword

During the first half century of genetics, coinciding with the first half of this century, geneticists dreamt of the repair of genetic disease by altering or replacing defective genes. H. J. Muller wrote of the great advantages of mutations, "nanoneedles" in his apt term, for delicately probing physiological and chemical processes. In the same spirit, genes could be used to provide treatments of needle point delicacy. Yet, during this period no realistic possibility appeared; it remained but a dream.

The situation changed abruptly at the half century. Microbial genetics and its offshoot, cell culture genetics, provided the route. Pneumococcus transformation showed that exogenous DNA could become a permanent part of the genome; yet attempts to reproduce this in animals produced a few tantalizing hints of success, but mostly failures. Transduction, using a virus as mediator, offered a better opportunity. The first reproducible in vivo gene therapy in a whole animal came in 1981. This was in Drosophila, with a transposable element as carrier. Flies were "cured" of a mutant eye color by incorporation of the normal allele, and the effect was transmissible, foreshadowing not only somatic, but germ line gene therapy.

At the same time, retroviruses carrying human genes were found to be extremely efficient in transferring their contents to the chromosomes of cultured cells. The viruses were simply doing what comes naturally and, as Dunckley and Dickson point out in this book, this activity seems not to be impaired by carrying all but the largest genes. By this time it was apparent that gene therapy would be developed; it was only a matter of time.

Gene therapy will be of greatest value, at least in the easily foreseeable future, for specific monogenic diseases. These, of course, are a small fraction of genetic disease, and a still smaller fraction of all disease. But it is an important fraction, because many of these diseases cause severe lifetime impairments, miserable for the person, distressing for the family, and expensive for society.

The technological advances that facilitate gene therapy will also lead to better treatments of other kinds. And they will lead to diagnosis at successively earlier ages, with corresponding ease of removing defective embryos. As with medicine in general, prevention is better than cure. Ironically, as it becomes increasingly effective, gene therapy may become of lesser importance. Ideally we would have

one generation of treatment for those diseases already existing, followed by prevention of new ones.

How useful will gene therapy be for complex, polygenic disease? This will be
much more difficult, although a high-resolution physical and linkage map will aid
in the discovery of the more important individual components. There are grounds
for optimism, as several articles in this volume attest.

For many monogenic diseases the time for gene therapy is here. Clinical
trials are underway. Ethical doubts have been properly raised, but are of decreasing intensity as well thought-out protocols provide more predictable and safer re-
lief for drastic disease. The humanitarian value of eliminating Duchenne muscular
dystrophy, in my view, strongly outweighs any slippery-slope fears. I cheer the
day that all existing Duchenne disease genes become extinct and we have ways of
early detection of new mutations.

Practical applications of molecular biology have been slow in coming, surprisingly slow, but they are making up for this by an explosive growth now. The
dream at the beginning of the century will become the reality at its end. How
different this fin de siècle is from the last, though perhaps not in spirit.

James F. Crow

Preface

The best theories are usually those that explain much in simple terms. There is a certain beauty to such ideas. Physicists in search of a "theory of everything," for example, like to admire the aesthetic qualities of their theoretical constructs.

The reasoning behind gene therapy is attractive for this very reason. It is simple: if a genetic disease is caused by a dysfunctioning gene, then the disease state can be corrected by giving the patient the normal, functioning gene.

Although gene therapy was initially formulated to treat single gene defects, it now holds promise for a wide range of disorders, including cancer, heart disease, and degenerative neurologic disorders. Potentially, it could be a "treatment of everything," or at least of many things.

Initial attempts at gene therapy involved the genetic modification of cells in culture, which were then transplanted back into the body. This is known as an indirect, or *ex vivo*, approach. The focus of this book is the simpler, *in vivo* approach that involves the direct introduction of genes into the body without cell transplantation.

The direct approach resembles conventional pharmaceutical delivery methods and promises to be much less expensive than the indirect, *ex vivo* approaches. There is a certain elegance to its simplicity.

Of course, patients care only for alleviation of their disease. They are concerned with risk versus benefit ratios, not with the aesthetics of the theoretical underpinnings of their treatment. Only the results of clinical trials will enable us to judge the clinical value of direct gene therapeutics. However, the tremendous progress reported in this book suggests that this approach has a very promising future.

The book is divided into three sections. The first provides a scientific background for the concepts involved in gene therapy that include a history of previous experiments, and the production of mouse genetic models. The basic tenets of expression are explored in one chapter that addresses transcription and another chapter that addresses the post-transcriptional elements of expression. The second section covers the spectacular new methodologies and how these systems work. The methods include naked DNA, oligonucleotides, calcium phosphate precipitation, polylysine-complexes, adenovirus-polylysine DNA complexes, liposomes, electroporation, and particle bombardment. The third section covers applications for specific organs and diseases. They encompass gene delivery to the CNS skeletal muscle, heart, liver, lung, thyroid and joints. Applications for cardiovascular disease, brain tumors, immunization, arthritis, cystic fibrosis, and Duchenne muscular dystrophy are discussed. Pharmacokinetic considerations are also covered in the chapter by Fred Ledley.

Jon A. Wolff

Contributors

Julie K. Andersen, Division of Neurogerontology, Ethel Percy Andrus Gereontology Center, 3715 McClintock Avenue, University of Southern California, Los Angeles, California 90080-0191, USA

Eliav Barr, Department of Medicine, University of Chicago, 5841 South Maryland Avenue, Chicago, Illinois 60637, USA

R. Michael Blaese, Cellulaur Immunology Section, Metabolism Branch, National Cancer Institute, National Institutes of Health, Building 10, Room 6B05, Bethesda, Maryland 20892, USA

Xandra O. Breakefield, Neuroscience Center, Massachusetts General Hospital, East, Building 149, 13th Street, Charlestown, Massachusetts 02129, USA

Gary Brewer, Department of Microbiology & Immunology, Bowman Gray School of Medicine, Medical Center Boulevard, Winston-Salem, North Carolina 27157-1064, USA

Patricia L. Chang, Department of Pediatrics, McMaster University, 1200 Main Street West, Hamilton, Ontario, Canada L8N 3Z5

Liang Cheng, Institute of Pathology, Case Western Reserve School of Medicine, University Hospitals of Cleveland, 2085 Adelbert Road, Cleveland, Ohio 44106, USA

E. Antonio Chiocca, Neuroscience Center, Massachusetts General Hospital - East, Building 149, 13th Street, Charlestown, Massachusetts 02129, USA

Henry C. Chiou, TargeTech, Inc., 290 Pratt Street, Meriden, Connecticut 06450, USA

James F. Crow, Professor Emeritus of Genetics, Genetics Department, University of Wisconsin, Madison, Wisconsin 53706, USA

Kenneth W. Culver, Human Gene Therapy Research Institute, Iowa Methodist Medical Center, 1415 Woodland Avenue, Suite 218, Des Moines, Iowa 50309, USA

David Curiel, University of Alabama at Birmingham, 1824 6th Avenue South, Lurleen B. Wallace Tumor Institute, Room 620, Birmingham, Alabama 35294-3300, USA

Neal A. DeLuca, Department of Molecular Genetics & Biochemistry, University of Pittsburgh, W1152 Biomedical Science Tower, Pittsburgh, Pennsylvania 15261, USA

Carolyn DeLuna, Agracetus, Inc., 8520 University Green, Middelton, Wisconsin 53562, USA

George Dickson, Department of Experimental Pathology, Guy's Hospital, London Bridge, London SE1 9RT, United Kingdom

Martin E. Dowty, The Procter and Gamble Company, Miami Valley Laboratories, P.O. Box 398707, Cincinnati, Ohio 45239-8707, USA

Matthew G. Dunckley, Department of Experimental Pathology, Guy's Hospital, London Bridge, London SE1 9RT, United Kingdom

Christopher H. Evans, The Ferguson Laboratory, Department of Orthopedic Surgery, University of Pittsburgh School of Medicine, Pittsburgh, Pennsylvania 15261, USA

Mark A. Findeis, TargeTech, Inc., 290 Pratt Street, Meriden, Connecticut 06450, USA

David J. Fink, Department of Neurology & VA Medical Center, University of Michigan Medical School, Ann Arbor, Michigan 48109-0618, USA

Stephen Furs, Department of Medicine, University of Connecticut School of Medicine, Farmington, Connecticut 06030, USA

Joseph C. Glorioso, Department of Molecular Genetics & Biochemistry, University of Pittsburgh, E1246 Biomedical Science Tower, Pittsburgh, Pennsylvania 15261, USA

William F. Goins, Department of Molecular Genetics & Biochemistry, University of Pittsburgh, E1251, Biomedical Science Tower, Pittsburgh, Pennsylvania 15261, USA

Leaf Huang, Department of Pharmacology, University of Pittsburgh School of Medicine, West 1351 Biomedical Science Tower, Pittsburgh, Pennsylvania 15261-2071, USA

Vadim A. Klenchin, University of Wisconsin, Laboratory of Molecular Biology, 1525 Linden Drive, Madison, Wisconsin 53706, USA

Joshua Lederberg, Rockefeller University, 1230 York Avenue, Suite 400, New York, New York 10021-6341, USA

Fred D. Ledley, Gene Medicine, Inc., 8080 North Stadium Drive, Houston, Texas 77054, **and** Departments of Cell Biology and Pediatrics, Baylor College of Medicine, One Baylor Plaza, Houston, Texas 77030, USA

Jeffrey M. Leiden, Department of Medicine and Pathology, Section of Cardiology, University of Chicago, MC 6080, 5841 South Maryland Avenue, Chicago, Illinois 60637, USA

Robert L. Martuza, Department of Neurosurgery, Georgetown University Medical Center, 3800 Reservoir Road N.W., Washington, DC 20007, USA

J. David McDonald, The Wichita State University, Department of Biological Sciences, 1845 Fairmount, Box 26, Wichita, Kansas 67260-0026, USA

June R. Merwin, TargeTech, Inc., 290 Pratt Street, Meriden, Connecticut 06450, USA

Elizabeth G. Nabel, Associate Professor of Internal Medicine, Interim Director, Cardiovascular Research Center, The University of Michigan, 1150 W. Medical Center Drive, 3560 MSRB II, Ann Arbor, Michigan, 48109-0688, USA

Gary J. Nabel, Associate Investigator, Howard Hughes Medical Institute and Professor, Internal Medicine and Biological Chemistry, The University of Michigan, 1150 W. Medical Center Drive, 4510 MSRB I, Ann Arbor, Michigan 48109-0650, USA

Leonard M. Neckers, Clinical Pharmacology Branch, Building 10, Room 12N22b, National Institutes of Health, National Cancer Institute, Bethesda, Maryland 20892, USA

Michel Perricaudet, Laboratoire de Genetique des Virus Oncogenes (CNRSUA 1301), Institut Gustave Roussy, 39 rue Camille Desmoulins, 94805 Villejuif Cedex, France

Gregory E. Plautz, Assistant Professor, Pediatrics, The University of Michigan, 1150 W. Medical Center Drive, A510C MSRB I, Ann Arbor, Michigan 48109-0684, USA

Paul D. Robbins, Departments of Molecular Genetics and Biochemistry, University of Pittsburgh School of Medicine, Pittsburgh, Pennsylvania 15261, USA

Arun Singhal, Department of Pharmacology, University of Pittsburgh School of Medicine, Biomedical Science Tower, West 1316, Pittsburgh, Pennsylvania 15261-2071, USA

George L. Spitalny, TargeTech, Inc., 290 Pratt Street, Meriden, Connecticut 06450, USA

Leslie D. Stratford-Perricaudet, Laboratoire de Genetique des Virus Oncogenes (CNRSUA 1301), Institut Gustave Roussy, 39 rue Camille Desmoulins, 94805 Villejuif Cedex, France

Sergei I. Sukharev, University of Wisconsin, Laboratory of Molecular Biology, 1525 Linden Drive, Madison, Wisconsin 53706, USA

Yoshiaki Takamiya, Department of Neurosurgery, Georgetown University Medical Center, 3800 Reservoir Road N.W., Washington, DC 20007, USA

Alexander V. Titomirov, Informax, Inc., P.O. Box 2926, Gaithersburg, Maryland 20886, USA

Robert G. Whalen, Institut Pasteur, Département de Biologie Moléculaire, Unité de Biochimie, 25 rue du Dr. Roux, 75724 Paris cedex 15, France

Jon A. Wolff, University of Wisconsin Medical School, Departments of Pediatrics, Medical Genetics and Neurology, Waisman Center, Room 607, 1500 Highland Avenue, Madison, Wisconsin 53705-2208, USA

George Y. Wu, Division of Gastroenterology-Hepatology, University of Connecticut School of Medicine, 263 Farmington Avenue, Farmington, Connecticut 06030, USA

Ning-Sun Yang, Agracetus, Inc., 8520 University Green, Middleton, Wisconsin 53562, USA

Part I

BACKGROUND

A HISTORY OF GENE TRANSFER AND THERAPY

Jon A. Wolff and Joshua Lederberg

INTRODUCTION

"Gene therapy" is generally thought of as a very new concept, but the notion that genes could be manipulated to treat human disease actually goes back several decades. Many of the pioneers of modern genetics realized that their discoveries eventually could lead to medical applications. Some even proposed gene transfer approaches decades ago that are still being explored today.

Perhaps the reason this history is little known is that progress in the science of gene therapy and transfer has been so slow in coming. However, the pace has accelerated in recent years, and many researchers are now embarking on clinical trials of very promising gene therapies. At this point, it seems useful to review the evolution of gene therapy's theoretical underpinnings and thereby gain insights into its medical, scientific, social, ethical, and economic implications. This historical perspective may be particularly useful for evaluation of the "prior art" in patent applications.

Several reviews have discussed some of the more recent advances in gene therapy (Miller, 1992; Friedmann, 1989) and in nonviral gene transfer methods (Felgner, 1990). One of the early proponents for gene therapy has recently reviewed its history (Friedmann, 1992).

GENETIC ENGINEERING

Since ancient times humans have bred animals and plants for specific purposes. We see the fruits of their labors when we eat corn, train a dog, race a horse, or smell a rose. Such selective breeding practices were the forerunners of the modern science of genetics, although the term "genetics" has come into use only relatively recently.

The "International Conference of Hybridization and on the Cross-Breeding of Varieties," held in 1899 in London, later came to be known as the "First International Congress of Genetics" (Crow, 1992). William Bateson suggested the use of the term "genetics" at the Third Congress in 1906. In the interim, H. de Vries and others had rediscovered Mendel's work, which originated the concept of the gene as a unit of hereditary.

Gene Therapeutics: Methods and Applications of Direct Gene Transfer
Jon A. Wolff, Editor • ©1994 *Birkhäuser Boston*

One of the first uses of the term "genetic engineering" was in a paper of that title presented at the "Sixth International Congress of Genetics" held in 1932 in Ithaca, New York (Crow, 1992). The term was used to mean "the application of genetic principles to animal and plant breeding." Nonetheless, Marxist commentators used the term "genetic engineering" for "eugenics" as contrast to the "social engineering" of the USSR (Lederberg, 1973).

THE PHARMACEUTICAL TRADITION

The term "gene therapy," coined in part to distinguish it from the somewhat Orwellian connotations of the term "human genetic engineering," can be defined as "the application of genetic principles to the treatment of human disease." Under this broad definition, the highly successful screening programs for phenylketonuria and Tay-Sachs disease could be included. Even many conventional medical and surgical therapeutic approaches, such as liver transplantation, might fall under this definition because they were founded on an understanding of their genetics and biochemistry, although they do not directly utilize genetic principles.

More specifically, however, the term "gene therapy" combines the concepts of pharmacotherapeutics with genetic principles. It implies the use of a substance to treat the disease state.

In 1878, Langley proposed the concept of the "receptor substance," now known simply as the "receptor" (Goodman, 1975). The hypothesis that interactions between a drug and its receptor are governed by the law of mass action was further developed by A.J. Clark in the 1920's. The molecular understanding of protein function and enzyme action led to development of rational drug design based on targeting the receptor, or active site (Perutz, 1992). Anti-sense and ribozyme gene therapies represent an extension of this concept.

Gene therapy approaches that involve gene addition or gene modification are conceptually similar to protein replacement therapies, such as those for diabetes mellitus and the hemophilias, in that a natural macromolecule of the human body is administered. Transient gene therapy approaches such as the use of artificial mRNA (Wolff, 1990) would also be similar to these protein replacement therapies. However, nontransient gene therapy approaches such as retroviral vectors differ in that the administered gene may be permanently incorporated into the cells' chromosomes. In this sense, gene therapy also resembles surgery, in which a tissue or organ is permanently modified.

THE GENE AS A PHYSICAL ENTITY

Avery, MacLeod, and McCarthy first showed that a gene could be transferred within nucleic acids (Avery, 1944). Their 1944 article begins with a sentence pertinent to gene therapy:

"Biologists have long attempted by chemical means to induce in higher organisms predictable and specific changes which thereafter could be transmitted in series as hereditary characters."

The ability for viruses to transmit genes was first demonstrated in Salmonella (Zinder and Lederberg, 1952). The idea that viral genomes could become a permanent part of cell genomes (i.e., prophages) was first discovered with bacteriophages (Lwoff, 1972; Lederberg, 1956) and then extended to animal viruses. For example, the ability of the Rous Sarcoma Virus to transform cells in culture, which in turn could produce new virus, led to the idea that the viral genes were responsible for the cells' transformation. Further studies of RSV infections in vitro led to the proviral hypothesis (Temin, 1976; Temin, 1971). Other studies demonstrated integration of SV40 viral DNA in SV40-transformed cells (Sambrook, 1968).

Watson and Crick's discovery of the structure of DNA and its implication concerning DNA's function had a revolutionary effect on biology (Watson, 1954). The history of the subsequent discoveries of mRNA and the formulation of the "central dogma" (genetic information flows from DNA to RNA to protein) is described in H. Judson's classic book entitled, "The Eighth Day of Creation" (Judson, 1979).

EARLY SPECULATIONS ON GENE THERAPY

Several key aspects of gene therapy were covered in a talk that Tatum gave in New York on May, 1966 (Tatum, 1966). One, that viruses could be used to transduce genes, is evident in his prediction that,

"Finally, it can be anticipated that viruses will be effectively used for man's benefit, in theoretical studies in somatic-cell genetics and possibly in genetic therapy... We can even be somewhat optimistic on the long-range possibility of therapy by the isolation or design, synthesis, and introduction of new genes into defective cells of particular organs."

He also speculated that since the basis of cancer is altered genes, treatment could be achieved "by modification and regulation of gene activities, or by means of gene repair or replacement." Tatum also anticipated indirect or *ex vivo* approaches towards gene therapy:

"Hence, it can be suggested that the first successful genetic engineering will be done with the patient's own cells, for example, liver cells, grown in culture. The desired new gene will be introduced, by directed mutation, from normal cells of another donor by transduction or by direct DNA transfer. The rare cell with the desired change will then be selected, grown into a mass culture, and reimplanted in the patient's liver. The efficiency of this process and its potentialities may be considerably improved by the synthesis of the desired gene according to the specifications of the genetic code and of the enzyme it determines, by in vitro enzymatic replication of this DNA, and by increasing the effectiveness of DNA uptake and integration by the recipient cells, as we learn more about the factors and conditions affecting these processes."

He was extremely confident that gene therapy would be feasible, given our understanding of the structure and function of genes.

One of us speculated about the possibility of gene therapy in an October 24, 1962 letter to Stanfield Rogers:

"it will only be a matter of time, and perhaps not a long time, before polynucleotide sequences can be grafted by chemical procedures onto a virus DNA."

These ideas were first published by Lederberg in a 1968 article that states,

"an attempt could then be made to transform liver cells of male offspring of haemophiliac ancestry by the introduction of carefully fractionated DNA carrying the normal alleles of the mutant haemophilia gene. This experiment would appear to be entirely analogous to the typical attempts at transforming bacterial forms. However, it is not clear whether one should regard this as a pure example of genetic engineering, since the practical outcome would probably be best achieved by influencing the nuclear consitution of somatic tissues rather than by direct tackling of the germ line. The precedent for this type of intervention would be the virus-mediated transduction of genetic characteristics that was also demonstrated in bacteria almost twenty years ago. The proposal, recently revived by Dr. S. Rogers, would require the discovery or artificial formation of cryptic viruses to which specified genetic information relevant to the cure of a genetic disease has been grafted. These viruses would then carry that information into the requisite cells of the host. Once the essential techniques for grafting segments of DNA from different sources onto that of a microbe have been perfected, experiments along these lines provide the most favourable opportunity to select those segments of DNA information which are needed. In this way it should not be extraordinarily difficult to obtain microbial DNA packets which are enriched with the gene, for example, for the synthesis of phenylalanine hydroxylase. One may of course argue that similar results could be achieved by the manipulation of tissue cells in culture as if they themselves were micro-organisms."

A. Kornberg's successful replication of DNA in a test tube was widely reported in the popular press as the "creation of life in a test tube." It sparked an article by Lederberg on gene therapy that was published in the Washington Post in January 13, 1968.

W. Szybalski (Szybalski, 1991; Szybalski, 1992) who performed one of the earliest mammalian gene transfer experiments (see below), stated at a presentation to the Poultry Breeder's Round Table,

"When presenting our data at seminars and symposia in 1962-1964, we coined the terms 'gene surgery' and 'gene therapy' to stress the clinical potential of our work, but there was little interest in our results (except among poultry breeders), probably because at that time prokaryotes, DNA synthesis, and the genetic code was the center of attention."

By the late 1960's and early 1970's, gene therapy became the subject of an increasing number of articles and meetings. Sinsheimer speculated on the prospect for "designed genetic change" of mankind (Sinsheimer, 1969). At an autumn, 1969 meeting (Aposhian, 1970), Aposhian proposed the use of pseudoviruses derived from the mouse virus, polyoma. He saw gene therapy arising from the pharmaceutical tradition.

"If one considers the purpose of a drug to be to restore the normal function of some particular process in the body, then DNA would be considered to be the ultimate drug."

In a 1970 *Science* article, B. Davis discussed human genetic engineering and explored the feasibility and ethics of several procedures, including somatic and germ cell alterations, cloning of humans, genetic modification of behavior, predetermination of sex, and selective reproduction (Davis, 1970). One of his major points was that "control of polygenic behavioral traits is much less likely than cure of monogenic diseases."

In 1971, a symposium on gene therapy was sponsored by the National Institute of Neurologic Disease and Stroke at the NIH and the Fogarty International Center (Publication, 1971). The first session entitled "Information transfer by mammalian viruses" included talks on recombinant SV40 viruses by D. Jackson and P. Berg and on RNA tumor viruses by H. Temin. The other sessions were entitled "Isolation of altered viruses with specific genes," "Information transfer by DNA," "Mammalian cellular systems," and "Immunologic and medical aspects." A discussion of gene therapy was offered in a 1972 *Science* article by Friedmann and Roblin (Friedmann, 1972). In 1976, gene therapy was the subject of another meeting sponsored by the New York Academy of Sciences (Morrow, 1976).

Obviously, then, the idea for gene therapy quickly occurred to several key researchers, once the basics of molecular genetics were established. However, despite these premonitions, Friedmann (Friedmann, 1990) observes that

"It has not always been quite so obvious as it is now that gene therapy is a rational and logically consistent approach to the treatment of some forms of human disease, from both the medical and scientific perspectives. Until fairly recently, the concept of gene therapy has been criticized by a sizable portion of the molecular biologic community as being remote and even improbable, possibly even unnecessary."

GENE TRANSFER INTO MAMMALIAN CELLS IN VITRO

Despite the unavailability of recombinant DNA and hybridization techniques, several studies attempted to demonstrate that mammalian cells were able to take up

DNA, just as bacteria do. Several studies in the late 1950's and early 1960's demonstrated that cultured cells took up radioactive DNA (Sirotnak, 1959; Schimizu, 1962; Gartler, 1960; Mathias, 1962; Kay, 1961; Hill, 1970; Gartler, 1959; Borenfreund, 1961; Rabotti, 1963; Azrin, 1961). Some of these studies also reported entry of the radioactive DNA into the nucleus of the cells.

The study of viruses has motivated several early efforts for transferring genes into mammalian cells. In the late 1950's and early 1960's, several studies demonstrated that naked, viral DNA or RNA can be infective when applied to cells. This was first discovered with plants and tobacco mosaic virus in 1956 and then quickly extended to poliomyelitis, Semliki Forest encephalitis, influenza and several other viruses in mammalian cells. These studies prompted a Science review article which discussed the infectious disease implications of these studies (e.g., "their release from infected tissues and resistance to antibodies may explain some anomalous conditions") (Herriott, 1961). The infectious entity presumed to be polynucleotides was obtained by phenol-extraction of the virus, was labile to nucleases, and was not neutralized by antibodies. For example, a phenol-extract of polio virus yields RNA that produces plaque-forming poliovirus when injected into embryonated eggs (Mountain, 1959) or when applied to monkey kidney tissue cultures (Dubes, 1961), (Klingler, 1959) mouse embryo cells (Weil, 1961), or HeLa cells (Alexander, 1958).

Another series of studies explored the effect of viral RNA concentration, solution composition, and temperature to cause infections of Mengo encephalomyelitis in mouse fibroblasts (Colter, 1957; Colter, 1961). They found that hypertonic saline and sucrose solutions increased the infectivity of the RNA. Another study also found that exposure of HeLa cells to hypertonic solutions increased the number of plaques formed from polioviral RNA (Koch, 1960). In 1960, it was reported that polioviral RNA uptake was enhanced by high concentrations of magnesium sulfate (2M) (Holland, 1960). In 1961, Dubes and Klinger reported increased efficiency of polioviral RNA plaque formation with the use of calcium depleted cells and "poorly soluble substances" such as $CaHPO_4 \cdot 2H_2O$ and Cr_2O_3, Al_2O_3, $CaCO_3$, $CaSO_4$, Fe_2O_3, MgF_2 (Dubes, 1961). A footnote reported that

> "Infection is also facilitated by the fine cloudly precipitate, very probably a calcium phosphate, formed when phosphate-buffered saline is made by mixing its ingredients before sufficient dilution with water."

Several early studies reported increased uptake of cellular or viral polynucleotides by complexing them with various proteins. Amos found that the uptake of radiolabelled E. coli RNA by cultured chick cells was enhanced by complexing it with protamine (Amos, 1961). Other polycations such as streptomycin, spermine, and spermidine did not increase uptake but were observed to protect the RNA from RNase and caused precipitates to form in some formulations (Amos, 1961). Smull and Ludwig, in 1962, reported that calf thymus histone or protamine enhanced the infectivity of polioviral and Coxsackie B_3 RNA in HeLa cells but did not protect the RNA from RNase digestion (Smull, 1962). Another study found that methylated albumin (a basic protein) protected DNA and RNA from nucleases and enhanced their uptake by HeLa cells (Cocito, 1962). Bensch and King's observations that L cells did not take up appreciable amounts of DNA but did phagocytose particles prompted them to incorporate DNA into particles (Bensch, 1961). Using the Feulgen stain, acridine organge, and radioactive DNA, they found that DNA complexed with charcoal or activated resin did not increase DNA's uptake. However, DNA incorporated into 0.5-50 μm-sized, gelatin particles entered the cytoplasm and nucleus of the L cells. Much later in 1975, Farber and co-workers reported that cultured Chinese hamster lung cells took up more radiolabelled genomic DNA when complexed with polyornithine than with DEAE-dextran, 125 mM $CaCl_2$, latex spheres, spermine, polylysine, and polyarginine (Farber, 1975).

Several studies in the early 1960's reported changes in cellular phenotype by the transfer of foreign genes. Kraus reported in *Nature* in 1961 that bone marrow cells in culture from a patient homozygous for sickle cell disease expressed the normal β-globin polypeptide (per electrophoresis) when the cells were exposed to DNA from normal bone marrow cells (Azrin, 1961). Weisburger reported in the *Proceedings of the National Academy of Science* that the transfer of ribonucleoprotein (resistant to DNase but sensitive to RNase and trypsin digestion) from a normal bone marrow or spleen caused the expression of normal hemoglobin in sickle cell bone marrow and reticulocytes as determined by electrophoresis, column chromatography and peptide digests (Weisberger, 1962). Also in the *Proceedings* in 1962, Kantoch and Bang reported that they were able to transfer genetic susceptibility to mouse hepatitis virus infection between macrophages of two different mouse strains (Kantoch, 1962). In their discussion, they reported that this transfer was blocked by incubating the extract with DNase. In 1962, French workers reported that they could modify the karyotype of chicken cells by exposing them to cow DNA (Frederic, 1962). Another study noted increased survival of irradiated, L cells if they were exposed to DNA from nonirradiated L cells (Djordjevic, 1962). Several negative results concerning DNA transfer were reported as well in the early 60's. Mathias and Fisher attempted to transfer amethopterin resistance in mouse leukemic cells without success (Mathias, 1962). The exposure of donor, bone marrow cells to naked and gelatin-complexed DNA from the host bone marow cells in isotonic and hypertonic solutions did not affect the success of bone marrow transplantation in mice (Floersheim, 1962). The premise was that transfer of histocompatibility genes would induce immunotolerance.

The development of cell lines containing defined enzymatic defects and selectable systems proved extremely useful in gene transfer studies and ushered in the modern era of gene transfer. W. and E. Szybalski developed HPRT-deficient cell lines and the HAT selection media. DNA isolated from HPRT+ cells was able to confer HAT-resistance to HPRT- cells. The DNA was transferred in a phosphate buffer containing spermine in order to bind the DNA and shield it from DNase activity (Szybalska, 1962). In Table I of their 1962 article, they showed a dose-dependent relationship between the amount of donor DNA and the number of transformants. Subsequent experiments indicated that the spermine contained 30% $CaCl_2$ and that the spermine could be replaced by $CaCl_2$ when used with phosphate buffers. Precipitates were observed during these experiments. These later experiments with $CaCl_2$ were reported in Table 2 of their paper in Proceedings of the 12th Annual Session National Poultry Breeder's Roundtable (Szybalski, 1963) in 1963:

> "It was noticed that only one of preparations of spermine was especially active in the transformation process. Addition of this spermine solution to the phosphate-buffered saline (PBS) resulted in clouding of the solution, both in the presence or absence of the transforming DNA and the cells. Since we found that the particular spermine preparation contained a high concentration of calcium, the precipitate was most probably the calcium phosphate."

Further chemical analysis indicated that the contaminant was in fact calcium (Szybalski, 1992). This finding was not widely disseminated because of the specialized nature of the publication in which it were reported, but Szybalski's early contribution to DNA-mediated gene transfer was recognized by Scangos and Ruddle in a 1981 review (Scangos, 1981). Also, in 1962, Bradley, Roosa, and Law used 8-azaguanine selection to demonstrate the cellular uptake of naked, genomic DNA (Bradley, 1962).

Despite these early observations concerning calcium phosphate precipitation, most workers used DEAE-dextran to transfer foreign DNA into mammalian cells as a result of a report by Vaheri and Pagano in 1965 that showed increased transfer of polio virus RNA with DEAE-dextran (Vaheri, 1965). This 1965 study compared the use of DEAE-dextran to that of hypertonic magnesium solutions. Burnett and Harrington also used DEAE-dextran to transfer polyoma virus DNA but indicated that this was not successful with adenoviral DNA (Burnett, 1968). Subsequently several other studies reported the successful use of DEAE-dextran. McCutchan and Pagano transferred SV40 DNA(McCutchan, 1968), Warden and Thorne transferred polyoma virus, (Warden, 1968), and Nicolson and McAllister transferred adenovirus 1 (Nicolson, 1972). Hill and Hillova produced infectious RSV after non-infected cells were transfected using DEAE-dextran with DNA from Rous sarcoma virus infected cell (Hill, 1972).

It was not until the detailed study of Graham and Van Der Eb on calcium phosphate-mediated transfection that this technique became widely used and accepted (Graham, 1973). They systematically explored the use of calcium or magnesium ions for transfection and determined that co-precipitates of DNA, calcium and phosphate were necessary for efficient transfection. They also explored several parameters, such as pH (6.9-7.4), incubation times, confluency of cells (60-90%) and adenoviral and carrier DNA concentration, in a systematic fashion. Because of this and the reproducible, 50- to 100-fold increase in efficiency over DEAE-dextran, this study had a major impact on the field and is widely cited as the primary source for the "calcium phosphate transfection" technique. After their initial publication in 1973, they modified the procedure further in 1974 (Graham, 1974),

EARLY ATTEMPTS AT DIRECT GENE TRANSFER IN VIVO

Perhaps the earliest predecessor of a direct in vivo approach was the use of vaccines, which permanently modify the body's response to infection. Vaccination with attenuated viruses may be viewed as a form of gene therapy, especially since the viral genomes may persist long-term. The ease of administration, relative cheapness, and long-lasting effect of vaccines are ideal qualities to which proponents of direct gene therapy aspire.

Another idea for direct, in vivo therapy was the notion of treating bacterial infections by the injection of bacteriophages. While this therapeutic approach was discussed in Sinclair Lewis' novel Arrowsmith, there were several actual reports of its successful use in animals and humans (d'Herelle, 1926). The negative results of well-controlled studies (Boyd, 1944) and the advent of antibiotics stopped its further investigation. Interestingly, there have been some recent reports of its exploration in animals (Reynaud, 1992; Soothill, 1992).

Several early studies reported the direct transfer of polynucleotides into tissues in vivo and in situ. Rieke reported that periotoneal malignant and normal cells in the peritoneum took up radioactive DNA (Rieke, 1962). Rabotti reported the uptake of radioactive DNA into tumors in vivo (Rabotti, 1963), but the foreign DNA demonstrated no functional activity. Radioactive DNA injected intravenously or intraperitoneally in rodents were taken up by spleen and bone marrow cells (Hudnik-Plevnik, 1959; Hill, 1961). Other studies reported the uptake of labelled DNA by cells in mice in vivo.

J. Benoit et al. reported beginning in 1956 that Peking ducklings injected intraperitoneally with DNA extract from Khaki Campbell ducks exhibited characteristics of the Khaki Campbell ducks in terms of body and head size, and that these effects were passed onto their progeny (Benoit, 1960; Benoit, 1960). Much to the dismay of paté manufactures and Chinese chefs who were expecting a culinary breakthrough, these results in Ducks have never been reproduced.

The Benoit studies in ducks attracted enough attention to prompt several other investigators to attempt phenotypic modifcation by DNA transfer in other species. The injection of rat DNA from a pigmented rat into an albino rat did not produce any change in skin color (Perry, 1958). Two other studies also reported the inability to produce pigmentary studies in albino rodents by injection of DNA from a pigmented rodent (Bearn, 1961), (Holoubek, 1961). In addition, the intraperitoneal injection of DNA from a normal rat did not correct the hyperbilirubinemic state of the CNH strain (noted to be deficient in glucuronyl transferase) (Perry, 1958). In chickens, the injection of a "Tyrode" solution or DNA in the Tyrode solution into the blood stream of young chicken embyros did not cause any morphological changes but did cause teratogenic malformations (Martinovitch, 1962).

In mice, another group observed that the intraperitoneal injection of DNA from breast cancers of agouti C_3H mice but not DNA from other organs caused cytological changes in the livers of white mice (Leuchtenberger, 1958). Two different groups noted that injection of DNA from one mouse strain caused weak transplantation immunity against skin grafts but raised the possiblity that contaminants may have been responsible for the effect (Haskova, 1958; Medawar, 1958).

In summary, the Benoit studies prompted many attempts to research DNA uptake by vertebrate cells. However, the study made the entire field of gene transfer into cells of higher organisms somewhat suspect (W. Szybalski, personal communication).

Other studies explored the ability of DNA to transfer the neoplastic state. In the early 1950's, it was reported that new tumors formed after injection of DNA from tumor cells into normal mouse tissues (Stasney, 1950), (Paschkis, 1955). One-third of rats subcutaneously injected with lymphosarcoma chromatin were said to have developed lymphosarcomas or leukemia, while approximately one-third of rats injected intrahepatically were said to have developed hepatomas. A subsequent report observed a similar phenomenon but concluded that it was the result of contaminating cancer cells (Klein, 1952). A 1958 report observed that the repeated, subcutaneous injections of herring-sperm DNA caused duodenal adenocarcinoma in two mice but this was not repeatable with a different batch of DNA (Meek, 1959). This report prompted a subsequent study that reported that repeated, subcutaneous injections of herring-sperm DNA caused intestinal carcinomas in cichlids (Stolk, 1960). The injection of *Drosophila melanogaster* DNA was also noted to be mutagenic in *Drosophila* (Fahmy, 1961). Only many years later was the phenotype for neoplastic transformation reliably transferred from mammalian DNA into cells in culture (Cooper, 1980; Shih, 1979). Nonetheless, several studies in the late 1950's and early 1960's reported neoplastic transformation by viral polynucleotides in vivo just as there was a flurry of reports at this time concerning the infectivity of viral polynucleotides. For example, phenol extracts of SE polyoma virus were able to cause infections and tumors in hamsters (DiMayorca, 1959). Also, phenol extracts of papillomatous tissue (Shope) of Cottontail rabbits, produced paillomas when injected into the skin of rabbits (Ito, 1960), (Ito, 1961).

The development of plasmid expression vectors, reporter genes, and better in situ detection systems prompted more recent attempts at direct, in vivo gene transfer. In 1983, large liposomes containing the rat preproinsulin gene within a plasmid were injected intravenously into rats (Nicolau, 1983). The injections caused a ~30% decrease in blood glucose and a ~50% increase in blood insulin.

Another early study involved the injection of calcium phosphate-precipitated polyoma viral DNA into mouse liver and spleen along with hyaluronidase and collagenase (Dubensky, 1984). The investigators reported the presence of the polyoma DNA in the tissues and inferred that the viral DNA had to replicate. Similar studies were also done with polyoma DNA and proteoliposomes (Mannino, 1988).

Another study involved the intraperitoneal injection of calcium phosphate-precipitated plasmids containing chloramphenicol acetyltransferase (CAT), hepatitis B surface antigen, human growth hormone, or mouse preproinsulin genes (Benvenisty, 1986). The investigators observed some CAT activity, immunohistochemical staining for the hepatitis antigen, insulin RNA, and growth hormone RNA in livers injected with the respective plasmids.

FIRST ATTEMPTS AT HUMAN GENE THERAPY

In the late 1960s, S. Rogers injected the Shope papilloma virus into patients with arginase deficiency, based upon his studies that indicated that the virus contained an arginase gene. His initial observation was that rabbit skin tumors induced by the Shope papilloma virus contained high levels of arginase activity (Rogers, 1963; Rogers, 1959). Since he did not find any arginase activity in normal rabbit skin, he concluded that the virus carried an arginase gene. He also reported that the virus induced a virus-specific arginase in fibroblasts from a patient with arginase deficiency (Rogers, 1973). A biochemical assay demonstrated increased arginase activity, and an immunohistochemical stain with anti-sera specific against the virus-specific arginase distinguished the virus-induced arginase from native arginase. Administration of the virus to animals caused no harmful effect and reduced blood arginase levels. However, other workers found arginase activity in normal skin (Rothberg, 1961; Orth, 1967). These other workers also showed that rabbit liver arginase and Shope had similar kinetic and antigenic properties and that papillomas induced by a carcinogen also contained arginase. They concluded that the Shope virus either induces arginase expression or leads to the preferential growth of cells with higher arginase activity. The final outcome to this controversy was that three siblings with arginase deficiency were injected with the Shope virus, without any effect on their arginine levels (Terheggen, 1975).

In a 1980 *Nature* report, Cline reported that DNA from a highly methotrexate-resistant Swiss 3T6 cell line (containing many copies of the DHFR gene) was calcium phosphate transfected into mouse bone marrow cells (Cline, 1980). The donor bone marrow cells had a different karyotype to distinguish them from the recipient bone marrow cells. The recipient mice were irradiated and treated with methotrexate before being injected with the transfected cells. After transplantation, the recipient animals were reported to have an increased percentage of marrow cells with the donor karyotype and increased DHFR enzymatic activity. A similar study was published in *Science* which used recombinant DNA containing the herpes TK gene in the pBR322 plasmid vector (Mercola, 1980). On the basis of this experimental data they attempted to calcium phosphate transfect the β-globin gene into human bone marrow cells, which were then transplanted into patients with thalasemia. Their clinical trial was criticized for both scientific and procedural reasons, and this led to Cline's censure by the NIH and by his university (Wade, 1980; Wade, 1981; Wade, 1981). As a result, the NIH decided that all future human gene therapy trials would have to be approved by the NIH Recombinant DNA Advisory Committee.

Unsound practices in these early studies in cell cultures, animals, and humans made both the experimental results and the entire approach of gene therapy seem suspect, even though some of the basic concepts and approaches upon which the studies were based were eventually proven correct.

THE DEVELOPMENT OF RECOMBINANT DNA TECHNOLOGY

It was not until early transfection techniques and selection systems for cultured cells were combined with recombinant DNA technology that major progress was made in gene transfer. The isolation of a single gene enabled both greater efficiency and better documentation of its transfer.

Using UV-irradiated herpes simplex virus, Munyon in 1971 showed that the thymidine kinase (TK) gene from herpes simplex could rescue TK- cells in HAT media (Munyon, 1971). Later in the 1970's, several groups used total herpes simplex DNA and calcium phosphate-transfection to transfer the herpes TK gene into TK- human cells (Wigler, 1977; Bacchetti, 1977; Maitland, 1977; Minson, 1978). Subsequently, sheared and restriction enzyme fragments of herpes simplex DNA were calcium phosphate transfected into mouse TK- cells. Wigler et. al. then provided definitive proof that the transformation occurred by transfer of the herpes TK gene (Wigler, 1978). Transformed TK+ cell lines contained herpes TK activity by isoelectric focusing electrophoresis and the herpes TK gene by Southern blot analysis. Transfection of total cellular DNA from the transformed TK+ cell line transferred TK activity to a TK-deficient cell.

Subsequently, other genes such as APRT and human HPRT were transferred (Wigler, 1979; Willecke, 1979; Graf, 1979; Pellicer, 1980). An advance was the transfer and selection for unlinked genes (Wigler, 1979). These studies demonstrated that any gene can be transferred into mammalian cells along with a selectable marker. By 1981, Scangos and Ruddle (Scangos, 1981) concluded:

"Thus, in the last two decades the field of DNA mediated gene transfer (DMGT) has progressed from relatively simple experiments in which the HAT selective system was developed and the feasibility of the technique was tested, through the development and refinement of the calcium-phosphate technique, to experiments in which many selectable and non-selectable genes have been transferred into mammalian cells."

DEVELOPMENT OF VIRAL VECTORS

One of the earliest attempts to produce a viral vector was that by Rodgers and Pfuderer in 1968 (Rogers, 1968). They enzymatically added a poly A sequence to Tobacco mosaic virus RNA and reported that plants infected with this modified virus contained increased amounts of polylysine. Other workers experimented with purifying polyoma viral capsid proteins to form pseudovirions (Aposhian, 1972; Friedmann, 1971).

In a series of studies, Berg and colleagues developed the first recombinant viral vector system based upon the papilloma simian virus (SV40). In 1972, lambda phage DNA and the E. coli galactose operon was ligated into DNA of SV40 DNA (Jackson, 1972). In 1976, recombinant SV40 vectors with lambda phage DNA were propagated in cultured monkey kidney cells (Goff, 1976). Hamer et al. similarly constructed an SV40 virus carrying an E. coli suppressor gene (Hamer, 1977).

After the full-length double-stranded cDNA for rabbit globin mRNA was synthesized in vitro using now standard techniques involving reverse transcriptase and DNA polymerase I (Maniatis, 1976), it was exchanged with the major capsid protein, VP1 of the SV40 virus. The recombinant vector expressed the rabbit β-globin protein in the infected cells (Mulligan, 1979). Other workers also found expression of β-globin protein from cells infected with SV40 recombinant viruses carrying the β-globin gene (Mulligan, 1979; Hamer, 1979; Hamer, 1979).

The development of retroviral vectors has been reviewed previously (Miller, 1989). Briefly, three groups independently developed the first retroviral vectors. Shimotohono and Temin made an avian retroviral vector derived from spleen necrosis virus that expressed the herpes thymidine kinase gene (Shimotohno, 1981). Wei et al constructed vectors derived from Harvey murine sarcoma virus, which also expressed the herpes TK gene (Wei, 1981). Tabin et. al. also used the herpes TK gene to construct a vector derived from Moloney leukemia virus (Tabin, 1982). These early developments in viral vectors culminated in a meeting at the Banbury Center of the Cold Spring Harbor Laboratory in 1982 that generated much enthusiasm and interest in conducting further research toward human gene therapy (Cold Spring Harbor Laboratory, 1983). Helper-free packaging cell lines were subsequently developed (reviewed in (Miller, 1989). After several disease-related genes were transferred into various cells in culture, the possibility of efficient gene transfer into mammalian cells for the purpose of gene therapy became widely accepted.

CONCLUSION

Although the discovery of the central dogma of molecular genetics quickly led to the idea for gene therapy, development of the field was hindered initially by several poorly designed studies. As the field has gained credibility in recent years, however, progress has accelerated. Central to this progress have been the development of basic genetic concepts in bacteria and bacteriophages and the extension of these concepts to mammalian cells, the development of recombinant DNA technology, and the development of mammalian gene transfer techniques, including viral vectors and physical-chemical methods.

The new field of gene therapy combines the advantages of pharmacology (namely, the ability to treat human disease with externally administered substances that have specific actions) and surgery (namely, the ability to permanently alter a tissue or organ). As such, it represents more than an extension of established medical practice. Rather, gene therapy is an entirely new branch of medicine, one that could potentially revolutionize the way we treat human disease.

REFERENCES

Alexander HE, Koch G, Mountain IM, Sprunt K, Van Damme O (1958): Infectivity of ribonucleic acid of poliovirus on HeLa cell monolayers. *Virology* 5:172-173

Amos H (1961): Protamine enhancement of RNA uptake by cultured chick cells. *Biochem Biophys Res Comm* 5:1-4

Anderson WF, Fletcher JC (1980): Gene therapy in human beings: when is it ethical to begin? *N Eng J Med* 303(22):1293-1297

Anderson WF, Killos L, Sanders-Haigh L, Kretschmer PJ, Diacumakos EG (1980): Replication and expression of thymidine kinase and human globin genes microinjected into mouse fibroblasts. *Proc Natl Acad Sci USA* 77(9):5399-5403

Aposhian HV (1970): The use of DNA for gene therapy—the need, experimental approach, and implications. *Perspectives in Biology and Medicine* 14:987-108

Aposhian HV, Qasba PK, Osterman JV, Waddell A (1972): Polyoma pseudovirions: an experimental model for the develpment of DNA for gene therapy. *Federation Proceedings* 31(4):1310-1325

Aposhian HV, Qasba PK, Osterman JV, Waddell A (1972): Polyoma pseudovirions: an experimental model for the develpment of DNA for gene therapy. *Federation Proceedings* 31(4):1310-1325

Avery OT, MacLeod CM, McCarty M (1944): Studies on the chemical nature of the substance inducing transformation of pneumococcal types. *Journal of Experimental Medicine* 79:137-158

Azrin NH (1961): Incorporation of heterologous deoxyribonucleic acid into mammalian cells. *Science* 133:381-383

Bacchetti S, Gaham FL (1977): Transfer of the gene for thymidine kinase to thymidine kinase-deficient human cells by prurified herpes simplex viral DNA. *Proc Natl Acad Sci USA* 74(4):1590-1594

Baltimore D (1970): Viral RNA-dependent DNA polymerase. *Nature* 226:1209-1211

Bearn JG, Kirby KS (1961): Failure of deoxyribonucleic acid to produce pigment changes in the albino rat. *Exp Cell Res* 17:547-549

Benoit J, Leroy P, Vendrely R, Vendrely C (1960): Experiments on pekin ducks treated with DNA from khaki campbell ducks. *Transaction of The New York Academy of Sciences* 22: 494-503

Benoit J, Leroy P,Vendrely R, Vendrely C (1960): Modifications de caracteres raciaux du canard pekin par l'acide desoxyribonucleique de canard khaki cambell et leur transmission a la descendance. *Biochemical Pharmacology* 4:181-194

Bensch KG, King DW (1961): Incorporation of heterologous deoxyribonucleic acid into mammalian cells. *Science* 133:381-382

Benvenisty N, Reshef L (1986): Direct introduction of genes into rats and expression of the genes. *Proc Natl Acad Sci USA* 83:9551-9555

Borenfreund E, Bendich A (1961): A study of the penetration of mammalian cells by deoxyrobonucleic acids. *The Journal of Biophysical and Biochemical Cytology* 9:81-91

Boyd JSK, Portnoy B (1944): Bacteriophage therapy in bacillary dysentery. *Trans R Soc Trop Med Hyg* 37:243-262

Bradley TR, Roosa RA, Law LW (1962): DNA transformation studies with mammalian cells in culture. *Journal of cellular and comparative physiology* 60:127-138

Burnett JP, Harrington JA (1968): Infectivity associated with Simian Adenovirus Type SA7 DNA. *Nature* 220:1245

Cline MJ, Stang H, Mercola K, Morse L, Ruprecht R, Browne J, Salser W (1980): Gene transfer in intact animals. *Nature* 284:422-5

Cocito C, Prinzie A, De Somer P (1962): Uptake by mammalian cells of nucleic acids combined with a basic protein. *Experientia* 18:218-220

Cold Spring Harbor Laboratory (1983): *Gene Therapy: Fact and Fiction*. Cold Spring Harbor, NY: Cold Spring Harbor Laboratory

Colter JS, Bird HH, Moyer AW, Brown RA (1957): Infectivity of ribonucleic acid isolated from virus-infected tissues. *Virology* 4:522-532

Colter JS, Ellem KAO (1961): Interaction of viral nucleic acids with mammalian cells. *Federation Proceedings* 20:650-655

Cooper GM, Okenquist S, Silverman L (1980): Transforming activity of DNA of chemically transformed and normal cells. *Nature* 284:418-421

Crow JF (1992): Anecdotal, Historical and Critical Commentaries on Genetics. *Genetics* 131:761-768

Cushman DW, Ondetti MA (1991): History of the design of captopril and related inhibitors of angiotensin converting enzyme. *Hypertension* 17(4):589-592

d'Herelle F (1926): *The bacteriophage and its behavior.* (Smith GH, Trans.). Paris: Balliere

Davis BD (1970): Prospects for Genetic Intervention in Man. *Science* q170:1279-1283

DiMayorca GA, Eddy BE, Stewart SE, Hunter WS, Friend C, Bendich A (1959): Isolation of infectious deoxyribonucleic acid from SE polyoma-infected tissue cultures. *Proc Natl Acad Sci USA* 45:1805-1808

Djordjevic O, Kostic L, Kanazir D (1962): Recovery of ultra-violet-irradiated L strain cells by means of highly polymerized deoxyribonucleic acid. *Nature* 195:614-615

Doehmer J, Barinaga M, Vale W, Rosenfeld MG, Verma IM, Evans RM (1982): Introduction of rat growth hormone gene into mouse fibroblasts via a retorviral DNA vector: Expression and regulation. *Proc Natl Acad Sci USA* 79:2268-2272

Dubensky TW, Campbell BA, Villarreal LP (1984): Direct transfection of viral and plasmid DNA into the liver or spleen of mice. *Proc Natl Acad Sci USA* 81:7529-7533

Dubes GR, Klingler EA (1961): Facilitation of Infection of Monkey Cells with Poliovirus "Ribonucleic Acid". *Science* 133:99-133

Fahmy OG, Fahmy MJ (1961): Induction of mutations by deoxyribonucleic acid in Drosophila melanogaster. *Nature* 191:776-779

Farber FE, Melnick JL, Butel JS (1975): Optimal conditions for uptake of exogenous DNA by chinese hamster lung cells deficient in hypoxanthine-guanosine phosphoribosyltransferase. *Biochim Biophys Acta* 390:298-311

Felgner PL (1990): Particulate systems and polymers for in vitro and in vivo delivery of polynucleotides. *Advanced Drug Delivery Reviews* 5:163-187

Floersheim GL (1962): System for the recognition of genetic transformation in haemopoietic cells. *Nature* 193:1266-1268

Fournier REK, Ruddle FH (1977): Microcell-mediated transfer of murine chromosomes into mouse, Chinese hamster, and human somatic cells. *Proc Natl Acad Sci USA* 74(1):319-323

Frederic J, Corin-Frederic J (1962): Modifications des chromosomes et du caryotype dans des cellules de Poulet cultivees in vitro en presence d'acides desoxyribonucleiques de veau. *C R Soc Biol* 156:742-745

Friedmann T (1971): In vitro reassembly of shell-like particle from disrupted polyoma virus. *Proc Natl Acad Sci USA* 68(10):2574-2578

Friedmann T (1976): The future for gene therapy—a reevaluation. *Annals New York Academy of Science* 265:141-152

Friedmann T (1989): Progress toward human gene therapy. *Science* 244:1275-1281

Friedmann T (1990): The Evolving Concept of Gene Therapy. *Human Gene Therapy* 1:175-181

Friedmann T (1992): A brief history of gene therapy. *Nature genetics* 2(october):93-98

Friedmann T, Roblin R (1972): Gene therapy for human genetic disease? *Science* 175(4025):949-955

Gartler SM (1959): Cellular uptake of deoxyribonucleic acid by human tissue culture cells. *Nature* 184:1505-1506

Gartler SM (1960): Demonstration of cellular uptake of polymerized DNA in mammalian cell cultures. *Biochem Biophys Res Comm* 3:127-131

Goff SP, Berg P (1976): Construction of hybrid viruses containing SV40 and gamma phage DNa segments and their propagation in cultured monkey cells. *Cell* 9:695-705

Goodman LS, Gilman A (Ed.). (1975): *The Pharmacologic Basis of Therapeutics*. New York: Macmillan Publishing Co

Graessmann M, Graessmann A (1976): "Early" simian-virus-40-specific RNA contains information for tumor antigen formation and chromatin replication. *Proc Natl Acad Sci USA* 73:366-370

Graf BH, Urlaub G, Chasin LA (1979): Transformation of the gene for hypoxanthine phophoribosyltransferase. *Somatic Cell Genetics* 5(6):1031-1044

Graham FL, Van Der Eb AJ (1973): A New technique for the assay of infectivity of human adenovirus 5 DNA. *Virology* 52:456-467

Graham FL, Van der Eb AJ, Heijneker HL (1974): Size and location of the transforming region in human adenovirus type 5 DNA. *Nature* 251:687-90

Green MR, Treisman R, Maniatis T (1983): Transcriptional Activation of Cloned Human Beta-Globin Genes by Viral Immediate-Early Gene Products. *Cell* 35:137-148

Hamer DH, Davoli D, Thomas CA, Fareed GC (1977): Simian virus 40 carrying an Escherichia coli Suppressor Gene. *Journal of Molecular Biology* 112:155-182

Hamer DH, Leder P (1979): Expression of the chromosomal mouse β^{maj}-globin gene cloned in SV40. *Nature* 281:35-40

Hamer DH, Smith KD, Boyer SH, Leder P (1979): SV 40 Recombinants Carrying Rabbit bet-Globin Gene Coding Sequences. *Cell* 17:725-735

Haskova V, Hrubesova M (1958): Part played by deoxyribonucleic acid in transplantation immunity. *Nature* 182:61-62

Herriott RM (1961): Infectious nucleic acids, a new dimension in virology. *Science* 134:256-260

Hershey AD, Burgi E (1965): Complementary structure of interacting sites at the ends of lambda DNA molecules. *Proc Natl Acad Sci USA* 53:325-328

Hill M (1961): Uptake of deoxyribonucleic acid (DNA): a special property of the cell nucleus. *Nature* 189:916-917

Hill M, Hillova J (1972): Virus Recovery in chicken Cells tested with Rous Sarcoma Cell DNA. *Nature New Biology* 237:35-39

Hill M, Huppert J (1970): Fate of exogenous mouse DNA in chicken fibroblasts in vitro non-conservative preservation. *Biochimica and Biophysica Acta* 213:26-35

Hill M, Jakubickova J (1962): Intercellular passage of DNA as revealed in bone marrow autoradiographs. *Exp Cell Res* 26:541-551

Holland JJ, Hoyer BH, McLaren LC, Syverton JT (1960): Enteroviral ribonucleic acid. I—Recovery from virus and assimilation by cells. *J Exp Med* 112:821-864

Holoubek V, Hnilica L (1961): The failure to produce somatic and immunologic changes in inbred AKR mice by specific deoxyribonocleic acid. *Can J Biochem Physio* 39:1478-1479

Hudnik-Plevnik T, Glisin VR, SImic MM (1959): Fate of the highly polymerized spleen deoxyribonucleic labelled with Phosphorus-32 injected intraperitoneally into rats. *Nature* 184:1818-1819

Ito Y (1960): A tumor-producing factor extracted by phenol from papillomatous tissue (Shope) of Cottontail Rabbits. *Virology* 12:596-601

Ito Y (1961): Heat-resistance of the tumorigenic nucleic acids of Shope papillomatosis. *Proc Natl Acad Sci USA* 47:1897-1900

Jackson DA, Symon RH, Berg P (1972): Biochemical method for inserting new genetic information into DNA of Simian Virus 40: Circular SV40 DNA molecules containing lambda phage genes and the galactose peron of Escherichia coli. *Proc Natl Acad Sci USA* 69(10):2904-2909

Judson HF (1979): *The Eighth Day of Creation: The makers of the revolution in biology*. New York: Simon and Schuster.

Kaneda Y, Iwai K, Uchida T (1989): Increased Expressio of DNA cointroduced with nuclear Protein in adult rat liver. *Science* 243:375-377

Kantoch M, Bang FB (1962): Conversion of genetic resistance of mammalian cells to susceptibility to a virus infection. *Proc Natl Acad Sci USA* 48:1553-1559

Kao F-T, Puck TT (1968): Genetics of somatic mammalian cells, VII. Induction and isolation of nutritional mutants in chinese hamster cells. *Proc Natl Acad Sci USA* 60:1275-1281

Kay ERM (1961): Incorporation of Deoxyribonucleic Acid by mammalian cells in vitro. *Nature* 191:387-388

Keating A, Toneguzzo F (1990). Gene tranfer by electroporation: a model for gene therapy. In S. Gross,A. P. Gee, D. A. Worthington-White (Eds.), *Bone Marrow Purging and Processing*. (pp. 491-498). New Yord: Wiley-Liss

Klein G (1952): The nature of mammalian lymphosarcoma transmission by isolated chromatin fractions. *Cancer Research* 12:589-590

Klingler E, Chapin M, Dubes GR (1959): Relationship between inactivation of poliovirus by phenol and appearance of ribonuclease-labile infectivity. *Proc Soc Exp Biol Med* 101:829-832

Kobernick SD, Toovey EW, Webster DR (1952): Effects of the Application of Carcinogens to exposed gastric mucosa in the rat. *Cancer Research* 12:591-593

Koch G, Koenig S, Alexander H (1960): Quantitative studies on the infectivity of ribonucleic acid from partially purified and highly purified poliovirus preparations. *Virology* 10:329-343

Kraus L (1961): Formation of different haemoglobins in tissue culture of human bone marrow treated with human deoxyribonucleic acid. *Nature* 192:1055-1057

Lederberg J (1956): Genetic transduction. *American Scientist* 44:264-280

Lederberg J (1973): The genetics of human nature. *Social Res* 40:375-406

Leuchtenberger C, Leuchtenberger R, Uyeki E (1958): Cytological and cytochemical changes in livers of white mice following intraperitoneal injections of DNA preparations from breast cancers of Agouti C3H mice. *Proc Natl Acad Sci USA* 44:700-705

Levine F, Friedmann T (1991): Gene therapy techniques. *Current Opinion in Biotechnology* 2:840-844

Lewis W, Srinivasan PR, Stokoe N, Siminovitch L (1980): Parameters governing the transfer of the genes for thymidine kinase and dihydrofolate reductase into mouse cells using metaphase chromosomes or DNA. *Somatic Cell Genetics* 6(3):333-347

Linnane AW, Lamb AJ, Christodoulou C, Lukins HB (1967): The biogenesis of mitochondria, VI. Biochemical basis of the resistance of saccharomyces cerevisiae toward antibiotics which specifically inhibit mitochondrial protein synthesis. *Proc Natl Acad Sci USA* 59:1288-1293

Lwoff A (1972). Interaction among virus, cell, and organism:Nobel lecture, December 11, 1965. In *Nobel Lectures in Physiology or Medicine, 1963-1970* (pp. 174-185). New York: Elsevier

Maitland NJ, McDougall JK (1977): Biochemical transformation of Mouse Cells by Fragments of Herpes Simplex Virus DNA. *Cell* 11:233-241

Mandel M, Higa A (1970): Calcium-dependent bacteriophage DNA Infection. *Journal of Molecular Biology* 53:159-162

Maniatis T, Kee SG, Efstratiadis A, Kafatos FC (1976): Amplification and characterization of a Beta-Globin Gene Synthesized in vitro. *Cell* 8:163-182

Mannino RJ, Gould-Fogerite S (1988): Liposome Meidated Gene transfer. *BioTechniques* 6(7):682-90

Martinovitch PN, Kanazir DT, Knezevitch ZA, Simitch MM (1962): Teratological changes in the offspring of chicken embryos treated with tyrode or with tyrode plus DNA. *J Embryol Exp Morph* 10:167-177

Mathias AP, Fischer GA (1962): Transformation experiments with murine lymphoblastic cells (L5178Y) grown in culture. *Biochemical Pharm* 11:69-78

McCutchan JH, Pagano JS (1968): Enhancement of the infectivity of Simian Virus 40 Deoxyribonucleic Acid with Diethylaminoethyl-Dextran. *Journal of the National Cancer Institute* 41(2):351-357

Medawar (1958): Part played by deoxyribonucleic acid in transplantation immunity. *Nature* 182:62

Meek ES, Hewer TF (1959): An intestinal carcinoma in mice following injeciton of herring-sperm deoxyribonucleic acid. *Brit J Cancer* 13:121-125

Mercola KE, Stang HD, Browne J, Salser W, Cline MJ (1980): Insertion of a new gene of viral origin into bone marrow cells of mice. *Science* 208:1033-1035

Miller A, Rosman G (1989): Improved retoviral vectors for gene transfer and expression. *BioTechniques* 7(9):980-990

Miller AD (1992): Human gene therapy comes of age. *Nature* 357:455-60

Miller AD, Law M-F, Verma EM (1985): Generation of helper-free amphotropic retroviruses that transduce a dominant-acting, methotrexate-resistant dihydrofolate reductase gene. *Molecular and Cellular Biology* 5(3):431-437

Minson AC, Wildy P, Buchan A, Darby G (1978): Introduction of the Herpes simplex virus thymidine kinase gene into mouse cells using virus DNA or transformed cell DNA. *Cell* 13:581-587

Morrow JF (1976): The prospects for gene therapy in humans. *Annals of the New York Academy of Sciences* 265:13-21

Mountain IM, Alexander HE (1959): Infectivity of ribonucleic acid (RNA) from type I poliovirus in embryonated egg. *Proc Soc Exp Biol Med* 101:527-532

Mulligan RC, Berg P (1980): Expression of a bacterial Gene in mammalian Cells. *Science* 209:1422-1427

Mulligan RC, Berg P (1981): Selection for animal cells that express the Escherichia coli gene coding for xanthine-guanine phosphoribosyltransferase. *Proc Natl Acad Sci USA* 78:2072-2076

Mulligan RC, Berg R (1981): Factors Governing the Expression of a bacterial Gene in Mammalian Cells. *Molecular and Cellular Biology* 1(5):449-459

Mulligan RC, Howard B, Berg P (1979): Synthesis of rabbit beta-globin in cultured monkey kidney cells following infection with a SV40 beta-globin recombinant genome. *Nature* 277:108-114

Munyon W, Kraiselburd E, Davis D, Mann J (1971): Transfer of thymidine kinase to thymidine kinaseless L cells by infection with Unltraviolet-irradiated herpes simplex virus. *Journal of Virology* 7(6):813-820

Neville R (1976): Gene therapy and the ethics of genetic therapeutics. *Annals of the New York Academy of Sciences* 265:153-169

Nicolau C, Le Pape A, Soriano P, Fargette F, Juhel M-F (1983): In vivo expression of rat insulin after intravenous administration of the liposome-entrapped gene for rat insulin I. *Proc Natl Acad Sci USA* 80:1068-1072

Nicolson MO, McAllister RM (1972): Infectivity of Human Adenovirus-1 DNA. *Virology* 48:14-21

Orth G, Vielle F, Changeux JP (1967): On the arginase of the shope papillomas. *Virology* 31:729-32

Paschkis KE, Cantarow A, Stansney J (1955): Induction of neoplasms by injection of tumor chromatin. *Journal of the National Cancer Institute* 15(5):1525-1532

Pellicer A, Robins D, Wold B, Sweet R, Jackson J, Lowy I, Roberts JM, Sim GK, Silverstien S, Axel R (1980): Altering genotype and phenotype by DNA-mediated gene transfer. *Science* 209:1414-1422

Perry TL, Walker D (1958): Failure of deoxyribonucleic acid to effect somatic transformation in the rat. *Proc Soc Exp Biol Med* 99:717-720

Perutz M (1992): *Protein Structure: New approaches to disease and therapy*. New York: W.H. Freeman and Co.

Philipson L, Lonberg-Holm K, Pettersson U (1968): Virus-receptor interaction in an adenovirus system. *Journal of Virology* 2(10):1064-1075

Publication N (1971). The prospects of Gene Therapy. In E. Freese (Ed.), *Fogarty International Center*, Bethesda, Maryland: DHEW Publication

Rabotti GF (1963): Incorporation of DNA into a mouse tumor in vivo and in vitro. *Experimental Cell Research* 31:562-565

Reynaud A, Cloastre L, Bernard J, Laveran H, Ackermann H-W, Licois D, Joly B (1992): Characteristics and diffusion in the rabbit of a phage for escherichia coli 0103. Attempts to use this phage for therapy. *Vet Microbiol* 30:203-212

Rieke WO (1962): The in vivo reutilization of lymphocytic and sarcoma DNA by cells growing in the peritoneal cavity. *J Cell Biol* 13:205-216

Rogers S (1959): Induction of arginase in rabbit epithelium by the Shope rabbit papilloma virus. *Nature* 183:1815-1816

Rogers S, Lowenthal A, Terheggen HG, Columbo JP (1973): Induction of arginase activity with the shope papilloma virus in tissue culture cells from an argininemic patient. *Journal of Experimental Medicine* 137:1091-1096

Rogers S, Moore M (1963): Studies of the mechanism of action of the shope rabbit papilloma virus. I. Concerning the nature of the induction of arginase in the infected cells. *J Exp Med* 117:521-542

Rogers S, Pfuderer P (1968): Use of viruses as carriers of added genetic information. *Nature* 219:749-751

Rothberg S, Van Scott EJ (1961): Localization of Arginase in Rabbit Skin. *Nature* 189:832-833

Sambrook J, Westphal H, Srinivasan PR, Dulbecco R (1968): The integrated state of viral DNA in SV40-transformed cells. *Proc Natl Acad Sci USA* 60:1288-1295

Scangos G, Ruddle FH (1981): Mechanisms and applications of DNA-mediated gene transfer in mammalian cells-a review. *Gene* 14:1-10

Schimizu T, Koyama S, Iwafuchi M (1962): Nuclear uptake of deoxyribonucleic acid by Ehrlich ascites-tunor cells. *Biochim Biophys Acta* 55:795-798

Seegmiller JE, Rosenbloom FM, Kelley WN (1967): Enzyme defect associated with a sex-linked human neurological disorder and excessive purine synthesis. *Science* 155:1682-1685

Shih C, Shilo B-Z, Goldfarb MP, Dannenberg A, Weinberg RA (1979): Passage of phenotypes of chemically transformed cells via transfection of DNA and chromatin. *Proc Natl Acad Sci USA* 76(11):5714-5718

Shimotohno K, Temin HM (1981): Formation of infections progeny virus after insertion of herpes simplex thymidine kinsase gene into DNA of an Avian Retrovirus. *Cell* 26:67-77

Sinsheimer RL (1969): The prospect for designed genetic change. *American Scientist* 57(1):134-142

Sirotnak FM, Hutchison DJ (1959): Absorption of deoxyribonucleic acid by mouse lymphoma cells. *Biochim Biophys Acta* 36:246-248

Smull CE, Ludwig EH (1962): Enhancement of the plaque-forming capacity of poliovirus ribonucleic acid with basic proteins. *J Bacteriol* 84:1035-1040

Soothill JS (1992): Treatment of experimental infections of mice with bacteriophages. *J Med Microbiol* 37:258-261

Spizizen J, Reilly BE, Evans AH (1966): Microbial transformation and transfection. *Ann Rev Microbiol*: 20:371-400

Stacey DW (1980): Expression of a subgenomic retroviral messenger RNA. *Cell* 21:811-820

Stasney J, Cantarow A, Paschkis KE (1950): Production of neoplasms by injection of fractions of mammalian neoplasms. *Cancer Research* 10:775-782

Stolk A (1960): Experimental carcinoma of the intestine in the Cichlid Aequidens maroni (Steindachner) following injection of herring-sperm deoxyribonucleic acid. *Naturwissenschafften* 47:88-89

Szybalska EH, Szybalski W (1962): Genetics of human cell lines, IV. DNA-mediated heritable transformation of a biochemical trait. *Proc Natl Acad Sci USA* 48:2026-2034

Szybalski W (1963). DNA-mediated Genetic Transformation of Human Cell Lines.

In *Round Table Discussion, Poultry Breeders of America Annuel Meeting*, .
McArdle Memorial Laboratory, UW-Madison:

Szybalski W (1991): A forerunner of monoclonal antibodies and human gene therapy. *Current Contents* 34:11

Szybalski W (1992): Use of the HPRT gene and the HAT selection Technique in DNA-mediated transformation of mammalian cells: first steps toward developing hybridoma techniques and gene therapy. *BioEssays* 14(7):495-500

Tabin CJ, Hoffmann JW, Goff SP, Weinberg RA (1982): Adaptation of a retrovirus as a eucaryotic vector transmitting the herpes simplex virus thymidine kinase gene. *Molecular and Cellular Biology* 2(4):426-436

Tatum EL (1966): Molecular biology, nucleic acids and the future of medicine. *Perspectives in Biology and Medicine* 10:19-32

Temin H (1976): The DNA provirus hypothesis. *Science* 192:1075-1080

Temin HM (1971): Mechanism of cell transformation by RNA tumor Viruses. *Annual Review of Microbiology* 25:609-648

Temin HM, Mizutani S (1970): RNA-dependent DNA Polymerase in Virions of rous sarcoma virus. *Nature* 226:1211-1213

Terheggen HG, Lowenthal A, Lavinha F, Colombo JP, Rogers S (1975): Unsuccessful Trial of gene Replacement in arginase deficiency. *The Journal of Experimental Medicine* 119:1-3

Topp WC, Lane D, Pollack R (1981). Transformation by SV40 and polyoma virus. In J. Tooze (Eds.), *DNA Tumor Viruses* (pp. 205-296). Cold Spring Harbor

Vaheri A, Pagano JS (1965): Infectious Poliovirus RNA: a sensitive method of assay. *Science* 175:434-436

Wade N (1980): UCLA gene therapy racked by friendly fire. *Science* 210:509-511

Wade N (1981): Gene therapy cought in more entaglements. *Science* 212:24-25

Wade N (1981): Gene therapy pioneer draws mikadoesque rap. *Science* 212:1253

Warden D, Thorne HV (1968): The infectivity of polyoma virus DNa for mouse embryo cells in the presence of Diethylaminoethyl-dextran. *Journal of General Virology* 3(371-):377

Watson JD, Crick FHC (1954): Genetical implications of the structure of deoxyribonucleic acid. *Nature* 171:737-739

Wei C-M, Gibson M, Spear PG, Scolnick EM (1981): Construction and isolation of a transmissible retrovirus containing the src Gene of harvey murine sarcoma virus and the thymidine kinase gene of herpes simplex virus type I. *Journal of Virology* 39(3):935-944

Weil R (1961): A quantitative assay for a subviral infective agent related to polyoma virus. *Virology* 14:46-53

Weisberger AS (1962): Induction of altered globin synthesis in human immature erthrocytes incubated with ribonucleoprotein. *Proc Natl Acad Sci USA* 48:68-80

Wigler M, Pellicer A, Silverstein S, Axel R (1977): Transfer of purified Herpes virus thymidine kinase gene to cultured mouse cells. *Cell* 11:223-232

Wigler M, Pellicer A, Silverstein S, Axel R (1978): Biochemical Transfer of Single-

Copy Eucaryotic Genes Using Total Cellular DNA as Donor. *Cell* 14:725-731

Wigler M, Pellicer A, Silverstein S, Axel R, Urlaub G, Chasin L (1979): DNA-mediated transfer of the adenine phosphoribosyltransferase locus into mammalian cells. *Proc Natl Acad Sci USA* 76:1373-1376

Willecke K, Klomfa BM, Mierau R, Dohmer J (1979): Intraspecies transfer via total cellular DNA of the Gene for Hypoxanthine phosphoribosyltransferase into cultured mouse cells. *Molecular and General Genetics* 170:179-185

Wolff JA, Malone RW, Williams P, Chong W, Acsadi G, Jani A, Felgner PL (1990): Direct gene transfer into mouse muscle in vivo. *Science* 247:1465-1468

Zinder ND, Lederberg J (1952): Genetic exchange in Salmonella. *J Bacteriology* 64:679-699

PRODUCING MOUSE GENETIC MODELS FOR HUMAN DISEASES

J. David McDonald

INTRODUCTION

The scientific literature is replete with examples of the contribution of laboratory animal models to biomedical research. Indeed, they have been invaluable to the basic research support of fields as wide-ranging as immunology, reproduction, oncology, nutrition, infectious diseases, transplantation, cardiology, and anesthesiology (Report of the Council on Scientific Affairs, 1989). Due to recent advances in the techniques required for somatic gene transfer and in the ability to produce desired models for human heritable diseases, the stage is now set to extend the range of these areas of biomedical impact to include somatic gene therapy.

Laboratory mice possess many qualities that render them highly useful for human disease model production. Their genetics, biochemistry, and physiology are well characterized and quite similar to humans. Reproductive characteristics and body size are especially favorable for studies requiring large numbers of animals. A gestation period of 19-20 days and sexual maturity at about 6 weeks combine to give a generation time of close to 60 days. During a females reproductive life she may give birth to as many as 8 litters with an average size of 6 to 8. Development has reached a high level of definition and all stages, notably including very early embryonic stages, are open to investigation. Tested animals can be easily and inexpensively maintained in a completely controlled environment. Due to a long and productive history of murine germline mutagenesis, the methods for producing desired mouse mutants are much more highly developed than for any other mammalian system. Genetically standardized inbred lines permit studies where the mutation in question is the sole difference between test and control animals. This allows the most direct comparison possible between normal and mutant phenotypes, providing the best situation for assessing the reconstitution of gene activity through somatic gene transfer. This also permits the option of pilot studies where gene activity is reconstituted through tissue transplantation from syngenic donors. Thus there can be an initial assessment of required reconstitution levels unencumbered by the complicating features of tissue rejection or immunosuppression. The availability of numerous inbred lines provides another benefit for effective disease model production. Occasionally, a given mutation elicits an unsuitable disease phenotype on a given genetic background. It is sometimes found that placing the mutation on a different genetic background yields a more clinically relevant phenotype. The ability to accomplish such an action quickly and easily is also a hallmark of the murine system.

Taking all of these beneficial qualities together, mice are arguably the organism of choice for mutant searches aimed at human disease model production. However, the murine system is not without its shortcomings for disease modeling (Erickson, 1989). In certain cases, it can be difficult or impossible to replicate the human disease in the murine system. Nevertheless, the typical finding is that analogous mutations in the murine system produce some or all of the disease manifestations seen in humans. Further, even a mouse strain that models only one of a number of possible pathological manifestations of a genetic disease can still provide an excellent opportunity for assessing the efficacy of somatic gene therapy. Therefore, the relatively few complete failures discovered amongst potential disease models are overshadowed by the many successes from the past and the great promise for future successes, both of which will be reviewed in this chapter. Among the set of models already produced, the level of pathology varies from some that exhibit only one or a few disease manifestations to others that apparently model the disease completely. As the goal of this chapter is to focus on to production of disease models useful for gene transfer experiments, no attempt is made to describe each model in detail. Their inclusion is principally to document the efficacy of the reviewed production methods.

MOUSE DISEASE MODEL PRODUCTION

Historically, mouse disease models have either been discovered in existing colonies or produced in different ways (Bulfield, 1981; Leiter et al., 1987; and Metsaranta and Vuorio, 1992). For successful somatic gene therapy efforts, the demands on the disease model are numerous and can exclude some types of existing models. Disease phenocopy models, where pathology is produced by transgene expression or chemical treatment, are generally excluded because they present no deficiency correctable by simple gene addition. Spontaneous, radiation- and insertion-induced mutations may yield disease models that are compromised because the underlying mutations are complex and not amenable to correction by gene therapy. Some other heritable disease models are currently excluded because the affected gene has yet to be cloned and therefore gene addition is not possible. These mutants are called models for human disease based on phenotypic considerations and often comparative mapping data (Darling and Abbott, 1992). It is quite likely that, after further characterization, many from this latter class will become useful for somatic gene therapy efforts.

The ideal mutation for somatic gene therapy efforts is a single gene mutation at a disease locus that has been cloned and characterized. The most direct means of producing such mutations is mutating predesignated disease genes. Two methods of mutagenesis, high efficiency germline mutagenesis with the mutagen N-ethyl-

N-nitrosourea (ENU) and targeted gene replacement in embryonal stem (ES) cells, have consistently proven their ability to produce such mutations. High efficiency germline mutagenesis induces a rate of mutation that, while random in nature, is sufficiently increased that one can recover mutations at a predesignated locus with reasonable frequency. Targeted gene replacement achieves the mutation of a predesignated locus through the site-specific process of homologous recombination.

Before leaving the topic of the ideal mutation for gene transfer experiments, it is important to note that, on occasion, the dual requirements of locus predesignation and previous gene characterization can be foregone. If the disease phenotype produced is of sufficient biomedical interest, mutation localization and gene characterization can occur later. The only concern that suffers is the immediacy of the subsequent gene transfer experiments. However, since the current set of recognized disease loci (McKusick et al., 1992) far exceeds the subset that have been cloned, such mutants represent a valuable reservoir for future gene transfer experiments. A large population of such mutants would shift the rate-limiting step from production of disease models to characterization, a process much nearer to utilization. The single subtraction feature of the mutation is less dispensable for gene therapy efforts. Deletion, or even perturbation in the expression, of more than one genetic locus can easily render the interpretation of somatic gene therapy studies uncertain.

HIGH EFFICIENCY GERMLINE MUTAGENESIS

Using a noncomplementation screen, ENU was discovered to induce the highest murine germline mutation rate of any known mutagen (Russell et al., 1979). Later it was discovered that ENU dose fractionation increased the mutagenic yield further (Russell et al., 1982a; Russell et al., 1982b; and Hitotsumachi et al., 1983). This induced mutation frequency is of such magnitude that one need examine on average only 500-1,000 offspring from treated males to recover one mutated at the predesignated locus. Another important facet of ENU mutagenesis is the type of lesion produced. Numerous researchers have presented evidence from other organisms documenting that ENU is a small lesion mutagen, nearly always producing single base changes (Vogel and Natarjan, 1979; Lee et al., 1987; Richardson et al., 1987; Batzer et al., 1988; Eckert et al., 1988; Pastink et al., 1988; Zeilenska et al., 1988; and Pastink et al., 1989). These findings have been confirmed by sequenced mouse mutations (Popp et al., 1983; Peters et al., 1985; Lewis et al., 1988; Peters et al., 1990; and Su et al., 1992). This mutagenic lesion is the least likely to affect the expression of more than one genetic locus but yet is capable of producing all classes of mutations (i.e., hypo-, hyper-, neo- and nulli-morphs). The high inducible mutation frequency, the localized effect of the lesion and the ability to produce all mutation classes, combine to make this protocol a powerful tool for disease model production. ENU mutagenesis lends itself most easily to phenotype-driven searches. This searching strategy, which selects as its endpoint the demonstration of some readily detectable disease phenotype feature, protects against the production of an analogous mutation that does not cause representative pathology.

ENU mutagenesis has enabled the isolation of such a large number of desired mouse mutations that reviewing them is beyond the scope of this article. Instead, those mutations showing promise for human disease modeling are highlighted in Table 1. The methods of identifying ENU-induced mutations have varied but have all been phenotype-driven in some respect. Some researchers have screened mice for alterations in protein electrophoretic mobility and activity, for others, aberrant organismic phenotypes revealed the presence of desired mutations. Occasionally, beneficial mutants were discovered while searching for unrelated mutations. In particular, Min, a serendipitously discovered mouse model for the human disease adenomatous polyposis coli (Moser et al., 1990 and Su et al., 1992), provides a cogent reminder that using a high efficiency random mutagen also allows the recovery of unplanned but ultimately very useful disease phenotypes.

There are also several shortcomings associated with ENU mutagenesis. Single base changes are the most difficult mutational lesion to characterize on a molecular level. This limitation can slow the utilization of disease models. However, some methods are consistently proving their ability to detect and characterize such point mutations. The chemical cleavage method (Cotton et al., 1988) can yield information about the location of single base changes and the specific change that occurred. The single strand conformation polymorphism method (Orita et al., 1989) can rapidly localize such a lesion and is readily amenable to automation with the polymerase chain reaction. One of the advantages of ENU mutagenesis can also be scored a disadvantage for some disease model pursuits. On occasion, preliminary knowledge of a genetic disease may indicate that the only mutant class capable of producing a pertinent disease phenotype is the null class. Single base changes can yield "leaky" mutations, those allowing enough residual activity to avoid some or all characteristic pathology in the mutant animal. If this information is known prior to the search, then ENU may not be the mutagen of choice.

An important future role for ENU mutagenesis stems from the fact that, of the two methods discussed here, it is the only option for producing disease models caused by mutation at uncloned loci. Although such models are not immediately eligible for gene transfer studies, their production represents an important advance in several respects. New mutations can quickly be localized in the mouse genome by genetic mapping. Such mapping information can be used to infer the human gene location through previously characterized linkage and synteny homologies between the human and murine genomes (Davisson et al. 1991). Thus, at a minimum, one can gain valuable information about the map location of the human gene. Further, one mapping method, the simple sequence length polymorphism (SSLP) mapping method (Dietrich et al., 1992), is proceeding toward a goal of sufficient marker density to permit positional cloning of the newly induced mutation (see O'Brien et al., 1993 for the most recently published SSLP map). The abilities to produce disease phenotypes caused by mutation in uncharacterized genes

TABLE 1. ENU-induced Mouse Genetic Disease Models

Deficiency Produced	Disease Modeled	Reference
Hemoglobin, α-chain	α-thalassemia	Popp et al. (1983)
Hemoglobin, ß-chain	ß-thalassemia	Peters et al. (1985)
Carbonic anhydrase II (CA-II)	CA-II deficiency syndrome	Lewis et al. (1988)
Triosephosphate isomerase (TPI)	TPI deficiency syndrome	Merkle and Pretsch (1989)
GTP-cyclohydrolase I	Tetrahydrobiopterin-deficient hyperphenylalaninemia	Bode et al. (1988)
Phenylalanine hydroxylase	Classical phenylketonuria	McDonald et al. (1990) Shedlovsky et al. (1992)
Dystrophin	Muscular dystrophy	Chapman et al. (1989)
Sarcosine dehydrogenase	Hypersarkosinemia	Harding et al. (1992)
Adenomatous polyposis coli protein	Adenomatous intestinal polyposis	Moser et al. (1990)
Glucose-6-phosphate dehydrogenase (G6PD)	G6PD deficiency syndrome	Pretsch et al. (1988)

and to quickly localize them by genetic mapping with positional cloning as its endpoint has the potential to greatly accelerate human disease gene characterization.

Disease model production by ENU mutagenesis can also be made more efficient by feeding possible mutants into wide-ranging phenotypic screens. By testing such animals for phenotypic manifestations common to many inborn errors of metabolism, such as organicacidemia, mutagenized gametes are much more thoroughly tested for disease mutations and useful disease models can be expected to emerge at a greatly enhanced rate.

TARGETED MUTAGENESIS

About a dozen years ago, ES cells were first successfully isolated from mouse blastocysts and cultured in vitro (Evans and Kaufman, 1981 and Martin, 1981). The intervening years have witnessed the increasingly sophisticated exploration of ES cell mutagenesis (reviewed in Capecchi, 1989; Robertson, 1991; and Koller and Smithies, 1992). It was discovered that ES cells could be manipulated in culture but remain sufficiently undifferentiated to allow colonization of all mouse tissues, including the germline, after injection back into blastocysts (Gossler et al., 1986 and Robertson et al. 1986). This allowed, for the first time, an interfacing of cell culture and organismic biology. Any mutations that were inducible by manipulation of cultured cells could then be much more thoroughly investigated by examining their effect at the organismic level in mutant mice. Early work involved selection for random mutations in cultured ES cells (Hooper et al., 1987 and Kuehn et al., 1987). Later, mutations were introduced into selectable genes by homologous recombination, a process which results in targeted gene replacement (Doetschman et al., 1987; Thomas and Capecchi, 1987; Doetschman et al., 1988; Koller et al., 1989; and Thompson et al., 1989). Still later, it became possible to identify replacement events in nonselected genes (Jasin and Berg, 1988, Kim and Smithies, 1988 and Johnson et al., 1989). Researchers were then able to disrupt a number of such genes: *B2m* (Koller and Smithies, 1988 and Zijlstra et al., 1989); *int-2* (Mansour et al., 1988); *en-2* (Joyner et al., 1989); c-*abl* (Schwartzberg et al., 1989); *Hox-1.1* (Zimmer and Gruss, 1989); *Hox-1.5* (Chisaka et al., 1991); *Hox-1.6* (Lufkin et al., 1991 and Chisaka et al., 1992); *Hox-2.6* (Hasty et al., 1991a); and *Hox-3.1* (Le Mouellic et al., 1992). Some of the this work included the additional refinement of the introduction of subtle mutations at the targeted locus (Koller et al., 1989, Schwartzberg et al., 1989 and Hasty et al., 1991a). Although, initially, mutations were mostly produced to study mammalian development, the impact of this new technology is now being felt in the field of disease model production (Table 2, and for a recent review see Smithies, 1993).

There are a number of significant benefits to using targeted mutagenesis for disease model production. Targeting events can be selected such that only one predetermined locus is mutated by a previously determined lesion. This lesion can completely abolish expression from that locus or more subtle mutations can be introduced. The ability to have total control over the location and type of mutation promises to revolutionize the production of biomedically useful mutants.

In the relatively short period since the inception of ES cell mutagenesis, some shortcomings have also become apparent. It is very technically demanding to obtain both targeted gene replacement in ES cells and germline colonization in the resultant chimeric animals. Further, the possibility exists that the homologous gene replacement event, or the presence of a selectable gene inserted into the replacement cassette, may perturb the expression of nearby genes. However, substantial research effort has been expended to optimize both the gene targeting process (Hasty et al., 1991b; Hasty et al., 1991c; Jeannotte et al., 1991; Zheng et al., 1991; Valancius and Smithies, 1991a; Valancius and Smithies, 1991b; Reid et al., 1991; Thomas et al., 1992; te Riele et al., 1992; Hasty et al., 1992; and Davis et al., 1992) and the cell culture conditions needed to maintain the totipotent nature of ES cells (Hogan, 1986 and Williams et al., 1988). With the protocol improvements that have come from such studies, the difficulties are beginning to be surmounted by the general scientific community. For the purposes of disease model production, some residual problems remain due to a more fundamental characteristic, the genotype-driven nature of this type of mutagenesis. The mutant strain ultimately pro-

TABLE 2. Targeting-induced Mouse Genetic Disease Models

Deficiency Produced	Disease Modeled	Reference
Apolipoprotein E	Atherosclerosis and hypercholesterolemia	Plump et al., 1992 Piedrahita et al., 1992 Zhang et al., 1992
Glucocerebrosidase	Gaucher's disease	Tybulewics et al., 1992
Cystic fibrosis transmembrane conductance protein	Cystic fibrosis	Koller et al., 1991 Snouwaert et al., 1992 Colledge et al., 1992 Dorin et al., 1992
c-src protein	Osteopetrosis	Soriano et al., 1991
p53 protein	Increased spontaneous tumors	Donehower et al., 1992
Immunoglobulin chain	B cell Immunodeficiency	Kitamura et al., 1991
V(D)J recombination activating protein	T and B Cell Immunodeficiency	Mombaerts et al., 1992

duced may not manifest the appropriate level of pathology necessary for optimal disease modeling because the induced mutation itself is inappropriate. In addition, in a genotype-driven mutant search, this result is only discovered after considerable time, energy, and resources have been spent in strain production.

In predicting the future of mouse disease model production by targeting, it is certain that there will be continued production as more disease loci are cloned and as the processes of gene targeting and germline colonization are further optimized. Moreover, an increasing number of targeted mutations will be analogous to human mutations as protocols for recovering subtle locus changes become more facile.

FUTURE DIRECTIONS

In considering the future of mouse disease model production in general, it would be wise if researchers stayed alert to the possibilities for synergy that are possible from the combinatorial use of these two techniques. The highly specific alteration at a predetermined locus that can be achieved by targeting can serve to generate a founder allele at the disease locus regardless of whether the resultant phenotype turns out to be germane. Crossing animals, either homo- or hetero-zygous for this founder allele, to an ENU-treated animal allows the identification of new mutations by noncomplementation and requires only a single cross. This incorporates a phenotype-driven nature to the mutant search, allowing the recovery of more pertinent phenotypes without the guesswork involved in the targeted introduction of subtle mutations. For example, the overly severe phenotype exhibited by the Gaucher's mouse model (Tybulewics et al., 1992) illustrates that the null mutation is not necessarily the desired class for a disease model. The next step for the targeter might be to introduce a subtle mutation, one analogous to that seen in the human disease. This is a large undertaking and assumes that the analogous mutation would produce pertinent pathology in the mouse. This assumption is not necessarily valid. The analogous mutation may also produce an inappropriate phenotype, or no phenotype at all. However, there may well be other mutations within the mouse gene capable of yielding more appropriate pathology. Incorporating a phenotype-driven aspect to the production of mutant alleles ensures that discovered mutations manifest some pertinent pathology.

Many experiments have recently been undertaken which examine somatic transfer of reporter gene constructs into nonmutant mice. These experiments have been important in beginning to establish parameters such as the best means of gene introduction and the persistence of transferred gene expression. Thus, meaningful knowledge about somatic gene therapy is already being obtained. What these studies have until now lacked is a transfer recipient that will manifest pathology unless the appropriate transferred gene is expressed at a certain critical level. Those types of experiments require the genetic disease model. Future specific disease models should allow for greater general optimization of transfer protocols as well as the improvement of individual protocols for particular diseases.

REFERENCES

Batzer MA, Tedeschi B, Fossett NG, Tucker, Kilroy G, Arbour P, Lee WR (1988): Spectra of molecular changes induced in DNA of *Drosophila* spermatozoa by 1-ethyl-1-nitrosourea and x-rays. *Mutat Res* 199:255-268

Bode VC, McDonald JD, Guenet J, Simon D (1988): *hph-1*: A mouse mutant with hereditary hyperphenylalaninemia induced by ethylnitrosourea mutagenesis. *Genetics* 118:299-305

Bulfield G (1981): Inborn errors of metabolism in the mouse. In: *Biology of the House Mouse*. Berry RJ, Ed. New York: Academic Press

Capecchi M (1989): The new mouse genetics: Altering the genome by gene targeting. *Trends Genet* 5:70-76

Chapman VM, Miller DR, Armstrong D, Caskey CT (1989): Recovery of induced mutations for X chromosome-linked muscular dystrophy in mice. *Proc Natl Acad Sci USA* 86:1292-1296

Chisaka O, Capecchi MR (1991): Regionally restricted developmental defects resulting from targeted disruption of the mouse homeobox gene *Hox-1.5*. *Nature* 350:473-479

Chisaka O, Muisu TS, Capecchi MR (1992): Developmental defects of the ear, cranial nerves and hindbrain resulting from targeted disruption of the mouse homeobox gene *Hox-1.6*. Nature 355:516-520

Colledge WH, Ratcliff R, Foster D, Williamson R, Evans MJ (1992): Cystic fibrosis mouse with intestinal obstruction. *Lancet* 340:680

Cotton RGH, Rodrigues NR, Campbell RD (1988): Reactivity of cytosine and thymine in single-base-pair mismatches with hydroxylamine and osmium tetroxide and its application to the study of mutations. *Proc Natl Acad Sci USA* 85:4397-4401

Darling SM, Abbott CM (1992): Mouse models of human single gene disorders I: Non-transgenic mice. *BioEssays* 14:359-365

Davis AC, Wims M, Bradley A (1992): Investigation of coelectroporation as a method for introducing mutations into embryonic stem cells. *Mol Cell Biol* 12:2769-2776

Davisson MT, Lalley PA, Peters J, Doolittle DP, Hillyard AL, Searle, AG (1991): Report of the comparative committee for human, mouse and other rodents. *Cytogenet Cell Genet* 58:1152-1189

Dietrich W, Katz H, Lincoln SE (1992): A genetic map of the mouse suitable for typing intraspecific crosses. *Genetics* 131:423-447

Doetschman T, Gregg RG, Maeda N, Hooper ML, Melton DW, Thompson S, Smithies O (1987): Targeted correction of a mutant *HPRT* gene in mouse embryonic stem cells. *Nature* 330:576-578

Doetschman T, Maeda N, Smithies O (1988): Targeted mutation of the *HPRT* gene in mouse embryonic stem cells. *Proc Natl Acad Sci USA* 85:8583-8587

Donehower LA, Harvey M, Slagle BL (1992): Mice deficient for p53 are developmentally normal but susceptible to spontaneous tumours. *Nature* 356; 215-221

Dorin JR, Dickinson P, Alton EWFW, Smith SN, Geddes OM, Stevenson BJ, Kimber WL, Fleming S, Clarke AR, Hooper ML, Anderson L, Beddington RSP, Proteous DJ (1992): Cystic fibrosis in the mouse by targeted insertional mutagenesis. *Nature* 359:211-215

Eckert KA, Ingle CA, Klinedirst DK, Drinkwater NR (1988): Molecular analysis of mutations induced in humans cells by *N*-ethyl-*N*-nitrosourea. *Mol Carcinogen* 1:50

Erickson RP (1989): Why isn't a mouse more like a man? *Trends Genet* 5:1-3

Evans MJ, Kaufman MH (1981): Establishment of pluripotential cells from mouse embryos. *Nature* 292:154-156

Gossler A, Doetschman T, Korn R, Serfling E, Kemler R (1986): Transgenesis by means of blastocyst-derived embryonic stem cell lines. *Proc Natl Acad Sci USA* 83:9065-9069

Harding CO, Williams P, Pflanzer DM, Colwell RE, Lyne PW, Wolff JA (1992): *sar*: A genetic mouse model for human sarcosinemia generated by ethylnitrosourea mutagenesis *Proc Natl Acad Sci USA* 89:2644-2648

Hasty P, Ramirez-Soliz R, Krumlauf R (1991a): Introduction of a subtle mutation into the *Hox-2.6* locus in embryonic stem cells. *Nature* 350:243-246

Hasty P, Rivera-Perez J, Bradley A (1991b): The length of homology required for gene targeting in embryonic stem cells. *Mol Cell Biol* 11:5586-5591

Hasty P, Rivera-Perez J, Chang C, Bradley A (1991c): Target frequency and integration pattern for insertion and replacement vectors in embryonic stem cells. *Mol Cell Biol* 11:4509-17

Hasty P, Rivera-Perez J, Bradley A (1992): The role and fate of DNA ends for homologous recombination in embryonic stem cells. *Mol Cell Biol* 12:2462-2474

Hitotsumachi S, Carpenter D, Russell WL (1983): Dose fractionation as a means of increasing the mutagenic effectiveness of ethylnitrosourea in mouse spermatogonia. *Environ Mutagen* 5:380-385

Hogan B, Constantini F, Lacy E (1986): *Manipulating the Mouse Embryo*. New York: Cold Spring Harbor Laboratory Press

Hooper M, Hardy K, Handyside A, Hunter S, Monk M (1987): HPRT-deficient (Lesch-Nyhan) mouse embryos derived from germline colonization by cultured cells. *Nature* 326:292-295

Jasin M, Berg P (1988): Homologous integration in mammalian cells without target gene selection. *Genes Dev* 2:1353-1363

Jeannotte L, Ruiz JC, Robertson EJ (1991): Low level of *Hox-1.3* gene expression does not preclude the use of promoterless vectors to generate a targeted gene disruption. *Mol Cell Biol* 11:5578-5585

Johnson RS, Sheng M, Greenberg ME, Kolodner RD, Papaioannou VE (1989): Targeting of nonexpressed genes in embryonic stem cells via homologous recombination. *Science* 245:1234-1236

Joyner AL, Skarnes WC, Rossant J (1989): Production of a mutation in mouse *En-2* gene by homologous recombination in embryonic stem cells. *Nature* 338:153-156

Kim H, Smithies O (1988): Recombinant fragment assay for gene targeting based on the polymerase chain reaction. *Nucleic Acids Research* 16:8887-8903

Kitamura D, Roes J, Kühn R, Rajewsky K (1991): A B cell-deficient mouse by targeted disruption of the membrane exon of the immunoglobulin chain gene. *Nature* 350:423-426

Koller BH, Smithies O (1989): Inactivating the $_2$-microglobulin locus in mouse embryonic stem cells by homologous recombination. *Proc Natl Acad Sci USA* 86:8932-8935

Koller BH, Hageman LJ, Doetschman T, Hageman JR, Huang S, Williams PJ, First NL, Maeda N, Smithies O (1989): Germline transmission of a planned alteration made in a hypoxanthine phosphoribosyl transferase gene by homologous recombination in embryonic stem cells. *Proc Natl Acad Sci USA* 86:8927-8931

Koller BH, Kim H, Latour AM, Brigman K, Boucher RC, Scambler P, Wainwright B, Smithies O (1991): Toward an animal model of cystic fibrosis: Targeted interruption of exon 10 of the cystic fibrosis transmembrane regulator gene in embryonic stem cells. *Proc Natl Acad Sci USA* 88:10730-10734

Koller BH, Smithies O (1992): Altering genes in animals by gene targeting. *Annu*

Rev Immunol 10:705-730

Kuehn MR, Bradley A, Robertson EJ, Evans MJ (1987): A potential animal model for Lesch-Nyhan syndrome through introduction of HPRT mutations into mice. *Nature* 326:295-298

Le Mouellic H, Lallemand Y, Brulet P (1992): Homeosis in the mouse induced by a null mutation in the *Hox-3.1* gene. *Cell* 69:251-264

Lee CS, Curtis D, McCarron M, Love C, Gray M, Bender W, Chovnick A (1987): Mutations affecting expression of the *rosy* locus in *Drosophilia melanogaster*. *Genetics* 116:55-66

Leiter EH, Beamer WG, Shultz LD, Barker JE, Lane PW (1987): Mouse models of genetic diseases. In: *Medical and Experimental Mammalian Genetics: A Perspective.* McKusick VA, Roderick TH, Mori J, Paul NW, eds. New York: Liss

Lewis SG, Erickson RP, Barnett LB, Venta PJ, Tasian RE (1988): *N*-ethyl-*N*-nitrosourea-induced null mutation at the mouse *Car-2* locus: An animal model for human carbonic anhydrase II deficiency syndrome. *Proc Natl Acad Sci USA* 85:1962-1966

Lufkin T, Dierich A, LeMeur M, Chambion P (1991): Disruption of the *Hox-1.6* homeobox gene results in defects in a region corresponding to its rostral domain of expression. *Cell* 66:1105-1119

Mansour SL, Thomas KR, Capecchi MR (1988): Disruption of the proto-oncogene *int-2* in mouse-derived stem cells: a general strategy for targeting mutations to non-selectable genes. *Nature* 336:348-352

Martin G (1981): Isolation of a pluripotential cell line from early mouse embryos cultured in medium conditioned by teratocarcinoma stem cells. *Proc Natl Acad Sci USA* 78:7634-7638

McDonald JD, Bode VC, Dove WF, Shedlovsky A (1990): Pah^{hph-5}: a mouse mutant deficient in phenylalanine hydroxylase. *Proc Natl Acad Sci USA* 87:1965-1967

McKusick VA, Francomano CA, Antonarakis SE (1992): *Mendelian inheritance in man: catalogs of autosomal dominant, autosomal recessive, and X-linked phenotypes, 10th edition.* Baltimore, Johns Hopkins University Press

Merkle S, Pretsch W (1989): Characterization of triosephosphate isomerase mutants with reduced enzyme activity in *Mus musculus*. *Genetics* 123:837-844

Metsaranta M, Vuorio E (1992): Transgenic mice as models for heritable diseases. *Ann Med* 24:117-120

Mombaerts P, Iacomini J, Johnson RS, Herrup K, Tonegawa S, Papaioannou VE (1992): RAG-1-deficient mice have no mature B, T lymphocytes. *Cell* 68:869-877

Moser A R, Pitot H C, Dove W F (1990): A dominant mutation that predisposes to multiple intestinal neoplasia in the mouse. *Science* 247:322-324

O'Brien SJ ed (1992): *Genetic maps: locus maps of complex genomes, 6th edition.* New York, Cold Spring Harbor Laboratory Press

Orita M, Suzuki Y, Sekiya T, Hayashi K (1989): Rapid and sensitive detection of point mutations and DNA polymorphisms using the polymerase chain reaction. *Genomics* 5:874-879

Pastink AC, Vrecken C, Vogel EW (1988): The Nature of *N*-ethyl-*N*-ethylnitrosourea-induced mutations at the white locus of *Drosophila melanogaster. Mutat Res* 199:47-53

Pastink AC, Vreeken C, Mivard MJM, Searles LL, Vogel EW (1989): Sequence analysis of *N*-ethyl-*N*-nitrosourea-induced *Vermilion* mutations in *Drosophila melanogaster. Genetics* 123:123-129

Peters J, Andrews SJ, Loutit JF, Clegg JB (1985): A mouse -globin mutant that is an exact model of hemoglobin Ranier in man. *Genetics* 110:709-721

Peters J, Jones J, Ball ST, Clegg JB (1990): Analysis of electrophoretically detected mutations induced in mouse germ cells by ethylnitrosourea. In: *Biology of Mammalian Germ Cell Mutagenesis*, Allen JW, Bridges BA, Lyon MF, Moses MJ, Russell LB, eds. New York, Cold Spring Harbor Laboratory Press

Piedrahita JA, Zhang SH, Hagaman JR, Oliver PM, Maeda N (1992): Generation of mice carrying a mutant apolipoprotein E gene inactivated by gene targeting in embryonic stem cells. *Proc Natl Acad Sci USA* 89:4471-4475

Plump AS, Smith JD, Hayek T, Aalto-Setälä K, Walsh A, Verstuyft JG, Rubin EM, Breslow JL (1992): Severe hypercholesterolemia and atherosclerosis in apolipoprotein E-deficient mice created by homologous recombination in ES cells. *Cell* 71:343-353

Popp RA, Bailiff EG, Skow LC, Johnson FM, Lewis SE (1983): Analysis of a mouse -globin gene mutation induced by ethylnitrosourea. *Genetics* 105:157-167

Pretsch W, Charles DJ, Merkle S (1988): X-linked glucose-6-phosphate dehydrogenase deficiency in *Mus musculus. Biochem Genet* 26:89-103

Reid LH, Shesely EG, Kim HS, Smithies O (1991): Cotransformation and gene targeting in mouse embryonic stem cells. *Mol Cell Biol* 11:2769-2777

Report of the Council on Scientific Affairs (1989): Animals in Research. *JAMA* 261 (24):3602-3606

Richardson KK, Richardson FC, Crosby RM, Swenberg JA, Skopek TR (1987): DNA base changes and alkylation following in vivo exposure of *Escherichia coli* to *N*-ethyl-*N*-nitrosourea. *Proc Natl Acad Sci USA* 84:344-348

Robertson EJ, Bradley A, Kuehn M, Evans M (1986): Germ-line transmission of genes introduced into cultured pluripotential cells by retroviral vector. *Nature* 323:445-447

Robertson EJ (1991): Using embryonic stem cells to introduce mutations into the mouse germline. *Biol Reprod* 44:238-245

Russell WL, Kelly EM, Hunsicker PR, Bangham JW, Maddux SC, Phipps EL (1979): Specific locus test shows ethylnitrosourea to be the most potent mutagen in the mouse. *Proc Natl Acad Sci USA* 76:5818-5819

Russell WL, Hunsicker PR, Raymer GD, Steele MH, Stelzner KF, Thompson HM (1982a): Dose response for ethylnitrosourea-induced-specific-locus mutations in mouse spermatogonia. *Proc Natl Acad Sci USA* 79:3589-3591

Russell WL, Hunsicker PR, Carpenter DA, Cornett CV, Guinn GM (1982b): Effect of dose fractionation on the ethylnitrosourea induction of specific-locus mutations in mouse spermatogonia. *Proc Natl Acad Sci USA* 79:3592-3593

Schwartzberg PL, Goff SP, Robertson EJ (1989): Germline transmission of a c-*abl* mutation produced by targeted gene disruption in ES cells. *Science* 246:799-803

Shedlovsky A, McDonald JD, Symula D, Dove WF (1992): Mouse models of human PKU. Submitted to *Genetics*

Smithies O (1993): Animal models of human genetic diseases. *Trends Genet* (In Press)

Snouwaert JN, Brigman KK, Latour AM, Malouf NN, Boucher RC, Smithies O, Koller BH (1992): An animal model for cystic fibrosis made by gene targeting. *Science* 257:1083-1088

Soriano P, Montgomery C, Geske R, Bradley A (1991): Targeted disruption of the c-src proto-oncogene leads to osteopetrosis in mice. *Cell* 64:693-702

Su L, Kinzler KW, Vogelstein B, Preisinger AC, Moser AR, Luongo C, Gould KA, Dove WF (1992): Multiple intestinal neoplasia caused by a mutation in the murine homolog of the APC gene. *Science* 256:668-670

te Riele H, Maandag ER, Berns A (1992): Highly efficient gene targeting in embryonic stem cells through homologous recombination with isogenic DNA constructs. *Proc Natl Acad Sci USA* 89:5128-5132

Thomas KR, Deng C, Capecchi MR (1992): High-fidelity gene targeting in embryonic stem cells by using sequence replacement vectors. *Mol Cell Biol* 12:2919-2923

Thomas KR, Capecchi MR (1987): Site-directed mutagenesis by gene targeting in mouse embryo-derived stem cells. *Cell* 51:503

Thompson S, Clarke AR, Pow AM, Hooper ML, Melton DW (1989): Germ line transmission and expression of a corrected HPRT gene produced by gene targeting in embryonic stem cells. *Cell* 56:313-321

Tybulewics VLJ, Tremblay ML, LeMarca ME, Willemsen R, Stubblefield BK, Winfield S, Zablorka B, Sidransky E, Martin BM, Huang SP, Mintzer KA, Westphal H, Mulligan RC, Ginns EI (1992): Animal model of Gaucher's disease from targeted disruption of the mouse glucocerebrosidase gene. *Nature* 357:407-410

Valancius V, Smithies O (1991a): Double-strand gap repair in a mammalian gene targeting reaction. *Mol Cell Biol* 11:4389-4397

Valancius V, Smithies O (1991b): Testing and "in-out" targeting procedure for making subtle modifications in mouse embryonic stem cells. *Mol Cell Biol* 11:1402-1408

Vogel E, Natarjan AJ (1979): The relation between reaction kinetics and mutagenic action of mono-functional alkylating agents in higher eukaryotic systems. I Recessive lethal mutations and translocations in *Drosophila*. *Mutation Res* 62:51-100

Williams Rl, Hilton DJ, Pease S, Willson TA, Stewart CL, Gearing DP, Wagner

EF, Metcalf D, Nicola NA, Gough NM (1988): Myeloid leukemia inhibitory factor maintains the developmental potential of embryonic stem cells. *Nature* 336:684-687

Zeilenska M, Beranek D, Guttenplan JB (1988): Different mutational profiles induced by *N*-nitroso-*N*-ethylurea: Effects of dose and error-prone DNA repair and correlations with DNA adducts *Environ Molec Mutagen* 11:473-485

Zhang SH, Reddick RL, Piedrahita JA, Maeda N (1992): Spontaneous hypercholesterolemia and arterial lesions in mice lacking apolipoprotein E. *Science* 258:468-471

Zheng H, Hasty P, Brenneman MA, Grompe M, Gibbs RA, Wison JH, Bradley A (1991): Fidelity of targeted recombination in human fibroblasts and murine embryonic stem cells. *Proc Natl Acad Sci USA* 88:8067-8071

Zijlstra M, Li E, Sajjadi F, Subramani S, Jaenisch R (1989): Germ-line transmission of a disrupted beta 2-microglobulin gene produced by homologous recombination in embryonic stem cells. *Nature* 342:435-438

Zimmer A, Gruss P (1989): Production of chimeric mice containing embryonic stem (ES): cells carrying a mutation of homoeobox *Hox 1.1* allele mutated by homologous recombination *Nature* 338:150-153

POST-TRANSCRIPTIONAL CONSIDERATIONS OF GENE EXPRESSION: TRANSLATION, MRNA STABILITY, AND POLY(A) PROCESSING

Gary Brewer

Many genes are regulated by switching their transcription on or off. However, the steady-state level of a protein depends not only upon the rate at which the mRNA is synthesized, but also upon the rates at which the mRNA is processed, transported and translated along with the rates at which the mRNA and protein are degraded. Therefore, each of these post-transcriptional processes is linked to "gene expression," and it is important to know how each contributes to the level or timing of expression of a given protein. The purpose of this review is to describe a number of considerations about post-transcriptional processes when the goal is to express a recombinant protein in a mammalian cell. I hope to demonstrate that achieving optimal synthesis of a recombinant protein might not be as simple as linking a transcriptional promoter to an open reading frame; considerations concerning the effects of RNA splicing, 3' end formation/polyadenylation, RNA localization, translation and stability of the cytoplasmic mRNA and protein all influence the production of a protein. In keeping with the purpose of this review, specific examples of each type of control will be described. Obviously, the examples will not be exhaustive but rather illustrative. Thus by necessity, the work of many research groups will not be described. Since this review is practical in nature, I will emphasize the cis-acting elements of a gene which control post-transcriptional RNA processing and translation; I will not discuss the trans-acting factors which must interact with the cis-elements to effect post-transcriptional and translational control. Recent evidence indicates that one process or element can affect several post-transcriptional processes. However, as much as possible, I will strive to discuss the cis-elements controlling gene expression in the temporal order in which they play a role. Finally, expression of recombinant proteins in mammalian cells is more art than science. That is, the cis elements in the gene construct for "optimal" production of one protein may not suffice for optimal production of a different protein. Thus, the requirements for production of proteins of interest should be considered for each protein.

Gene Therapeutics: Methods and Applications of Direct Gene Transfer
Jon A. Wolff, Editor • ©1994 *Birkhäuser Boston*

SEQUENCES AFFECTING 3' END FORMATION AND POLY(A) PROCESSING

Promoter Elements

Many constructs containing promoters which drive transcription efficiently in mammalian cells are available either commercially or through generous research laboratories. However, a little appreciated fact is that a promoter element can affect the post-transcriptional processing of the homologous gene, albeit in rare cases. Three examples are the U1 snRNA gene, immunoglobulin μ genes and the long terminal repeat (LTR) of human immunodeficiency virus type 1 (HIV-1), which is included in these examples because retroviral LTRs are frequently employed as promoters in mammalian cells. The U1 gene is transcribed by RNA polymerase II, just as genes encoding mRNA are (Hernandez and Weiner, 1986; Neuman de Vegvar et al., 1986). However, 3' end formation of the snRNA precursors requires the snRNA promoter; promoters for genes encoding mRNAs cannot substitute. For the immunoglobulin μ gene, an intron is required for its expression when transcription is driven by the V_H promoter/enhancer (Neuberger and Williams, 1988). The requirement for an intron is obviated by substitution of a different promoter. (More discussion of intron requirements in gene expression will be presented below.) The U3 region of the HIV-1 proviral LTR drives transcription of the HIV-1 genome. A sequence known as the TAR element is located at the extreme 5' end of HIV-1 mRNAs. TAR is believed to both activate the transcription of the HIV-1 genome and control translation of viral mRNAs. Braddock et al. (1990) found that the U3 region of the HIV-1 LTR was responsible for the low expression potential of the mRNA, since RNAs of identical structure were efficiently translated when transcription was driven by a heterologous cytomegalovirus immediate-early (CMV-IE) promoter. One rationale for these post-transcriptional promoter effects is that transcription, RNA processing and RNA transport in the nucleus might be coupled in a spatially organized process dictated by nuclear structure (Blobel, 1985; Mattaj, 1990). In conclusion, it is important to be aware that transcriptional promoter elements can have effects on post-transcriptional gene expression in addition to driving transcription of the DNA of interest.

Introns

Introns of course are removed during processing of the primary transcript by RNA splicing. Introns provide a means of controlling gene expression. For example, alternative splicing can create two or more functional forms of mRNA. This also permits stage- and cell-specific gene expression (reviewed in Baker, 1989 and Maniatis, 1991). Additionally, a transcript can be rendered functional by removal of all introns or kept nonfunctional by retaining at least part of an intron (reviewed in Kozak, 1988). However, in addition to these well-known effects, introns can have drastic consequences for RNA polyadenylation and transport. This was first observed in early studies of gene expression using DNA viruses such as SV40 and adenovirus. Several studies revealed that splicing was required for the production of detectable steady-state levels of cytoplasmic 16S, 19S and small t-antigen mRNAs (Huang and Gorman, 1990; Ryu and Mertz, 1989 and references therein). The intron did not have to be of viral origin; an intron from a β-globin gene would also suffice. Thus, it was thought that splicing was required for gene expression in general in mammalian cells. However, other groups found that adequate levels of mRNA could be achieved without introns and splicing (Simonson and Levinson, 1983; Treisman et al., 1981), and indeed, several animal cell and virtually all yeast genes lack introns altogether.

As a result, several groups initiated studies to examine gene expression from plasmid vectors containing cDNAs with or without an inserted intron (Buchman and Berg, 1988; Huang and Gorman, 1990; Ryu and Mertz, 1989; Yu et al., 1991). The upshot of these studies was that introns can increase the levels of steady-state cytoplasmic mRNA by 2- to 500-fold; however, transcribed sequences vary greatly in their dependence on an intron for high levels of mRNA production. The sequence of the intron between the 5' and 3' splice sites was not important, nor was the position of the intron within the transcribed portion of the gene (Buchman and Berg, 1988). An intron requirement is sometimes promoter dependent, sometimes promoter independent. For example, in the case of IgH gene expression described above, the requirement for an intron was promoter dependent. In the case of β-globin, neither the β-globin promoter, nor the herpes simplex virus type 1 thymidine kinase promoter, nor the CMV-IE promoter relieved the intron requirement for cytoplasmic accumulation of β-globin mRNA (Yu et al., 1991). From a practical point of view then, inclusion of an intron is a reasonable strategy for maximizing gene expression in mammalian cells. In the cases where an intron is clearly important, the intron is thought to affect the nuclear stability, polyadenylation and transport of the mRNA. Support for a connection between introns/splicing and polyadenylation comes from studies which indicate that polyadenylation is stimulated by an upstream intron (Huang and Gorman, 1990; Niwa et al., 1990; Ryu and Mertz, 1989), and mutation of the AAUAAA polyadenylation signal depresses in vitro splicing (Niwa and Berget, 1991).

3' End Formation And Polyadenylation Signals

Mammalian poly(A) signals are fairly well defined as is the biochemistry of polyadenylation (for reviews, see Proudfoot, 1991 and Wickens, 1990). Polyadenylation serves to control transcription of a gene (i.e., its termination) and processing of the primary RNA transcript (Proudfoot, 1988). Just as important, the poly(A) tract endows mRNAs with the essential properties of stability and translatability (for reviews, see Peltz et al., 1990 and Sachs, 1990). Translation and mRNA stability will be discussed in separate sections below.

The minimal, mammalian poly(A) signal is composed of an AAUAAA motif 20-30 nucleotides 5' to a GU-rich sequence (GU-box). Cleavage of the precursor

RNA generally occurs between these sequence motifs (Proudfoot, 1991). Thus the GU-box may not be present in the mature mRNA, and hence cDNA. One consequence of this is that transcription of a mammalian expression vector containing a cDNA only may lack the signals for optimal 3' end formation. Elements upstream of the poly(A) site can also influence its efficiency. For example, upstream sequences increase the efficiency of both the SV40 late and adenovirus L1 poly(A) sites in mammalian cells. Furthermore, from the discussion in the previous section, introns stimulate polyadenylation in vitro (Niwa et al., 1990; Niwa and Berget, 1991) and in vivo (Huang and Gorman, 1990; Ryu and Mertz, 1989).

In addition to the canonical polyadenylation signals described above, mRNAs contain information which leads to developmental, cell-specific or stimulus-specific lengthening or shortening of the poly(A) tract. Lengthening of the poly(A) tract tends to control mRNA translation and increases the stability of mRNA. Shortening of the poly(A) tract tends to lead to degradation of the mRNA. These properties of mRNAs will be described in later sections.

SEQUENCES THAT AFFECT TRANSLATION

The Initiation Codon

Initiation is a rate limiting step in translation and is controlled by four features of mRNA sequence: (1) context of the AUG initiation codon; (2) the position of the AUG codon(s); (3) secondary structure 5' and 3' to the AUG; and (4) length of the 5' untranslated region (5'UTR) (reviewed in Kozak, 1991). The requirements for specific nucleotide sequences surrounding the AUG codon, i.e. context, for efficient initiation have been identified in detail. Translation of most mammalian mRNAs is initiated by the binding of the 40S ribosomal subunit, along with associated factors, to the 5' end and scanning to the first AUG, where the 60S ribosomal subunit joins, and the first peptide bond is formed (Kozak, 1991). (Apparent exceptions to the scanning mechanism will be described later.) Experiments involving mutagenesis of nucleotides surrounding the AUG and transfection into COS cells revealed that the optimal context for initiation is 5'-GCC(A/G)CCAUGG-3', where the A of the AUG codon is designated the +1 nucleotide. The most critical residues controlling the efficiency of initiation are a purine at -3, usually A^{-3}, and G^{+4}. Deviations from this optimal context can have drastic effects on the codon chosen for initiation, such that the 40S subunits can bypass the first AUG and initiate at a downstream AUG. An example of the effect of multiple AUG codons on initiation is illustrated by the proto-oncogene c-lck mRNA. This mRNA has four AUG codons in the sequence,

5'-CCAAUGG....AGGAUGU....CUGAUGU...AUCAUGG....-3',

where the fourth lies in an optimal context and is the true initiation codon (Marth et al., 1988). The upstream AUG codons are in contexts ranging from weak to good. Their presence serves to suppress the efficiency of initiation at the fourth

AUG codon, since their deletion increases translation initiation approximately 9-fold. For some proto-oncogenes, this low level of translation is essential for their proper control. It also illustrates how upstream AUG codons can be used to temper the expression of proteins whose overexpression can have deleterious effects on the cell or organism.

Approximately 90% of vertebrate mRNAs are initiated at the first AUG codon in a good context, as defined above (Kozak, 1991). Position of the AUG codon relative to the 5' end is as important as context, since some ribosomes initiate at the first AUG even in a weak context. In fact, an A^{-3} at the first AUG codon will usually result in its selection for initiation, especially if the mRNA possesses secondary structure downstream from the AUG codon. Secondary structure, in the form of a hairpin 12-15 nucleotides downstream of an initiation codon, causes the 40S subunit to stall momentarily which facilitates initiation. Downstream secondary structure apparently serves two roles in translation initiation (Kozak, 1990). (1) It minimizes "leaky" initiation; 97% of vertebrate mRNAs have a purine at -3, but few have the full 5'-GCC(A/G)CCAUGG-3' consensus sequence. (2) It may permit control of translation from weak AUG codons and from rare non-AUG codons. There are a growing number of mammalian mRNAs that use alternative codons as an adjunct to an AUG codon. An advantage of this is that one mRNA can encode multiple polypeptides which may have very different properties from one another. For example, the subcellular localization of the mouse Int-2 oncoprotein, a fibroblast growth factor-related product, is determined by the choice of initiation codon (Acland et al., 1990). Int-2 initiated at the AUG codon localizes to the secretory pathway while Int-2 initiated at an upstream, in-frame CUG codon localizes to the nucleus. The requirements for initiation at a CUG or ACG are (A/G)$^{-3}$, G^{+4} and downstream secondary structure (Kozak, 1990; 1991). In conclusion, the context of the AUG codon is a major determinant of its selection as the translation start site, and modest secondary structure downstream of an AUG or non-AUG codon can have a positive effect on translation initiation.

Secondary Structure Within The 5'UTR

Secondary structure, i.e. hairpins, between the 7-methyl guanosine cap at the 5' end of the mRNA and the AUG codon do not facilitate initiation (Kozak, 1991). Negative effects of secondary structure in the 5'UTR depend on the position and free energy of the hairpin. For example, a hairpin with G = -30 kcal/mol severely inhibits translation when located within the first 12 nucleotides of the 5' end but has no effect 52 nt from the cap (Kozak, 1986;1989). In general, a 5'UTR containing a hairpin with G > -50 kcal/mol will severely inhibit translation in vivo and in vitro, since the 40S subunit and associated factors are unable to unwind secondary structures with this stability (Kozak, 1991).

However, secondary structure in the 5'UTR can be useful as a control mechanism for translation. One example is the iron-responsive element (IRE) located in the 5'UTR of mRNAs encoding ferritin, the iron storage protein (reviewed in Theil,

1990). In the presence of low intracellular levels of iron, the IRE serves to inhibit the translation of ferritin mRNAs; in high levels of iron, ferritin mRNAs are efficiently translated. A 5' hairpin from the IRE consisting of 32 nt with the following structure appears necessary and sufficient to confer iron-regulated translation upon heterologous mRNAs to which it is linked (Rouault et al., 1988).

Regulation by iron is controlled by an IRE-binding protein, known variously as IRE-BP, IRF or IRP (Leibold and Munro, 1988; Müllner et al., 1988; Rouault et al., 1988; Walden et al., 1988). In low iron this protein binds the IRE which is thought to stabilize its secondary structure thus blocking 40S subunits from the AUG codon. Koeller et al. (1991) have used constructs containing the IRE in the 5'UTR to control in vivo translation of heterologous mRNAs. Translation of a heterologous mRNA can be activated by treating cells with an iron source such as hemin without global effects on protein synthesis; translation is repressed when cells are treated with an iron chelator such as desferrioxamine.

Secondary structure in the 5'UTR may also have a role in regulating translation in developmental systems, such as oogenesis and early development. During oogenesis, the eggs of many animal species accumulate large pools of maternally derived poly(A+) mRNA. Most of this mRNA is translationally inactive until the egg is fertilized, after which specific mRNAs become translationally activated during various stages of early development (Fu et al., 1991). The mechanisms of differential translation are beginning to be identified. For example, mRNAs containing a stable 25 basepair (bp) hairpin in the 5'UTR were translated at 3% the efficiency as the homologous mRNA lacking a hairpin during oogenesis (Fu et al., 1991). The relative translational potential of the hairpin mRNA reached 100% in the newly fertilized egg and returned to 3% after the midblastula transition. Thus 5' secondary structure can be used to provide regulatory control over translation.

Length Of The 5'UTR

The length of the 5'UTR is another useful variable for controlling the efficiency of translation. At a minimum, around 20 nt of 5'UTR are required for initiation at an AUG codon in a favorable context (Kozak, 1991). In vitro, the efficiency of translation is proportional to a length of 17-80 nt. The effectiveness of the 5'UTR requires that it contain few G residues to ensure that secondary structure does not form. From a practical standpoint, several groups have used the β-globin 5'UTR to maximize translation of heterologous mRNAs both in vitro (Annweiler et al., 1991) and in vivo (Malone et al., 1989). The in vivo effect was about 9-fold in NIH 3T3 cells.

Internal Initiation Mediated By 5'UTR Sequences

As detailed above, the scanning model for translation initiation states that the 40S ribosomal subunit and associated factors bind the 5' end of an mRNA in a cap-dependent manner and scan linearly in a 5' to 3' direction to the first AUG codon in a good context for initiation (Kozak, 1991). As a corollary to this, translation at a downstream cistron of a dicistronic mRNA would be inefficient, since few ribosomes would continue to scan into the intercistronic spacer. However, in 1988 several groups reported that picornaviruses such as poliovirus and encephalomyocarditis (EMC) virus could initiate translation of viral mRNAs internally without first scanning from the 5' end (Jang et al., 1988; Pelletier and Sonenberg, 1988; Trono et al., 1988). Apparently, many picornaviruses are capable of this type of translational initiation (reviewed in Herman, 1989; Jackson, 1988; Jackson et al., 1990; and Sonenberg, 1991). The fact that internal initiation of picornavirus mRNAs did not require virally encoded proteins begged for the existence of cellular mRNAs which could also initiate internally. Indeed, two examples have been identified. The first was the mRNA encoding the human immunoglobulin heavy-chain binding-protein, known as BiP or GRP 78, glucose-regulated protein of relative molecular mass 78,000 (Macejak and Sarnow, 1991). The second example of internal initiation was the *Antennapedia* (ANTP) mRNA of *Drosophila melanogaster* (OH et al., 1992). The ANTP gene is involved in segment formation during development. For both the picornavirus and eukaryotic mRNAs which can initiate internally, the sequences responsible are located in the 5'UTR and are often referred to as ribosome landing pads (RLP) or internal ribosome entry sites (IRES). The mechanism(s) of internal initiation remain unknown, though binding of a cellular 57-kD RNA-binding protein to the IRES of EMC virus and binding of a 52-kD protein to the RLP of poliovirus have been implicated in the mechanism of internal initiation (Jang and Wimmer, 1990; Meerovitch et al., 1989). For excellent reviews of the sequence and structural features of a 5'UTR which permit internal initiation, see Jackson et al (1990) and Meerovitch and Sonnenberg (1990). Briefly, however, the major features appear to be a polypyrimidine tract set amidst secondary structure motifs.

Placement of an IRES between two open reading frames (ORF) permits the creation of a bicistronic mRNA in mammalian cells; both ORFs appear to be translated with equal efficiency. Indeed, Kim et al. (1992) used the IRES from EMC virus to create a bifunctional mRNA (5' neomycin resistance, 3' β-galactosidase) in chimeric mouse embryos. In their study, more than half of the embryonic stem cells made G418-resistant by their bicistronic construct also stained positive for β-galactosidase. As Kim et al. pointed out, the bicistronic vector system will provide the tools to obtain temporally and spatially coordinated expression of two genes driven by a single promoter in a single cell.

Sequences In The 3'UTR Which Affect Translation

The 3'UTR can control translation by means not as well understood as those by which 5'UTR sequences or AUG codon context control initiation. (For an excellent review of the role of the 3'UTR in translation, see Jackson and Standart, 1990). The 3'UTR controls translation in many ways, such as its efficiency, inducibility, its temporal control during gametogenesis and development, subcellular localization of mRNA and translational incorporation of alternative amino acids such as selenocysteine.

The 3'UTR appears to modulate translation in vivo rather than serve as an indispensable element for it. For example, some lymphokine mRNAs, such as those encoding β-interferon, granulocyte-macrophage colony-stimulating factor (GM-CSF) and cachectin/tumor necrosis factor (TNF) contain translation inhibitory sequences in their 3'UTRs (reviewed in Kruys et al., 1990). The inhibitory sequences map to the AU-rich elements (ARE), motifs characterized by one or more copies of AUUUA usually in a U-rich context (Caput et al., 1986; Shaw and Kamen, 1986). The ARE is inhibitory in reticulocyte lysates and in Xenopus oocytes (Kruys et al., 1987; 1988; 1989). Its effect on translation in somatic cells is less certain. One exception, however, is the ARE in TNF mRNA. Endotoxin-activated macrophages synthesize 10,000-fold more TNF than control macrophages, and this response appears to be due, in part, to a translational response mediated by the ARE (Han et al., 1990). Conceivably, the ARE of TNF could confer endotoxin-responsive translational control onto heterologous coding regions in macrophage cell lines (Beutler, 1992). In most cases, however, the ARE in particular and 3'UTR sequences in general appear to mediate mRNA stability (which will be discussed in a later section). Thus the 3'UTR can control the level of a protein by controlling mRNA stability.

Temporal control of translation is an important mechanism regulating the timed synthesis of proteins from mRNAs stored as an inactive mRNP in the absence of transcription of the gene. An excellent example of this type of control is exemplified by the temporal activation of protein synthesis in spermatids during spermatogenesis (Braun et al., 1989). Many of these proteins are not synthesized until days after transcription ceases, and a selective mechanism exists to activate specific mRNAs. The mouse protamine 1 (mP1) mRNA is stored as an inactive mRNP in the cytoplasm of the round spermatid up to one week before it is translated in elongating spermatids; 156 nt of 3'UTR is necessary and sufficient for its temporal activation. This sequence element is also required for the proper intracellular localization of mP1.

Selective localization of mRNA provides an efficient means for targeting proteins to specific compartments in the cell or organism. Localization permits a mechanism for constructing cellular domains with different protein compositions (reviewed in Gottlieb, 1990; Kleinman et al., 1990 and Singer, 1992). Differential distributions of mRNAs exist in, among others, Xenopus and Drosophila oocytes and embryos, during spermatogenesis, migrating fibroblasts, muscle fibers, oligodendroglial cells and neurons such as hippocampal neurons, sympathetic neurons and photoreceptors (Braun et al., 1989; Bruckenstein et al., 1990; Kleinman et al., 1990; Macdonald and Struhl, 1988; Masucci et al., 1990; Merlie and Sanes, 1985; Pollock et al., 1990; Singer, 1992; Wilkins, 1990; Yisraeli and Melton, 1988). For example, β-actin mRNA is localized along the leading edge of migrating fibroblasts (Singer, 1992); the mRNA encoding the morphogen *bicoid* (*bcd*) is localized at the anterior pole of the egg during oogenesis in Drosophila (Macdonald and Struhl, 1988); and the mRNA for the growth factor homolog *decapentaplegic* (*dpp*) is localized to imaginal disks during Drosophila development (Masucci et al, 1990).

The subcellular localization of an mRNA can be determined by sequences in the mRNA itself or by the nascent polypeptide. Targeting by mRNA sequences appears to be important for localization of many non-membrane associated proteins, examples of which were listed above. So far, mRNA-targeting sequences have been localized to the 3'UTR; this does not, however, preclude the existence of mRNAs whose targeting sequences are located in other regions of the mRNA. Three examples of mRNAs containing 3'UTR localization sequences are β-actin, *bicoid* and *decapentaplegic* , described above. These sequences probably interact with protein chaperons to effect localization (Singer, 1992). This mechanism also leads to the conclusion that mRNA can contain spatial positioning information in addition to protein encoding information (Singer, 1992). Targeting of mRNAs, encoding secretory precursor proteins, to the endoplasmic reticulum by the nascent polypeptide is usually translational and involves proteins that are localized both to membranes and cytosol (reviewed in Nunnari and Walter, 1992).

In some cases the 3'UTR is essential simply for the synthesis of the encoded protein. For example, the translational insertion of selenocysteine into mammalian selenoproteins such as glutathione peroxidase (GPX), selenoprotein P and Type I iodothyronine 5' deiodinase (5'DI) is dependent on a 200 nt region in the 3'UTR of each mRNA which can form phylogenetically conserved secondary structures (Berry et al., 1991; Gesteland et al., 1992). Selenocysteine is encoded by a UGA codon, which normally signals translation termination. The 200 nt stem-loop structure in the 3'UTR is essential for coding of a UGA as selenocysteine rather than a stop codon, since its mutation reduces or eliminates translation of selenoproteins. Therefore, the 200 nt sequence is referred to as a "selenocysteine-insertion sequence" (Berry et al., 1991).

Messenger RNA Stability

The half-life of an mRNA determines the length of time that molecule can function to synthesize protein (reviewed in Peltz et al., 1991). Hargrove and Schmidt (1989) have suggested that elements that govern stabilities of protein and mRNA have co-evolved so that the relative stabilities of an mRNA and the encoded protein are similar; that is, labile proteins tend to be encoded by labile mRNAs. Messenger RNA half-lives in mammalian cells vary from several minutes for selected oncogenes and cytokines to more than 100 hours for stable mRNAs. The average half-life is 10-20 hours. However, the half-life of an mRNA may not always be constant. For example, during induction or repression of a protein's synthesis, alterations in stability of the mRNA can result in a rapid change of several orders of magnitude in the concentration of the mRNA. These changes in concentration can, in some cases, occur in the absence of any alterations in the transcription rate.

Thus mRNA stability serves to fine tune the levels of some proteins. Two excellent reviews describing a mathematical treatment of the roles of mRNA and protein stability in gene expression have been presented (Hargrove and Schmidt, 1989; Hargrove et al., 1991).

So far, rapid *intrinsic* mRNA turnover in mammalian cells has been shown to result from cis-acting instability elements in an mRNA, rather than an absence of stabilizing sequences. This does not, of course, preclude the existence of stabilizing sequences in mammalian mRNAs. Thus a stable mRNA like β-globin can be rapidly degraded in cells if an instability element, such as an AU-rich element, is linked in cis (e.g., Shaw and Kamen, 1986). One of the best characterized mammalian instability determinants is the class of AU-rich elements or ARE. These sequences were first noticed in the 3' end of some cytokine and proto-oncogene cDNAs (Caput et al., 1986). Shortly afterwards, their role as a signal for rapid mRNA degradation was demonstrated by linking a 58 bp AT-rich sequence from the human GM-CSF gene to the 3' end of the rabbit β-globin gene. β-globin mRNA is normally very stable (Ross and Pizarro, 1983; Ross and Sullivan, 1985). However, the GM-CSF sequence motif resulted in the rapid degradation of the chimeric mRNA (Shaw and Kamen, 1986). The precise sequence requirements for an ARE are not known, however, the pentameric motif AUUUA in a U-rich context is frequently sufficient for ARE function (Vakalopoulou et al., 1991). It is also noteworthy that the ARE of proto-oncogene mRNAs such as c-myc and c-fos tend to have one or more AUUUA motifs within a U-rich context while cytokine mRNAs tend to have multiple repeats of AUUU in tandem (Vriz and Mèchali, 1989). This might be important because under some circumstances, such as T-cell activation, in which lymphokine mRNAs are transiently stabilized, proto-oncogene mRNAs such as c-myc and c-fos are not (Lindsten et al., 1989; Schuler and Cole, 1988). In this regard, the 58 nucleotide ARE of GM-CSF mRNA is sufficient to transiently stabilize a chimeric β-globin/ARE mRNA in fibroblasts stimulated to produce GM-CSF by phorbol esters (Akashi et al., 1991).

Transient induction of many mRNAs containing an ARE is made possible by the fact that the mRNA is unstable in the first place. Under some circumstances, it might be desirable to simply maximize expression of the protein without concerns for inducibility. Given the discussion of the ARE as a destabilizing element, the first inclination would be to delete the ARE and replace it with the β-globin 3'UTR for example. Thus deletion of the ARE from B-cell-stimulating factor-2 results in its stabilization (Tonouchi et al., 1989). However, this may not always work, since mRNAs containing an ARE can also have distinct instability elements in their coding region. For example, in some cases deletion of the ARE from c-myc mRNA has little effect on its half-life (Bonnieu et al., 1990; Laird-Offringa et al., 1991; Wisdom and Lee, 1991), since it contains an additional instability determinant at the C-terminal end of the coding region (Bernstein et al., 1991; Wisdom and Lee, 1991). Indeed, the coding region determinant appears to be necessary and sufficient for the post-transcriptional regulation of c-myc mRNA during myogenesis (Wisdom and Lee, 1990). Coding region instability determinants have also been identified in mRNA encoding the alpha subunit of the IL-2 receptor, c-fos mRNA and β-interferon mRNA (Kabnick and Housman, 1988; Kanamori et al., 1990; Shyu et al. 1989; Whittemore and Maniatis, 1990). Undoubtedly, others will be discovered. Obviously, if the mRNA encoding a protein of interest contains a coding region instability determinant, it is not possible to delete it unless that portion of the encoded protein is not necessary for its function. It is also important to be aware that an mRNA containing an ARE is not always unstable. For example, rearrangements of the c-myc gene, which produce an altered c-myc mRNA with exon 1 removed and IVS 1 sequence inserted as part of the mature transcript, result in an altered c-myc mRNA which is 3- to 10-fold more stable than wild-type mRNA (Piechaczyk et al., 1985). Additionally, comparison of chimers of v-/c-fos revealed that an optional intron in the 5'UTR could increase the mRNA half-life compared to mRNA lacking the optional 5' sequence (Roy et al, 1992). The common denominator to these two studies is that sequences at the 5' end of the mRNA can override the destabilizing function of the ARE. In summary, it may not be a simple matter to create a stable mRNA from an unstable one, and thus requires consideration on a case by case basis. On the other hand, one way to create an unstable mRNA which can be transiently induced is to link to it a cytokine ARE.

Two other systems are also available for creating mRNAs whose stability is inducible. One is the iron-responsive element or IRE described in the section on translational control; the other are glucocorticoid-responsive elements. As described in the section on translational regulation, an IRE located in the 5'UTR permits efficient translation of ferritin or heterologous mRNAs only upon treatment of cells with hemin, a source of iron. But an IRE located in the 3'UTR, such as occurs with transferrin receptor mRNA, does not regulate translation. Rather, a 3' IRE induces rapid mRNA degradation upon treatment of cells with hemin (Klausner and Harford, 1989; Müllner and Kuhn, 1988). A conveniently inducible mRNA decay system would be to link a 3' IRE to a heterologous mRNA; the mRNA would be stable under normal conditions, and its instability could be induced with hemin. Thus the IRE can regulate translation or mRNA stability when located in the 5' or 3'UTR, respectively.

Hormones, particularly steroids, are involved in regulation of mRNA stability (reviewed in Shapiro et al., 1987). For example, phosphoenolpyruvate carboxykinase (PEPCK) mRNA contains a glucocorticoid-responsive element in its 3'UTR (Petersen et al., 1989). When linked to a heterologous mRNA, the 3' UTR of PEPCK can stabilize the mRNA at least 4-fold when cells are treated with dexamethasone. From a practical point of view, it is also important to keep in mind that in systems for the induction of protein production, a combination of both inducible transcription *and* mRNA stability will have a combinatorial effect on production of the protein (Hargrove and Schmidt, 1989; Hargrove et al., 1991).

In conclusion, the stability of an mRNA is an important determinant of its steady-state level. Messenger RNA stability can be modulated by a variety of sequence elements designed to enhance either its degradation or stability upon an appropriate stimulus, permitting fine-tuning of protein levels.

Protein Stability

Similar to mRNA stability, the stability of a protein determines its steady-state level (reviewed in Hargrove and Schmidt, 1989). Most cellular proteins are relatively stable. However, proteolysis confers short half-lives on proteins whose concentrations vary with time or alterations in physiological status of the cell (Varshavsky, 1992). There are many intracellular proteases, and excellent reviews of their structure and function have been published (Bond and Butler, 1987; Goldberg and Rock, 1992; Hershko, 1988; Hershko and Ciechanover, 1982). Proteins are degraded either by cytosolic, ATP-dependent pathways that do or do not require ubiquitination or by lysosomal pathways (Dice, 1990). The contribution of each pathway depends upon the cell type and physiological status. Three characterized paradigms for predicting rapid proteolysis will be described. These are the N-end rule for the ATP-ubiquitin-dependent proteolytic system, PEST elements and peptide sequences that target proteins for cytoslic or lysosomal turnover.

The ATP-ubiquitin-dependent proteolytic system is the best characterized. Its substrates appear to be proteins with basic or hydrophobic N-terminal amino acids. This system does not readily degrade polypeptides with blocked N-terminal ends. A formalization of the rules governing rapid proteolysis by the ubiquitin system is known as the N-end rule (Bachmair et al., 1986). Bachmair et al. created a chimeric gene encoding a ubiquitin-β-galactosidase fusion protein that was efficiently deubiquitinated. However, depending on the identify of the N-terminal residues, X-βgal proteins were either long or short lived. In mammals, the N-end rule predicts that proteins with N-terminal glycine, valine, proline or methionine will be stable, whereas proteins with any other N-terminal amino acids would undergo more rapid proteolysis. In regard to N-end amino acids, it is also important to point out that the initiator methionine is frequently cleaved off proteins by Met aminopeptidase if the second amino acid is serine, alanine, glycine or valine (Boissel et al., 1985). Thus the specificity of Met aminopeptidase may be involved in determining a protein's half-life in mammalian cells. For example, given the considerations concerning the N-end rule and the specificity of Met aminopeptidase, a polypeptide with serine as the penultimate amino acid should be unstable, whereas one with a penultimate glycine should be stable. In summary, the N-terminal residue in a protein appears to mediate its stability and thus the potential for regulation of its stability.

There is also a correlation between lability of a protein and the presence of so-called PEST regions [proline (P), glutamic acid (E), serine (S) and threonine (T); Rogers et al., 1986]. These PEST regions are frequently flanked by clusters containing several positively charged amino acids. Algorithms (e.g., PEST-SCORE; Rogers et al., 1986) for identifying PEST regions are available in many software packages for analyzing nucleic acid and protein sequences.

Finally, lysosomes take up and degrade intracellular proteins in cultured cells both constitutively and in response to serum withdrawal and in tissues during starvation (reviewed in Dice, 1990). Examination of amino acid motifs in proteins that were degraded more rapidly during serum withdrawal lead to the identification of the following pentameric amino acid motif:

(lys,	phe,	glu,	X)	gln
arg	ile	asp		
his	leu			
	val			

Parentheses indicate the sequence of amino acids is not important; X is any amino acid and conservative substitutions are allowed for lys, phe and glu. A protein referred to as peptide recognition protein of 73 kD (prp73) is thought to facilitate transfer of the protein to be degraded into lysosomes.

It may be possible to create a stabilized protein which maintains function by selective removal of motifs described above which target a protein for rapid degradation. For example, the C-terminal end of ornithine decarboxylase (ODC) determines its lability (Ghoda et al., 1989). Truncation of this region has no effect on the enzymatic activity of ODC. However, a strategy such as this would have to be tested for the protein of interest.

SUMMARY

The steady-state level of a protein depends not only upon the rate at which the mRNA is synthesized, but also upon the rates at which the mRNA is processed, transported and translated along with the rates at which the mRNA and protein are degraded. Therefore, each of these post-transcriptional processes is linked to gene expression and are important processes contributing to the level or timing of expression of a given protein. This review has described a number of post-transcriptional processes that should be considered when the goal is to express a recombinant protein in a mammalian cell. Achieving "optimal" synthesis of a protein may require considerations concerning the effects of RNA splicing, 3' end formation/polyadenylation, RNA transport, translation and stability of the cytoplasmic mRNA and protein. Since expression of proteins in mammalian cells is more art than science, the cis elements in the gene construct for "optimal" production of one protein may not suffice for optimal production of a different protein. Thus, the requirements for production of proteins of interest should be considered for each protein.

ACKNOWLEDGMENT

I wish to thank Drs. Doug Lyles, Griffith Parks and Greg Shelness for very helpful comments on the manuscript.

REFERENCES

Acland P, Dixon M, Peters G, Dickson C (1990): Subcellular fate of the Int-2 oncoprotein is determined by the choice of initiation codon. *Nature* 343:662-665

Akashi M, Shaw G, Gross M, Saito M, Koeffler HP (1991): Role of AUUU sequences in stabilization of granulocyte-macrophage colony-stimulating factor RNA in stimulated cells. *Blood* 78:2005-2012

Annweiler A, Hipskind RA, Wirth T (1991): A strategy for efficient in vitro translation of cDNAs using the rabbit β-globin leader sequence. *Nuc Acids Res* 19:3750

Atwater JA, Wisdom R, Verma IM (1990): Regulated mRNA stability. *Annu Rev Genet* 24:519-541

Bachmair A, Finley D, Varshavsky A (1986): In vivo half-life of a protein is a function of its amino-terminal residue. *Science* 234:179-186

Baker BS (1989): Sex in flies: the splice of life. *Nature* 340:521-524

Bernstein PL, Herrick DJ, Prokipcak RD, Ross J (1992): Control of c-myc mRNA halflife in vitro by a protein capable of binding to a coding region stability determinant. *Genes Dev* 6:642-654

Berry MJ, Banu L, Chen Y, Mandel SJ, Keiffer JD, Harney JW, Larsen PR (1991): Recognition of UGA as a selenocysteine in Type I deiodinase requires sequences in the 3' untranslated region. *Nature* 353:273-276

Beutler B (1992): Application of transcriptional and posttranscriptional reporter constructs to the analysis of tumor necrosis factor gene regulation. *Am J Med Sci* 303:129-133

Blobel G (1985): Gene gating: a hypothesis. *Proc Natl Acad Sci USA* 82:8527-8529

Boissel J-P, Kasper TJ, Shah SC, Malone JI, Bunn HF (1985): Amino-terminal processing of proteins: hemoglobin South Florida, a variant with retention of initiator methionine and N-acetylation. *Proc Natl Acad Sci USA* 82:8448-8452

Bond JS, Butler PE (1987): Intracellular proteases. *Ann Rev Biochem* 56:333-364

Bonnieu A, Roux P, Marty L, Jeanteur P, Piechaczyk M (1990): AUUUA motifs are dispensable for rapid degradation of the mouse c-myc RNA. *Oncogene* 5:1585-1588

Braddock M, Thorburn AM, Kingsman AJ, Kingsman SM (1991): Blocking of Tatdependent HIV-1 RNA modification by an inhibitor or RNA polymerase II processivity. *Nature* 350:439-441

Braun RE, Peschon JJ, Behringer RR, Brinster RL, Palmiter RD (1989): Protamine 3'-untranslated sequences regulate temporal translational control and subcellular localization of growth hormone in spermatids of transgenic mice. *Genes Dev* 3:793-802

Bruckenstein DA, Lein PJ, Higgins D, Fremeau Jr RT (1990): distinct spatial localization of specific mRNAs in cultured sympathetic neurons. *Neuron* 5:809-819

Buchman AR, Berg P (1988): Comparison of intron-dependent and intron-independent gene expression. *Mol Cell Biol* 8:4395-4405

Caput D, Beutler B, Hartog K, Thayer R, Brown-Shimer S, Cerami A (1986): Identification of a common nucleotide sequence in the 3'-untranslated region of mRNA molecules specifying inflammatory mediators. *Proc Natl Acad Sci USA* 83:1670-1674

Dice JF (1990): Peptide sequences that target cytosolic proteins for lysosomal proteolysis. *Trends Biochem Sci* 15:305-309

Fu L, Ye R, Browder LW, Johnston RN (1991): Translational potentiation of messenger RNA with secondary structure in Xenopus. *Science* 251:807-810

Gesteland RF, Weiss RB, Atkins JF (1992): Recoding: reprogrammed genetic recoding. *Science* 257:1640-1641

Ghoda L, Van Daalen Wetters T, Macrae M, Sherman D, Coffino P (1989): Prevention of rapid intracellular degradation of ODC by c-terminal truncation. *Science* 243:1493-1495

Goldberg AL, Rock KL (1992): Proteolysis, proteosomes and antigen presentation. *Nature* 357:375-379

Gordon DA, Shelness GS, Nicosia M, Williams DL (1988): Estrogen-induced destabilization of yolk precursor protein mRNAs in avian liver. *J Biol Chem* 263:2625-2631

Gottlieb E (1990): Messenger RNA transport and localization. *Curr Opin Cell Biol* 2:1080-1086

Han J, Brown T, Beutler B (1990): Endotoxin-responsive sequences control cachectin/tumor necrosis factor biosynthesis at the translational level. *J Exp Med* 171:465-475

Hargrove JL, Schmidt FH (1989): The role of mRNA and protein stability in gene expression. *FASEB J* 3:2360-2370

Herman RC (1989): Alternatives for the initiation of translation. *Trends Biochem Sci* 14:219-222

Hernandez H, Weiner AM (1986): Formation of the 3' end of U1 snRNA requires compatible snRNA promoter elements. *Cell* 47:249-258

Hershko A (1988): Ubiquitin-mediated protein degradation. *J Biol Chem* 263:15237-15240

Hershko A, Ciechanover A (1982): Mechanisms of intracellular protein breakdown. *Ann Rev Biochem* 51:335-364

Hernandez H, Weiner AM (1986): Formation of the 3' end of U1 snRNA requires compatible snRNA promoter elements. *Cell* 47:249-258

Huang MTF, Gorman CM (1990): Intervening sequences increase efficiency of RNA 3' processing and accumulation. *Nucl Acids Res* 18:937-947

Jackson RJ (1991): Initiation without an end. *Nature* 353:14-15

Jackson RJ (1988): Picornaviruses break the rules. *Nature* 334:292-293

Jackson RJ, Howell MT, Kaminski A (1990): The novel mechanism of initiation of picornavirus RNA translation. *Trends Biochem Sci* 15:477-483

Jackson RJ, Standart N (1990): Do the poly(A) tail and 3' untranslated region control mRNA translation? *Cell* 62:15-24

Jang SK, Kräusslich H-G, Nicklin MJH, Duke GM, Palmenberg AC, Wimmer E (1988): A segment of the 5' nontranslated region of encephalomyocarditis virus RNA directs internal entry of ribosomes during in vitro translation. *J Virol* 62:2636-2643

Jang SK, Wimmer E (1990): Cap-independent translation of encephalomyocarditis virus RNA: Structural elements of the internal ribosomal entry site and involvement of a cellular 57-kD RNA-binding protein. *Genes Dev* 4:1560-1572

Kabnick KS, Housman DE (1988): Determinants that contribute to cytoplasmic stability of human c-fos and beta-globin mRNAs are located at several sites in each mRNA. *Mol Cell Biol* 8:3244-3250

Kanamori H, Suzuki N, Siomi H, Nosaka T, Sato A, Sabe H, Hatanaka M, Hohjo T (1990): HTLV-1 p27^{rex} stabilizes human interleukin-2 receptor chain mRNA. *EMBO J* 9:4161-4166

Kim DG, Kang HM, Jang SK, Shin H-S (1992): Construction of a bifunctional mRNA in the mouse by using the internal ribosome entry site of the encephalomyocarditis virus. *Mol Cell Biol* 12:3636-3643

Klausner RD, Harford JB (1989): Cis-trans models for post-transcriptional gene regulation. *Science* 246:870-872

Kleinman R, Banker G, Steward O (1990): Differential subcellular localization of particular mRNAs in hippocampal neurons in culture. *Neuron* 5:821-830

Koeller DM, Horowitz JA, Casey JL, Klausner RD, Harford JB (1991): Translation and the stability of mRNAs encoding the transferrin receptor and c-fos. *Proc Natl Acad Sci USA* 88:7778-7782

Kozak M (1986): Influences of mRNA secondary structure on initiation by eukaryotic ribosomes. *Proc Natl Acad Sci USA* 83:2850-2854

Kozak M (1988): A profusion of controls. *J Cell Biol* 107:1-7

Kozak M (1989): Circumstances and mechanisms of inhibition of translation by secondary structure in eucaryotic mRNAs. *Mol Cell Biol* 9:5134-5142

Kozak M (1990): Downstream secondary structure facilitates recognition of initiator codons by eukaryotic ribosomes. *Proc Natl Acad Sci USA* 87:8301-8305

Kozak M (1991): Structural features in eukaryotic mRNAs that modulate the initiation of translation. *J Biol Chem* 266:19867-19870

Kruys V, Wathelet M, Poupart P, Contreras R, Fiers W, Content J, Huez G (1987): The 3' untranslated region of the human interferon-β mRNA has an inhibitory effect on translation. *Proc Natl Acad Sci USA* 84:6030-6034

Kruys V, Marinx O, Shaw G, Deschamps J, Huez G (1989): Translational blockade imposed by cytokine-derived UA-rich sequences. *Science* 245:852-855

Kruys V, Beutler B, Huez G (1990): Translational control mediated by UA-rich sequences. *Enzyme* 44:193-202

Laird-Offringa IA, Elfferich P, van der Eb AJ (1991): Rapid c-myc mRNA degradation does not require (A+U)-rich sequences or complete translation of the mRNA. *Nucl Acids Res* 19:2387-2394

Leibold EA, Munro HN (1988): Cytoplasmic protein binds in vitro to a highly conserved sequence in the 5' untranslated region of ferritin heavy- and light-subunit mRNAs. *Proc Natl Acad Sci USA* 85:2171-2175

Lindsten T, June CH, Ledbetter JA, Stella G, Thompson CB (1989): Regulation of lymphokine messenger RNA stability by a surface-mediated T cell activation pathway. *Science* 244:339-342

Macdonald PM, Struhl G (1988): Cis-acting sequences responsible for anterior localization of bicoid mRNA in Drosophila embryos. *Nature* 336:595-598

Macejak DG, Sarnow P (1991): Internal initiation of translation mediated by the 5' leader of a cellular mRNA. *Nature* 353:90-94

Malone RW, Felgner PL, Verma IM (1989): Lipofectin mediated RNA transfection. *Proc Natl Acad Sci USA* 86:6077-6081

Maniatis T (1991): Mechanisms of alternative pre-mRNA splicing. *Nature* 251:33-34

Marth JD, Overell RW, Meier KE, Krebs EG, Perlmutter RM (1988): Translational activation of the lck proto-oncogene. *Nature* 332:171-173

Masucci JD, Miltenberger RJ, Hoffmann FM (1990): Pattern-specific expression of the Drosophila decapentaplegic gene in imaginal disks is regulated by 3' cis-regulatory elements. *Genes Dev* 4:2011-2023

Mattaj IW (1990): Splicing stories and poly(A) tales: An update on RNA processing and transport. *Curr Opin Cell Biol* 2:528-538

Meerovitch K, Pelletier J, Sonenberg N (1989): A cellular protein that binds to the 5'noncoding region of poliovirus RNA: implications for internal translation initiation. *Genes Dev* 3:1026- 1034

Merlie JP, Sanes JA (1985): Concentration of acetylcholine receptor mRNA in synaptic regions of adult muscle fibers. *Nature* 317:66-68

Müllner EW, Kuhn LC (1988): A stem-loop in the 3' untranslated region mediates iron-dependent regulation of transferrin receptor mRNA stability in the cytoplasm. *Cell* 53:815-825

Müllner EW, Neupert B, Kuhn LC (1989): A specific mRNA-binding factor regulates the iron-dependent stability of cytoplasmic transferrin receptor mRNA. *Cell* 58:373-382

Neuberger MS, Williams GT (1988): The intron requirement for immunoglobulin gene expression is dependent upon the promoter. *Nuc Acids Res* 16:6713-6724

Neuman de Vigvar HE, Lund E, Dahlberg JE (1986): 3' end formation of U1 snRNA precursors is coupled to transcription from snRNA promoters. *Cell* 47:259-266

Nicholson R, Pelletier J, Le S-Y, Sonenberg N (1991): Structural and functional analysis of the ribosome landing pad of poliovirus type 2: In vivo translation studies. *J Virol* 65:5886-5894

Niwa M, Berget SM (1991): Mutation of the AAUAAA polyadenylation signal depresses in vitro splicing of proximal but not distal introns. *Genes Dev* 5:2086-2095

Niwa M, Rose SD, Berget SM (1990): In vitro polyadenylation is stimulated by the presence of an upstream intron. *Genes Dev* 4:1552-1559

Nunnari J, Walter P (1992): Protein targeting to and translocation across the membrane of the endoplasmic reticulum. *Curr Op Cell Biol* 4:573-580

OH SK, Scott MP, Sarnow P (1992): Homeotic gene Antennapedia mRNA contains 5'noncoding sequences that confer translational initiation by internal ribosome binding. *Genes Dev* 6:1643-1653

Pelletier J, Sonenberg N (1988): Internal initiation of translation of eukaryotic mRNA directed by a sequence from poliovirus RNA. *Nature* 334:32-35

Peltz SW, Brewer G, Bernstein P, Hart PA, Ross J (1991): Regulation of mRNA turnover in eukaryotic cells. *Crit Rev Euk Gene Expression* 1:99-126

Petersen DD, Koch SR, Granner DK (1989): 3' noncoding region of phosphoenolpyruvate carboxykinase mRNA contains a glucocorticoid-responsive mRNAstabilizing element. *Proc Natl Acad Sci USA* 86:7800-7804

Piechaczyk M, Yang J-Q, Blanchard JM, Jeanteur P, Marcu K (1985): Posttranscriptional mechanisms are responsible for accumulation of truncated c-myc RNAs in murine plasma cell tumors. *Cell* 42:598-597

Pollock JA, Ellisman MH, Benzer S (1990): Subcellular localization of transcripts in Drosophila photoreceptor neurons chaoptic mutants have an aberrant distribution. *Genes Dev* 4:806-821

Proudfoot N (1988): How RNA polymerase II terminates transcription in higher eukaryotes. *Trends Biochem Sci* 14:105-110

Proudfoot N (1991): Poly(A) signals. *Cell* 64:671-674

Rogers S, Wells R, Rechsteiner M (1986): Amino acid sequences common to rapidly degraded proteins: the PEST hypothesis. *Science* 234:364-368

Ross J, Pizarro A (1983): Human beta and delta globin messenger RNAs turn over at different rates. *J Mol Biol* 167:607-617

Ross J, Sullivan TD (1985): Half-lives of beta and gamma globin messenger RNAs and of protein synthetic capacity in cultured human reticulocytes. *Blood* 66:1149-1154

Rouault TA, Hentze MW, Caughman SW, Harford JB, Klausner RD (1988): Binding of a cytosolic protein to the iron-responsive element of human ferritin messenger RNA. *Science* 241:1207-1210

Roy N, Laflamme G, Raymond V (1992): 5' untranslated sequences modulate rapid mRNA degradation mediated the 3' AU-rich element in v-/c-fos recombinants. *Nucl Acids Res* 20:5753-5762

Ryu WS, Mertz JE (1989): Simian virus 40 late transcripts lacking excisable intervening sequences are defective in both stability in the nucleus and transport to the cytoplasm. *J Virol* 63:4386-4394

Sachs AB (1990): The role of poly(A) in the translation and stability of mRNA. *Curr Opin Cell Biol* 2:1092-1098

Schuler GD, Cole MD (1988): GM-CSF and oncogene mRNA stabilities are independently regulated in trans in a mouse monocytic tumor. *Cell* 55:1115-1122

Shapiro DJ, Blume JE, Nielsen DA (1987): Regulation of messenger RNA stability in eukaryotic cells. *BioEssays* 6:221-226

Shaw G, Kamen R (1986): A conserved AU sequence from the 3' untranslated region of GM-CSF mRNA mediates selective mRNA degradation. *Cell* 46:659-667

Shyu A-B, Greenberg ME, Belasco JG (1989): The fos transcript is targeted for rapid decay by two distinct mRNA degradation pathways. *Genes Dev* 3:60-72

Simonson CC, Levinson A (1983): Isolation and expression of an altered mouse dihydrofolate reductase cDNA. *Proc Natl Acad Sci USA* 80:2495-2499

Singer RH (1992): The cytoskeleton and mRNA localization. *Curr Opin Cell Biol* 4:15-19

Sonnenberg N (1991): Picornavirus RNA translation continues to surprise. *Trends Genet* 7:105-106

Sonnenberg N, Meerovitch K (1990): Translation of poliovirus mRNA. *Enzyme* 44:278-291

Theil E (1990): Regulation of ferritin and transferrin receptor mRNAs. *J Biol Chem* 265:4771-4774

Tonouchi N, Miwa K, Karasuyama H, Matsui H (1989): Deletion of 3' untranslated region of human BSF-2 mRNA causes stabilization of the mRNA and high level expression in NIH 3T3 cells. *Biochem Biophys Res Comm* 163:1056-1062

Treisman R, Novak J, Favaloro, Kamen R (1981): Transformation of rat cells by an altered polyoma virus genome expressing only middle-T protein. *Nature* 292:595-600

Trono D, Andino R, Baltimore D (1988): An RNA sequence of hundreds of nucleotides at the 5' end of poliovirus RNA is involved in allowing viral protein synthesis. *J Virol* 62:2291-2299

Vakalopoulou E, Schaack J, Shenk T (1991): A 32-kilodalton protein binds to AU-rich domains in the 3'-untranslated regions of rapidly degraded mRNAs. *Mol Cell Biol* 11:3355-3364

Varshavsky A (1992): The N-end rule. *Cell* 69:725-735

Vriz S, Mèchali M (1989): Analysis of 3'-untranslated regions of seven c-myc genes reveals conserved elements prevalent in post-transcriptionally regulated genes. *FEBS Let* 251:201-206

Walden WE, Daniels-McQueen S, Brown PH, Gaffield L, Russell DA, Bielser D, Bailey LC, Thach RE (1988): Translational repression in eukaryotes: Partial purification and characterization of a repressor of ferritin mRNA translation. *Proc Natl Acad Sci USA* 85:9503-9507

Whittemore L-A, Maniatis T (1990): Postinduction turnoff of beta-interferon gene expression. *Mol Cell Biol* 10:1329-1337

Wickens M (1990): How the messenger got its tail: Addition of poly(A) in the nucleus. *Trends Biochem Sci* 15:277-281

Wilkins AS (1990): Localizing and sequestering mRNAs in oocytes. *BioEssays* 12:129-130

Wisdom R, Lee W (1990): Translation of c-myc mRNA is required for its post-transcriptional regulation during myogenesis. *J Biol Chem* 265:19015-19021

Wisdom R, Lee W (1991): The protein-coding region of c-myc mRNa contains a sequence that specifies rapid mRNA turnover and induction by protein synthesis inhibitors. *Genes Dev* 5:232-243

Yisraeli JK, Melton DA (1988): The maternal mRNA Vg1 is correctly localized following injection into Xenopus oocytes. *Nature* 336:592-595

Yu XM, Gelembiuk GW, Wang CY, Ryu W-S, Mertz JE (1991): Expression from herpesvirus promoters does not relieve the intron requirement for cytoplasmic accumulation of human β-globin mRNA. *Nuc Acids Res* 19:7231-7134

PROMOTERS, ENHANCERS, AND INDUCIBLE ELEMENTS FOR GENE THERAPY

Robert G. Whalen

INTRODUCTION

If the field of gene therapy of human diseases is in its infancy, attempts to modulate the expression of transferred genes is an endeavor which is still in gestation. The midwives to the birth of this area are those molecular biologists who are actively involved in the study of the control of gene expression. In particular, the tremendous surge of the last several years in understanding of the promoter elements and the protein factors involved in transcriptional regulation are beginning to find application to problems of gene therapy.

In this chapter, I will review some of the basic features of gene and promoter structure that are relevant to the design of vectors to be used for gene therapy. Of the examples to be given, some will be quite schematic, in order to illustrate simply the possible approaches to the confection of the promoters, minigenes and inducible elements that might allow some measure of modulation of gene expression in the therapeutic setting. By modulation, I mean the necessity of attaining, in the first instance, a high enough level of expression to effect a change in the target cells. However, it is worth considering already to what extent the level of expression can be more finely tuned, since in the long run this will surely be desirable in some instances.

THE CANONICAL TRANSCRIPTION UNIT

The term "structural gene," as defined since the time of Jacob and Monod (1961), refers to that DNA unit which can be decoded into the specific structure of the polypeptide chain. The terms "regulator" and "operator" used by those authors are today usually replaced by references to promoters, enhancers and so-called *trans*-acting factors, the latter being protein transcription factors in most cases. The expression of a structural gene for the purposes of gene therapy requires assembling a transcription unit containing the DNA coding sequences to be expressed, and the promoter and enhancer elements required for driving transcription of the gene and on which those *trans*-acting factors will impact.

Gene Therapeutics: Methods and Applications of Direct Gene Transfer
Jon A. Wolff, Editor • ©1994 *Birkhäuser Boston*

This canonical transcription unit is schematically dissected into its compo-nent parts in Figure 1 for the purpose of simplifying the discussion. The read-out of the structural gene into a primary RNA transcript by the RNA polymerase en-zyme begins at position +1 of the structural gene *per se*. The vast majority of eukaryotic structural genes are not a contiguous coding sequence which will be read out co-linearly into messenger RNA, but rather they are composed of an alter-nating array of blocks of coding sequences, called exons. They are separated by intervening DNA stretches called introns, which do not encode a protein sequence for the structural gene in question. The simplest pattern of RNA processing leads to the formation of a messenger RNA transcript as shown in Figure 1: all introns are removed and the exons are joined in a head-to-tail fashion. The exonic RNA sequences are joined together in their final linear arrangement in the gene by an exquisitely precise mechanism mediated by the splicing machinery in the nucleus (Weiner, 1993).

One caveat to this description of the read-out of the structural gene must be immediately introduced. DNA which is an intron in one gene may indeed serve a coding or exonic function for another gene, an overlapping one for example. Alter-natively, in many genes the "intronic" DNA may become exonic DNA if the splic-ing machinery has the option of including those sequences in the processed transcript. This is one result of the process known as alternative splicing (McKeown, 1992). A choice of exons may also occur during processing; exons may be in-cluded or excluded, or two exons may be used in a mutually exclusive fashion.

The mRNA transcript thus faithfully reflects the sequence of the exonic DNA in the structural gene. However, several features of the final processed transcript need to be remarked on (Alberts et al., 1989). The first is that certain of the se-quences in the transcript do not serve a protein coding function. At the level of the mRNA, they comprise what are known as the 5'- and 3'-untranslated regions (UTR). At the 5' end, the UTR precedes the initiator codon (ATG in Figure 1) and prob-ably plays a role in directing the protein synthesis machinery to the initiation site with a certain efficiency, depending on the nature of the 5'-UTR sequences. The most 5' nucleotide of the transcript is usually modified post-transcriptionally by the addition of a methylated G residue linked by a 5'-to-5' triphosphate bridge; this unusual feature is known as the "Cap" structure. The 5' Cap is essential for effi-cient initiation of protein synthesis. Thus, the 5'-UTR can be a determinant in the control of protein synthesis. The 3'-UTR, defined as the mRNA sequences follow-ing the termination codon (e.g. TAA in Figure 1) is commonly thought to play a potential role in mRNA transcript stability, again providing a determinant of mRNA levels and thus of the extent of protein synthesis.

Another remarkable feature of the mRNA transcript is the poly(A) tail. This homopolymeric stretch of A residues is added to the primary transcript by the nuclear processing mechanism ("poly-adenylation" in Figure 1), that is, it is not part of the structural gene but rather is added post-transcriptionally. A polyadenylation signal (AATAAA in Figure 1) is however found in the structural gene sequence, and it is near this signal that the primary transcript becomes trun-

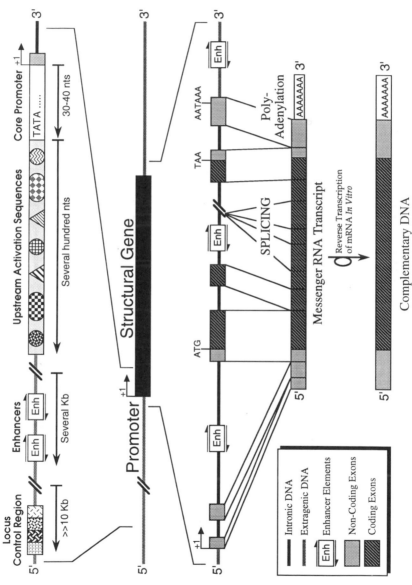

cated during processing. The 5'- and 3'-UTRs and the poly(A) tail all contributed to mRNA stability and/or translatability.

The construction of a transcription unit for gene therapy will need to take into account these features of gene structure and read-out, and constraints can easily be placed to obtain the desired result by appropriate construction of mini-genes. Often the sequences to be expressed are obtained in the form of complementary DNA (cDNA). This is a cloned DNA copy of the mRNA transcript (thus containing the joined exons) which can be transcribed directly (see Figure 1). Building the synthetic gene may however require leaving some introns in their place, to be removed during processing of the primary transcript, since the presence of introns during processing can in some cases lead to great increases in cytoplasmic messenger RNA levels (see the discussion by Brewer, this Volume, page 40).

PROMOTERS, ACTIVATORS, ENHANCERS, AND LCRS

Returning to the transcription unit *per se*, the DNA sequences immediately 5' to the start of transcription (at position +1 in Figure 1) are collective referred to as the promoter. This function of this entity is to control the rate of initiation of transcrip-

FIGURE 1. Schematic representation of a canonical eukaryotic transcription unit. In the upper middle part of the diagram, the unit is shown in its simplest form with an indication of the STRUCTURAL GENE (in solid black) and the flanking extragenic DNA containing the PROMOTER (see Legend, bottom left). The position marked +1 corresponds to the nucleotide at which initiation of RNA transcription of the gene begins; this defines the start of the structural gene. The promoter is further dissected into component parts in the upper part of the figure. The core promoter, upstream activation sequences (UAS), enhancers, and locus control region are all discussed in the text. The symbols (circles, ovals and triangles) in the UAS region represent DNA sequence motifs for the interaction of different DNA-binding proteins. The bi-directional arrows on the enhancer indicate that they can function in either orientation. The locus control region is composed of several types of activator elements, as indicated schematically. In the lower half of the figure, the detailed organization of the structural gene is shown. Since enhancers can also be found on the 3' side of the promoter (see text), two are indicated within the introns of the structural gene, and a third is placed beyond the 3' end of the structural gene. In most cases, the RNA transcript (starting at +1) begins at a sequence which serves a non-coding function in the final mRNA product (see text). The initiator codon ATG (encoding the first methionine residue) is thus found downstream from position +1, either in the first exon but frequently in the second or third exon as depicted. Protein coding sequences terminate at the TAA codon (one of several Stop codons that are used in different genes). Further 3' non-coding exons are usually included in the transcript, and the sequence AATAAA (or a variant thereof) is a signal for termination of the transcript and for the addition of polyA residues, which is a post-transcriptional event. Splicing of the primary RNA transcript joins the different exons in a precise head-to-tail fashion. Capping of the 5' end and polyadenylation give rise to the final messenger RNA transcript (see text). At the very bottom of the figure is shown the process of reverse transcription, which is carried out experimentally from isolated cellular mRNA for the purposes of cloning the coding exons in the form of complementary DNA for use in preparing gene expressing vectors (see text).

promoter. This function of this entity is to control the rate of initiation of transcription of the structural gene. Indeed, the ultimate success of any gene transfer protocol will rely critically on how efficiently, and for how long, transcription of the transferred structural gene is initiated. Modulation of the rate of initiation may also be crucial to achieve a positive therapeutic effect of gene expression. The promoter DNA sequence, and its associated regulatory sequence elements, will thus be responsible for this process since manipulation of these regulator sequences will provide a means of modulating expression of the introduced foreign genes.

Although the definitions are not always strict and one feature may blend into another, the promoter/regulatory elements can be considered at four different levels: (i) the core promoter, (ii) the adjacent upstream activator sequences, (iii) the enhancer or enhancers, and for some genes, (iv) a locus control region, or LCR (see the top of Figure 1). These terms are quite convenient for discussion of the current knowledge, and to an extent they do represent discrete functional entities. One way to view the regulatory unit to consider each of these regulatory elements as quite modular, and this modularity will be evident in examples discussed later.

In fact, DNA sequence motifs, from a few to up to tens of nucleotides in length, can be regarded as the building blocks of genetic regulatory elements. This can be understood in that the DNA sequence of the promoter has no coding function or intrinsic meaning on its own, but rather serves as sites for interaction with components of the transcriptional machinery, in most cases proteins. The protein-DNA interactions require the specificity afforded by the DNA sequence. The point of contact of the protein with the DNA strand is the sequence motif, hence the necessarily modular nature of the regulatory elements. This modularity means that a considerable degree of flexibility is available when deciding on the design of the promoter/regulatory elements to be used to control gene expression. For example, enhancers or other sequence motifs can be combined with heterologous promoters, that is, promoters with which they are not naturally associated. Thus it is often possible to combine the regulatory features of several genes in one functional, although artificial, transcription unit.

THE PROMOTER AND ITS ACTIVATOR ELEMENTS

The core promoter (see Figure 1, top) is defined here as the 30 or 40 nucleotides just 5' to the start site of transcription initiation (+1 in the Figure). Within this relatively short element one finds in most promoters a sequence motif known as the TATA box, which are variations on the theme of $TAT(^A/_T)(^A/_T)(^A/_T)(^A/_T)$ for example. Even though on its own it may not be very transcriptionally active, this TATA-box-containing core promoter thus has one of the minimal elements necessary for transcription initiation. A protein called TBP (TATA-binding protein) (Nikolov et al., 1992) interacts with this sequence and also with other proteins called TAFs (TBP-associated factors; see Greenblatt, 1992). The protein complex built up around TBP (referred to as TFIID) is quite large (300-700,000 daltons; see

Timmers and Sharp, 1991). Therefore TFIID is likely to provide multiple points of interaction with factors binding to other regulatory elements capable of interacting with the TAFs of the core promoter protein-DNA complex (Gill and Tjian, 1992). In conjunction with other transcription factors brought to this site, TFIID will help to position the RNA polymerase molecule in the vicinity of the start site so that accurate initiation can take place (for a review, see Roeder, 1991). TFIID is considered one of the basal transcription factors along with TFIIB, TFIIE and TFIIF, but they are not all general factors since TFIIE is not required for basal transcription activity of all promoters (Parvin et al., 1992).

Other regulatory elements (i.e. protein-binding DNA motifs) are located, in the simplest case, immediately upstream (i.e. to the 5' side) of the core promoter, and they are collectively referred to here as Upstream Activation Sequences, or UAS (Figure 1). These sequences can be found within several hundred nucleotides upstream from the promoter, however just where these sequences begin and end and other types of regulatory elements begin is difficult to define with precision. However, consideration of these UAS provides a rich source of information since many DNA sequence motifs and DNA-binding proteins have been identified in recent years which are contained in this region and which appear to be major players in stimulating transcription by interaction with core promoter elements.

It is now apparent that different classes of DNA-binding proteins exist which can be differentiated based on features of the protein structure which account either for their interaction with DNA or for the interactions of the proteins in the formation of multimers, often dimers (for review see Harrison, 1991). For example, the homeodomain proteins (as well as most of the prokaryotic transcriptional regulatory proteins) contain domains with a helix-turn-helix motif. Another class of factors contain zinc as a structural element which coordinates the polypeptide chain and forms a structure known as a Zinc-finger. These two types of domains participate directly in the DNA-protein interactions. Multimerization occurs in the case of the proto-oncogene transcription factors *jun* and *fos* through a dimerization motif known as the "leucine zipper" (Alber, 1992). This is found adjacent to a basic region which interacts with DNA. Dimerization is an important feature of these factors, since in the case where heterodimers can be formed, such as *jun-fos* in the AP1 transcription factor complex, there is the potential for a combinatorial increase in the possible regulatory elements formed. This also applies to a group of proteins containing a "helix-loop-helix" (HLH) segment also located adjacent to a basic region. While the latter binds to DNA, the HLH motif participates in protein-protein interactions leading to dimer, and particularly heterodimer, formation among members of this class of transcription factors. Examples of the basic HLH group include the proto-oncogene *c-myc*, the ubiquitous factors produced from the E2A gene, the myogenic regulatory factors of the MyoD family (for reviews, see Weintraub et al., 1991, Blackwood et al., 1992 and Wright, 1992), and many others. Some proteins contain no basic region but still retain the HLH motif; this is the case for the protein Id (inhibitor of differentiation; Jen et al., 1992). Clearly then, the interactions through the HLH motif provide a means for obtaining numerous combinations of individual HLH proteins, thus resulting in the formation of heterodimers with potentially different functionalities.

MODULARITY IN THE ORGANIZATION OF PROMOTER REGULATORY ELEMENTS

In many promoters, one can discern multiple sites for binding of transcription factors in the UAS region. The protein factors can be of different structural types (e.g. leucine zipper, HLH, etc.), as represented at the top of Figure 1 by circles, ovals and triangles. However each structural class of factor can be represented by several different proteins, or different multimeric combinations; this diversity of a given class (represented by circles for example) is illustrated by different shadings within the circles. This schematic diagram also emphasizes the linear arrangement of binding sites within the UAS region. The precise arrangement and nature of the sites will contribute greatly to the overall level and tissue-specificity of the transcriptional activity driven from the core promoter. Most current models illustrate the interaction of the transcription factors with the TBP and TAF complex by invoking bending of the DNA to bring all the necessary factors into contact. Thus the actual linear sequence of binding sites in the UAS may not be the crucial determinant of activity or specificity.

Two examples of upstream sequences containing recognizable binding sites can serve as illustration of the above principles. One example concerns the immediate-early gene of human cytomegalovirus (CMV), which contains one of the most highly active promoters and enhancers known, and the second is a strictly tissue-specific promoter driving an adult form of skeletal muscle myosin heavy chain.

CMV promoter-gene constructs are active in a large number of cell types when at least 600 base pairs of promoter sequence are present (Boshart et al., 1985). Inspection of this sequence reveals a relatively dense arrangement of binding sites for known transcription factors, especially for those which are found in most cell types (see Figure 2). There are seven GC-rich sites, several of which conform to the consensus binding site of the ubiquitous transcription factor SP1 (Berg, 1992). In addition, seven sites are found for the cAMP response element binding (CREB) protein (Brindle and Montminy, 1992), four binding sites for NF-κB factor are present (Nolan and Baltimore, 1992), and four binding sites (called E-boxes) are found for the basic HLH family of transcription factors. This large number of binding sites for protein transcription factors of widespread cellular distribution probably accounts for at least some of the transcriptional properties of this viral promoter.

Another example of modularity in the arrangement of promoter DNA sequence motifs is seen in the gene encoding the muscle-specific heavy chain subunit of myosin (MyHC) expressed specifically in a certain subpopulation of fast-contracting mammalian skeletal muscle fibers called type IIB (Takeda et al., 1992a). In this case, some of the promoter motifs and the factors which bind to them are also

```
- 603                             RSRF
ATGTTGACATTGATTATTGACTAGTTATTAATAGTAATCAATTACGGGGTCATTAGTTC


       CArG/SRF                                   GC-rich
ATAGCCCATATATGGAGTTCCGCGTTACATAACTTACGGTAAATGGCCCGCCTGGCTGA


 SP1          SP1/AP2      CREB         CREB
CCGCCCAACGACCCCCGCCCATTGACGTCAATAATGACGTATGTTCCCATAGTAACGCC


      NFκB          CREB                              E - Box
AATAGGGACTTTCCATTGACGTCAATGGGTGGAGTATTTACGGTAAACTGCCCACTTGG


      E - Box    E - Box         GC-rich      CREB     CREB
CAGTACATCAAGTGTATCATATGCCAAGTACGCCCCCTATTGACGTCAATGACGGTAAA


 GC-rich                                   NFκB
TGGCCCGCCTGGCATTATGCCCAGTACATGACCTTATGGGACTTTCCTACTTGGCAGTA


CATCTACGTATTAGTCATCGCTATTACCATGGTGATGCGGTTTTGGCAGTACATCAATG


                             NFκB                      CREB
GGCGTGGATAGCGGTTTGACTCACGGGGGATTTCCAAGTCTCCACCCCATTGACGTCAAT


                             NFκB                   Long SP1
GGGAGTTTGTTTTGGCACCAAAATCAACGGGACTTTCCAAAATGTCGTAACAACTCCGC


(SP1)  CREB E - Box SP1                    TATA-Box
CCCATTGACGCAAATGGGCGGTAGGCGTGTACGGTGGGAGGTCTATATAAGCAGAGCTC


      +1 ---> mRNA Transcript
GTTTAGTGAACCG TCAGATCGCCTGGAGACGCCATCCACGCTGTTTTGACCTCCATAG
```

FIGURE 2. Part of the DNA sequence (upper strand only) of the human cytomegalovirus genome is presented, showing 603 bp of the promoter and the first part of the transcribed sequence of the immediate-early gene (starting at +1). The sequence is taken from Hennighausen and Fleckenstein (1986), and corresponds to GenBank accession number X03922. The putative binding sites in the promoter DNA sequence for a number of transcription factors is shown by single and.double underlining and single overlining. A brief explanation of the sites is: TATA-Box: Generic motif found in most eukaryotic promoters; site for binding of the transcription factor complex TFIID; the consensus sequence is TAT(A/T)$_{2-4}$. CArG/SRF: "C, A/T-rich, G" site; identical to Serum Response Factor site; consensus binding site is CC(A/T)$_6$GG. RSRF: Related to Serum Response Factor; consensus binding site is (C/T)TA(A/T)(A/T)(A/T)(A/T)TA(A/G). E-Box: Enhancer Box; binding site for proteins containing the basic-helix-loop-helix domain; consensus binding site is CANNTG. GC-rich: A minimum of six G or C nucleotides; potential binding site for SP1. SP1: Factor binding to GC-rich site of the form GGGCGG; long form of this motif is (T/G)GGGCGG(A/G)(A/G)(C/T). AP2: Activator Protein which binds to sequences of the form C(C/G)CC(A/C)N(C/G)(C/G). CREB: Cyclic AMP Response Element Binding factor; binds to the sequence TGACG (short form) or TGACGTCA (inverted repeat). NFκB: Nuclear Factor kappa-B; binds to sequences of the form GGG(A/G)(A/C/T)T(C/T)(C/T)(A/C/T)C.

characteristic of muscle tissue. First of all, the proximal 200 bp of the IIB MyHC promoter from mouse contain six regions which are highly conserved with a family of MyHC promoters in the avian genome (Takeda et al., 1992b). It is remarkable that these motifs are so similar: 96% identity between the mouse IIB and the chicken embryonic MyHC gene promoters (see Figure 3A). This can be interpreted as a conservation of sequences which originated in the ancestral promoter and are involved in transcriptional functions common to the present day family of MyHC promoters. Randomization of the sequences between the conserved motifs has apparently occurred during the 300 million years since the separation of the two species. Two "myosin AT-rich" sequences called mAT1 and mAT2 harbor binding sites for the muscle-specific transcription factor MEF2 (Martin et al., 1993) and for the mesodermal homeodomain protein MHox (Cserjesi et al., 1992). The "CArG box" is typical of many muscle gene promoters, but not totally specific (Treisman, 1992). The extended mCArG motif is however characteristic of the MyHC promoters. An E-box, the consensus sequence of which is CANNTG, is found in the mouse promoter but not the chicken one (not shown in Figure 3A). This motif can potentially bind a myogenic basic-HLH transcription factor such as MyoD. A canonical TATA box motif is found in a majority of eukaryotic promoters, but the nine bp CTATAAAAG sequence found in the IIB and embryonic MyHC promoters, called mTATA, is typical of the skeletal MyHC genes.

The distribution of a number of DNA-binding sites for muscle-specific proteins, along with other sites for more typical DNA-binding proteins, in a relatively small region near the site of transcription initiation suggests that the different binding proteins interact to form a proximal initiation complex (Roeder, 1991). In the case of the MyHC gene promoters, this initiation complex could contain several muscle-specific factors and thus be specific to myogenic cells. As mentioned above, the large protein complex called TFIID, which is one of several basal transcription factors, binds to the TATA box region via TBP. In muscle cells, this basal factor might conceivably contain muscle-specific components, or at least interact in a specific way with the factors such as MEF2, MHox, MyoD, etc. These ideas are summarized in the cartoon shown in Figure 3B, in which the existence of specific Myogenic-Initiation-Complex factors is postulated.

THE USE OF TISSUE-SPECIFIC REGULATORY ELEMENTS FOR GENE THERAPY

One of the most obvious uses for promoter modulatory elements is to confer tissue specificity such that the transferred gene is transcribed only in the tissue which requires the physiological effect of the protein to be made from the resulting mRNA transcript. It should be noted that this will not always be a desired feature, since many proteins play a role in cell physiology in numerous tissues. Even a protein which at first sight would seem to be important only for the predominantly afflicted tissue, such as the protein dystrophin which is missing from muscle fibers in Duchenne muscular dystrophy, has turned out to be expressed in the brain in

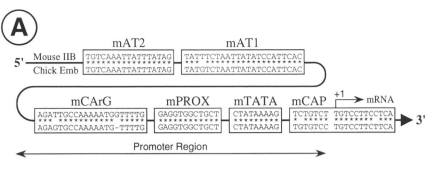

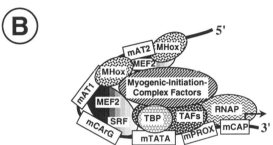

FIGURE 3. A comparison of evolutionarily conserved DNA sequence motifs in the promoters of myosin heavy chain genes expressed in mouse and chicken skeletal muscle, and a hypothetical view of protein interactions in a myogenic preinitiation complex. In Panel A, the conserved sequences found in the mouse type IIB MyHC promoter (top strand) and the chicken embryonic promoter (lower strand) are compared (see Takeda et al., 1992a, b). The conserved motifs are found in the first 200 base pairs of promoter sequence. The sequences between the motifs have diverged and there is no significant homology between the two promoters. The significance of the different motifs is explained in the text. Panel B represents the proteins that can bind to the MyHC proximal promoter, and shows in what way the interactions among the muscle-specific factors MEF2 and MHox, the TFIID complex (TBP plus TAFs) and putative Myogenic-Initiation-Complex factors could take place. This schematic representation is purely hypothetical and serves to suggest one way in which the protein-binding DNA motifs could cause a muscle-specific, active preinitiation complex to be formed.

normal individuals (Boyce et al., 1991). Furthermore, a shorter protein expressed from this same gene (but by use of from an internal promoter) is found in numerous non-muscle cell types including brain whereas it is absent from muscle tissue (Lederfein et al., 1992).

Many promoters for cell-specific genes have been studied, and their tissue-restricted activity has been documented by transfection into cells in culture, or more importantly by the production of transgenic mice. The results from transgenic animals are the most persuasive since the gene is incorporated into the genome and thus present in all cell types. As a consequence, the finding of a cell type-specific activity has considerable physiological meaning provided that the introduced transgene is expressed according to a certain tissue-restricted pattern independently of the site of integration into the host genome. In practice this means obtaining the same result in at least two different transgenic lines since the site of the transgene in the genome is virtually certain to be different due to the independent integration events.

Nonetheless, the fact that integration of the foreign gene into the host genome as a heritable transgene does not necessarily make it a good model for all types of gene therapy protocols. Although the use of retroviruses, for example, will lead to integration of the viral genome into the host DNA (since this is a natural feature of retroviral infection), this is not the case with adenovirus, for which the viral genome does not integrate to a high frequency. Likewise, when pure plasmid DNA is injected into muscle tissue, the DNA remains extrachromosomal in the nuclei of the transfected muscle fibers (Wolff et al., 1992). It is therefore possible that regulatory promoter elements of the promoter DNA sequences will not behave identically in all cellular and genomic contexts. There is at least two examples which indicate that this can indeed be the case.

The CMV promoter is one of the most active promoters of many tested (including those for muscle genes) when injected as a plasmid vector into mouse skeletal muscle tissue where it remains extrachromosomal (Manthorpe et al., 1993). In contrast, when present as a transgene in the mouse genome it is a very poor promoter in skeletal muscle but, surprisingly, it exhibits the highest activity in the heart, which is also a striated muscle (Schmidt et al., 1990). Although rather few examples of this sort are currently available, largely due to a paucity of comparative studies using the same promoter sequences as a transgene or as a viral- or plasmid-based element, it is nonetheless difficult to predict the activity of a given cloned promoter element in different tissue types or even to extrapolate from one experimental model to another. To state it another way, the combination of promoter and activator elements that are required for a certain type of expression or regulation pattern may depend on the type of vector into which they are put.

In the second example, the cDNA gene encoding dystrophin was introduced as a transgene into the *mdx* mouse mutant (Lee et al., 1993). This mutant is the murine model of Duchenne muscular dystrophy in which, like the human disease, the dystrophin gene is mutated, leading in both cases to a deficit of dystrophin. The transgene was expressed under the control of the mouse muscle creatine kinase gene promoter linked to two enhancers from the creatine kinase gene. Although expression was indeed confined to muscle tissue (skeletal and cardiac), the extent of expression varied between muscle types; in particular, dystrophin was virtually absent in the diaphragm muscle of the *mdx* transgenic mice. This may or may not be a special case due to the different types of skeletal muscle fibers. However, since experimental gene therapy of dystrophin is well advanced, these models can alert us to some of the potential problems that could be encountered with muscle, but potentially for other tissue types as well.

One very successful experimental application of the use of muscle-specific regulatory elements has been reported by Dai et al. (1992). They produced a defective retroviral vector expressing canine factor IX cDNA in which the CMV promoter was combined with a muscle gene enhancer, derived once again from the mouse creatine kinase gene. This vector was used to infect primary mouse myoblasts which were then grafted into the hindlimb muscles of mice; the levels of canine factor IX found in the mouse plasma were stable for over 6 months. In contrast, use of the CMV promoter without the muscle enhancer gave only transient expression. In summary, an appropriate choice of promoters and enhancers offers promise not only for obtaining high-level tissue-specific expression *per se* but also for taking advantage of regulatory elements to confer other advantages such as longevity of expression as in the case of the factor IX experiments.

MODULATORY ELEMENTS

A number of physiological influences regulate gene expression, and some of these could, at least in principle, be harnessed to modulate the expression of promoters in gene therapy protocols. One of these physiological influences would be the process of differentiation itself. Therefore the regulation of genes as a function of the stage of tissue maturation would most likely require the use of developmentally regulated promoters and/or enhancer elements, similar to the model discussed in the previous section.

Hormonal regulation is another form of physiological influence that could be put to use to modulate expression of transferred genes. The following examples will serve to illustrate some of the possibilities. Remarkable progress has been achieved in the last several years concerning the molecular mechanisms of regulation achieved by steroid hormones, thyroid hormone, retinoic acid and vitamin D_3, all of which bind to receptors belonging to the same family of genes (Evans, 1988; Leid et al., 1993; Reichel and Jacob, 1993). Indeed, these ligands all bind to receptors which are DNA-binding proteins capable of activating transcription from target genes. Moreover, the natural DNA sequences to which these receptors bind are similar: they are most often constituted of a "half-site" of the sequence AGGTCA (or closely related sequences) which can be repeated two or three times in different orientations. A synthetic thyroid hormone response element can be made from a palindromic repeat of this half-motif: the sequence AGGTCATGACCT serves as a binding site for the receptor, and it will mediate a stimulatory response to both thyroid hormone T3 as well as the hormone estrogen (Glass et al., 1988).

In a particularly elegant example of the molecular basis for physiological hormone regulation, Umesono et al. (1991) and Näär et al. (1991) showed that hormone response elements can be constructed of two half-motifs arranged as a direct repeat with a separation between the two halves of either 3, 4 or 5 base pairs (comprised of any of the four nucleotides at each position). If the separation is three bp, the response element interacts with the Vitamin D_3 receptor, if it is four bp then it serves as a T3 responsive element, and if the separation is five bp the it becomes a retinoic acid response element. Thus the half-site spacing plays a critical role in achieving the selective hormonal response. The molecular definition of the hormonal response elements thus allows a choice of DNA sequence elements which can serve to regulate heterologous promoters which would then be potentially subject to modulation by certain natural or synthetic pharmacoactive molecules, which could be easily administered.

One final example of a physiological influence, using one of the simplest types of modulator that can be envisioned, concerns regulation by a metal ion. It has been shown, principally from studies on the metallothionein gene promoter, that heavy metals can regulate the transcription of this class of genes. A heavy-metal regulatory region was delineated and a synthetic 12 bp conserved sequence was shown to confer metal regulation on heterologous genes (Stuart et al., 1985). The use of heavy metals is another way of achieving promoter-based regulation of genes in most types of tissues where the metal-binding transcriptional activator proteins are found.

LOCUS CONTROL REGIONS

The chromosomal locus containing the several genes encoding the human β-globin proteins offers a tantalizing and elegant example of the sort of regulatory functions which coordinate the expression of a multigene locus. The five genes of this locus are expressed in a tissue-specific and developmentally regulated fashion as the site of erythropoiesis shifts during development (Enver and Greaves, 1991; Crossley and Orkin, 1993). The embryonic ε-globin gene is located at the 5' end of the locus, with the other four genes arranged in the order 5'- γ^G - γ^A - δ - β -3'. Between 6 and 18 kilobase pairs to the 5' side of the embryonic gene lies a regulatory region responsible for controlling activation and high-level expression of the various genes of the locus. If long-range coordinate regulation by LCRs turns out to be a general feature of many gene loci, then these types of control elements will be useful and possibly necessary features of expression systems for gene therapy approaches.

The regulatory DNA sequences that make up this Locus Control Region, or LCR, of the β-globin complex are being extensively investigated. The β-globin LCR was initially discovered as a series of accessible or "open" chromatin sites found upstream of the human locus, and the function of this chromosomal region has been extensively studied by the introduction of these DNA sequences, along with the human globin promoters and coding regions, as transgenes in mice. Among the DNA sequence motifs present in the LCR are binding sites for the erythroid-specific proteins GATA-1 and NF-E2 (Andrews et al., 1993), as well as numerous widely distributed proteins including the transcription factor SP1. As pointed out by Crossley and Orkin (1993), one striking feature of the β-globin LCR is its relative simplicity, considering the apparent function of the elements. The protein factors involved are all transcriptional activators in erythroid cells, and the LCR thus seems to be constituted by DNA motifs, the combination of which might be novel, but which themselves do not bind proteins whose unique function concerns the LCR.

Several models have been proposed to account for the effect of the LCR on coordinated regulation of the β-globin multigene locus. One point is that, to a first approximation, the LCR affects the different genes in a polar fashion. When the human locus is introduced into transgenic mice, the ε and γ genes are found to be activated during development before the adult β-globin gene (Strouboulis et al, 1992). If a new promoter is experimentally introduced close to the LCR of the endogenous human locus of a cultured mouse/human hybrid erythroid cell line by homologous DNA recombination, then the introduced promoter is activated after the induction of differentiation and in these cells the endogenous β-globin gene remains inactive (Kim et al, 1992). Thus, placing a foreign promoter nearer to the LCR than any of the globin genes (actually within the LCR in the case of Kim et al.) leads to activation of the nearest gene, at the expense of the endogenous gene which would normally be induced.

A correlate to the idea of polarity is that there is competition for the activating effect of the LCR (Peterson and Stamatoyannopoulos, 1993). To explain the gene switching phenomenon then, it is postulated that the developmental genes ε and γ are actively repressed as erythroid differentiation proceeds. When this occurs, the β-globin gene can come under the influence of the LCR. In the absence of active repression, for example in early development, how is selectivity of gene expression achieved by the LCR? Hanscombe et al (1991) have proposed a model whereby the distance of the LCR from the individual genes could suffice to explain the polar effect of the LCR on any given gene within the locus (represented schematically in Figure 4). In the absence of further information on three-dimensional chromatin structure involving this locus, one point concerning this sort of model is that the effect of the LCR in a volume, might vary inversely as the cube of the distance, which if true would amplify the distance effect among the regulatory elements of the locus. Peterson and Stamatoyannopoulos (1993) have however argued, based on results of elegant experiments, that the individual promoters compete for the activating effects of the LCR and that distance plays a minor role.

Although the precise explanation of the LCR effect on gene expression remains to be found, such a regulatory element might be crucial for gene transfer and expression in some situations. The concept which arises from the experimental evidence with transgenic mice is that the LCR confers position- and copy number-independent expression on the genes placed under its control. In other words, the LCR-promoter-gene complex functions as an independent regulatory unit. Since virtually all gene therapy approaches will involve expression of genes which are either unintegrated or integrated into the host genome at unnatural positions, the incorporation of LCR-type elements will become important for high level expression and appropriate regulation.

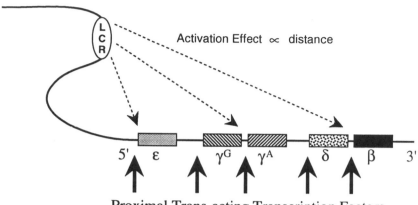

FIGURE 4. A schematic illustration of two explanations for the mechanism of action of the Locus Control Region (LCR) of the human β-globin multigene complex. The polar effect on expression of the different globin genes during development could be explained by an activator effect of the LCR which is proportional to the distance from the individual promoters. According to this model, distal genes would become active during development by active repression of proximal genes (see text). Another possible explanation is that the differential expression of genes within the locus is due to competition for the activator effect of the LCR by the different trans-acting factors associated with each promoter. The two explanations are not necessarily mutually exclusive.

CONCLUDING REMARKS

The structure and organization of regulatory elements in eukaryotic promoters shows a great deal of modularity. It is thus possible to envisage unnatural, but effective, combinations of promoter, enhancer and even LCR modules to build regulatory elements to accomplish specific tasks in a gene therapy protocol. These tasks might be simply achieving high-level expression, but very likely would also include generating tissue-restricted expression to avoid unwanted side effects of the gene products. Some measure of developmental regulation could be necessary, and the modulation of expression by other physiological stimuli or by adminis-tered drugs could also be a desirable feature. Some principles which could govern future work in this area are given in Table 1, although they are, at the very least, simply a starting point for future guidelines.

The molecular biological tools required to test various combinations of regu-latory modules are certainly available, and our knowledge concerning the various regulatory elements in play is constantly increasing. In order to fully test the mul-titude of possibilities, we must have the means, at least for the experimental preclinical stages of the work, of introducing the genetic vectors in a simple way. While transgenic animals, grafting of transfected cells, or the use of viral vectors will play an important role in the development of therapeutic approaches (Miller,

TABLE 1. Principles regarding use of expression vectors for gene therapy protocols

1. Promoters, activators sequences, enhancers and LCRs are composed of modular elements that bind individual transactivation protein factors.

2. The modular regulatory elements can be combined with promoters in many different ways. Heterologous combinations are by all means worth trying.

3. Several types of modulatory elements are currently available, and those based on hormone response elements would appear quite suitable for the purpose of influencing the expression of introduced genes.

4. The context in which the introduced regulatory elements find themselves within the host nucleus or genome can have a major influence on the expression pattern seen.

5. Extrapolation from results obtained with one vector system to another (transgenic mice, viral vectors, extrachromosomal plasmid constructs) may be difficult if not impossible; first principles count little when confronted with the results.

6. Trial and error may supersede scientific logic in finding the most appropriate expression system for a given gene therapy protocol; experimental models of human diseases are a necessity.

7. Methodology allowing the rapid testing of many experimental parameters will be of great benefit. More emphasis should be placed on the use of plasmid DNA constructs for gene therapeutic purposes and methods for direct delivery of such plasmids should be developed further.

1992), they are nonetheless uniformly lengthy procedures which might not only limit the speed of development of therapeutic approaches but also the range. However, the discovery of the unexpected ability of tissues to directly take up and express plasmid DNA, either in the pure form or complexed with lipids (Wolff et al., 1990; Davis et al., 1993a,b; Zhu et al., 1993), will greatly simplify this work. The development of genetic vaccines, for example, will be facilitated since plasmid DNA becomes the vaccinating molecule (Davis et al., 1993c; Ulmer et al., 1993; Wang et al., 1993). Given the complexity of what needs to be accomplished, these latter methods for introducing DNA combined with the relative ease of modifying plasmid DNA vectors, should make important contributions to the development of gene therapeutic paradigms.

ACKNOWLEDGEMENTS

I am particularly grateful to Dr. Heather L. Davis for our ongoing conversations on gene therapy and for her helpful comments on this chapter. I also thank Melissa

Lakich, Thierry Diagana and Dr. Shin'ichi Takeda for many fruitful discussions. The author is Director of Research in the French Centre National de Recherche Scientifique. This laboratory is supported by the Pasteur Institute and the Centre National de Recherche Scientifique, and the research is financed by grants from the Association Française contre les Myopathies, the Institut National de la Santé et de la Recherche Médicale, the French Ministry of Research and NATO.

REFERENCES

Alber T (1992): Structure of the leucine zipper. *Curr Opin Genet Dev* 2:205-210

Alberts B, Bray D, Lewis J, Raff M, Roberts K, Watson J (1989): *Molecular Biology of the Cell.* New York: Garland Publishing, Inc., pp. 528ff

Andrews NC, Erdjument-Bromage H, Davidson MB, Tempst P, Orkin SH (1993): Erythroid transcription factor NF-E2 is a haematopoietic-specific basic-leucine zipper protein. *Nature* 362:722-728

Berg JM (1992): Sp1 and the subfamily of zinc finger proteins with guanine-rich binding sites. *Proc Natl Acad Sci USA* 89:11109-11110

Blackwood EM, Kretzner L, Eisenman RN (1992): Myc and Max function as a nucleoprotein complex. *Curr Opin Genet Dev* 2:227-235

Boshart M, Weber F, Jahn G, Dorsch-Häsler K, Fleckenstein B, Schaffner W (1985): A very strong enhancer is located upstream of an immediate early gene of human cytomegalovirus. *Cell* 41:521-530

Boyce FM, Beggs AH, Feener C, Kunkel LM (1991): Dystrophin is transcribed in brain from a distant upstream promoter. *Proc Natl Acad Sci USA* 88:1276-1280

Brindle PK, Montminy MR (1992): The CREB family of transcription activators. *Curr Opin Genet Dev* 2:199-204

Cserjesi P, Lilly B, Bryson L, Wang Y, Sassoon DA, Olson EN (1992): MHox: a mesodermally restricted homeodomain protein that binds an essential site in the muscle creatine kinase enhancer. *Development* 115:1087-1101

Crossley M, Orkin SH (1993): Regulation of the β-globin locus. *Current Opinion in Genetics and Development* 3:232-237

Dai Y, Roman M, Naviaux RK, Verma IM (1992): Gene therapy via primary myoblasts: long-term expression of factor IX protein following transplantation in vivo. *Proc Natl Acad Sci USA* 89:10892-10895

Davis HL, Whalen RG, Demeneix BA (1993a): Direct gene transfer into skeletal muscle in vivo: Factors affecting efficiency of transfer and stability of expression. *Hum Gene Ther* 4:151-159

Davis HL, Demeneix BA, Quantin B, Coulombe J, Whalen RG (1993b): Plasmid DNA is superior to viral vectors for direct gene transfer in adult mouse skeletal muscle. *Hum Gene Ther* 4:733-740

Davis HL, Michel ML, Whalen RG (1993c): DNA-based immunization for Hepatitis B induces continuous secretion of antigen and high levels of circulating antibody. *Hum Molec Genet* 2:1847-1851

Enver T, Greaves DR (1991): Globin gene switching: a paradigm or what? *Current Opinion in Biotechnology* 2:787-795

Evans RM (1988): The steroid and thyroid hormone receptor superfamily. *Science* 240:889-895

Gill G, Tjian R (1992): Eukaryotic coactivators associated with the TATA box binding protein. *Curr Opin Genet Dev* 2:236-242

Glass CK, Holloway JM, Devary OV, Rosenfeld MG (1988): The thyroid hormone receptor binds with opposite transcriptional effects to a common sequence motif in thyroid hormone and estrogen response elements. *Cell* 54:313-323

Greenblatt J (1992): Riding high on the TATA box. *Nature* 360:16-17

Hanscombe O, Whyatt D, Fraser P, Yannoutsos N, Greaves D, Dillon N, Grosveld F (1991): Importance of globin gene order for correct developmental expression. *Genes and Dev* 5:1387-1394

Harrison SC (1991): A structural taxonomy of DNA-binding domains. *Nature* 353:715-715

Hennighausen L, Fleckenstein B (1986) Nuclear factor 1 interacts with five DNA elements in the promoter region of the human cytomegalovirus major immediate early gene. *EMBO J* 5:1367-1371

Jacob F, Monod J (1961): Genetic regulatory mechanisms in the synthesis of proteins. *J Mol Biol* 3:318-356

Jen Y, Weintraub H, Benezra R (1992): Overexpression of Id protein inhibits the muscle differentiation program: in vivo association of Id with E2A proteins. *Genes and Dev* 6:1466-1479

Kim CG, Epner EM, Forrester WC, Groudine M (1992): Inactivation of the human β-globin gene by targeted insertion into the β-globin locus control region. *Genes and Dev* 6:928-938

Lederfein D, Levy Z, Augier N, Mornet D, Morris G, Fuchs O, Yaffe D, Nudel U (1992): A 71-kilodalton protein is a major product of the Duchenne muscular dystrophy gene in brain and other nonmuscle tissues. *Proc Natl Acad Sci USA* 89:5346-5350

Lee CC, Pons F, Jones PG, Bies RD, Schlang AM, Leger JJ, Caskey CT (1993): *Mdx* transgenic mouse: restoration of recombinant dystrophin to the dystrophic muscle. *Hum Gene Ther* 4:273-281

Leid M, Kastner P, Chambon P (1992): Multiplicity generates diversity in the retinoic acid signalling pathways. *Trends Biochem Sci* 17:427-433

Manthorpe M, Cornefert-Jensen F, Hartikka J, Felgner J, Rundell A, Margalith M, Dwarki V (1993): Gene therapy by intramuscular injection of plasmid DNA: Studies on firefly luciferase gene expression in mice. *Human Gene Ther* (In Press)

Martin JF, Schwarz JJ, Olson EN (1993): Myocyte enhancer factor (MEF) 2C: a tissue-restricted member of the MEF-2 family of transcription factors. *Proc Natl Acad Sci USA* 90:5282-5286

McKeown M (1992): Alternative mRNA splicing. *Annu Rev Cell Biol* 8:133-155

Miller AD (1992): Human gene therapy comes of age. *Nature* 357:455-460

Näär AM, Boutin J-M, Lipkin SM, Yu VC, Holloway JM, Glass CK, Rosenfeld MG (1991): The orientation and spacing of core DNA-binding motifs dictate selective transcriptional responses to three nuclear receptors. *Cell* 65:1267-1279

Nikolov DB, Hu S-H, Lin J, Gasch A, Hoffman A, Horikoshi M, Chua N-H, Roeder RG, Burley SK (1992): Crystal structure of TFIID TATA-box binding protein. *Nature* 360:40-46

Nolan GP, Baltimore D (1992): The inhibitory ankyrin and activator Rel proteins. *Curr Opin Genet Dev* 2:211-220

Parvin JD, Timmers HThM, Sharp PA (1992): Promoter specificity of basal transcription factors. *Cell* 68:1135-1144

Peterson KR, Stamatoyannopoulos G (1993): Role of gene order in developmental control of human γ- and β-globin gene expression. *Mol Cell Biol* 13:4836-4843

Reichel RR, Jacob ST (1993): Control of gene expression by lipophilic hormones. *FASEB J* 7:427-436

Roeder RG (1991): The complexities of eukaryotic transcription initiation: regulation of preinitiation complex assembly. *Trends Biochem Sci* 16:402-408

Schmidt EV, Christoph G, Zeller R, Leder P (1990): The cytomegalovirus enhancer: a pan-active control element in transgenic mice. *Mol Cell Biol* 10:4406-4411

Strouboulis J, Dillon N, Grosveld F (1992): Developmental regulation of a complete 70-kb human β-globin locus in transgenic mice. *Genes and Dev* 6:1857-1864

Stuart GW, Searle PF, Palmiter RD (1985): Identification of multiple metal regulatory elements in mouse metallothionein-I promoter by assaying synthetic sequences. *Nature* 317:828-831

Takeda S, North DL, Lakich MM, Russell SD, Whalen RG (1992): A possible regulatory role for conserved promoter motifs in an adult-specific muscle myosin gene from mouse. *J Biol Chem* 267:16957-16967

Takeda S, North DL, Lakich MM, Russell SD, Kahng LS, Whalen RG (1993): Evolutionarily conserved promoter motifs and enhancer organization in the mouse gene encoding the IIB myosin heavy chain isoform expressed in adult fast skeletal muscle. *Comptes Rendus Acad Sci Paris* 315:467-472

Timmers HThM, Sharp PA (1991): The mammalian TFIID protein is present in two functionally distinct complexes. *Genes and Dev* 5:1946-1956

Treisman R, Ammerer G (1992): The SRF and MCM1 transcription factors. *Curr Opin Genet Dev* 2:221-226

Ulmer JB, Donnelly JJ, Parker SE, Rhodes GH, Felgner PL, Dwarki VJ, Gromkowski SH, Deck RR, DeWitt CM, Friedman A, Hawe LA, Leander KR, Martinez D, Perry HC, Shiver JW, Montgomery DL, Liu MA (1993): *Science* 259:1745-1749

Umesono K, Murakami KK, Thompson CC, Evans RM (1991): Direct repeats as selective response elements for the thyroid hormone, retinoic acid, and vitamin D_3 receptors. *Cell* 65:1255-1266

Wang B, Ugen KE, Srikantin V, Agadjanyan MG, Dang K, Refaeli Y, Sato AI, Boyer J, Williams WV, Weiner DB (1993): *Proc Natl Acad Sci USA* 90:4156-4160

Weiner AM (1993): mRNA splicing and autocatalytic introns: distant cousins or the products of chemical determinism? *Cell* 72:161-164

Weintraub H, Davis R, Tapscott S, Thayer M, Krause M, Benezra R, Blackwell TK, Turner D, Rupp R, Hollenberg S, Zhuang Y, Lassar A (1991): The myoD gene family: nodal point during specification of the muscle cell lineage. *Science* 251:761-766

Wolff JA, Malone RW, Williams P, Chong W, Acsadi G, Jani A, Felgner PL (1990): Direct gene transfer into mouse muscle in vivo. *Science* 247:1465-1468

Wolff JA, Ludtke JJ, Acsadi G, Williams P, Jani A (1992): Long-term persistence of plasmid DNA and foreign gene expression in mouse muscle. *Hum Molec Genet* 1:363-369

Wright WE (1992): Muscle basic helix-loop-helix proteins and the regulation of myogenesis. *Curr Opin Genet Dev* 2:243-248

Zhu N, Liggitt D, Debs R (1993): Systemic gene expression after intravenous DNA delivery into adult mice. *Science* 261:209-211

Part II

METHODS AND MECHANISMS

POSSIBLE MECHANISMS OF DNA UPTAKE IN SKELETAL MUSCLE

Martin E. Dowty and Jon A. Wolff

INTRODUCTION

Somatic gene therapy promises to be a revolutionary advance in the medical treatment of both acquired and genetic disease states. The major obstacle for the full realization of gene therapy is currently the ability to transfer the appropriate gene into enough target cells which will result in sufficient levels of protein expression to control the biological disorder. A number of methods to transfer genes into cells are currently being explored and include viral (Miller, 1990), physical (Capecchi, 1980; Chu et al., 1987; Wu and Wu, 1988; Wolff et al., 1990; Mirzayans et al., 1992), and chemical (Benvenity and Reshef, 1986; Felgner et al., 1987; Felgner and Ringold, 1989; Yang et al., 1990) techniques. With each of these methods, the gene needs to traverse the cell membrane and, subsequently, enter the nucleus where it can be expressed. The processes involved in the transfer of DNA across biological membranes are, at this time, mostly speculative and require more research to fully define the processes involved in polynucleotide transport. This chapter will discuss what is known about the uptake of naked foreign DNA by muscle cells after intramuscular injection or implantation as well as speculate as to the possible mechanism of cellular uptake based on current data. An understanding of the mechanism by which a polynucleotide traverses the external lamina and sarcolemma of a myofiber, and subsequently enters the nucleus, should allow for the refinement of methods to deliver foreign DNA to muscle cells. It would also increase our knowledge of basic muscle physiology to learn whether there is an intrinsic property of muscle cells which allows them to take up DNA or whether it is a vagary of the delivery method.

FOREIGN GENE EXPPRESSION BY INTRAMUSCULAR INJECTION OF PLASMID DNA: BASICS OF THE PHENOMENON

It has been shown that intramuscular injection of plasmid DNA expression vectors in rodent and nonhuman primates results in the cellular uptake of the plasmid and subsequent expression of the protein encoded by the vector (Wolff et al., 1990; Acsadi et al., 1991b; Jiao et al., 1992a; Jiao et al., 1992b). Since the plasmid DNA expression vectors contain type II RNA polymerase promoters, it may be assumed that the plasmid DNA expression vectors entered the nuclei of muscle cells in order to be transcribed. Foreign plasmid DNA has been shown to remain and express in skeletal muscle of mice for at least 19 months (Wolff et al., 1992a). In addition, the methylation pattern of the injected vector was the same as its bacterial form indicating that the foreign DNA did not undergo replication in the muscle cells (Wolff et al., 1992a). Furthermore, experiments involving the bacterial electroporation of total cellular DNA from injected muscle demonstrated that the plasmid DNA was maintained episomally (Wolff et al., 1992a).

Various conditions such as needle type, speed of injection, volume and type of the injection fluid, dosage form, muscle innervation and contraction, and animal age have been evaluated with regards to the efficiency of gene delivery after intramuscular injection (Wolff et al., 1991). These types of experiments provide some indirect evidence as to the mechanism of DNA uptake or at least exclude some possibilities. Plasmid DNA delivered in normal saline consistently resulted in greater expression compared with various sucrose, glycerol, dextrose, and cell culture solutions. Less damage to myofibers was evident with normal saline injections relative to sucrose solutions which may have accounted for the greater expression seen with the former solution. Solution osmolarity, up to twice physiologic osmolarity, and buffer capacity of the solution did not significantly affect gene expression suggesting myofiber uptake of DNA is not related to an osmotic phenomena. The speed of injection and volume of the injection solution did not significantly affect gene expression suggesting that different stretching or pressures created in these experiments is not important for myofibers to take up DNA. In fact, DNA pellets implanted into muscle with fine-tipped forceps, which do not cause the same types of pressures as a solution, resulted in similar or greater gene expression. The needle type used in single plasmid DNA injections did not affect expression, however, it appears that increased damage occurs with repetitive needle injections and, subsequently, results in less efficient gene delivery. Sustained muscle contractions prior to injection, which may also cause myofiber damage, decreases DNA uptake as well. This data suggests that DNA is not likely to express in grossly damaged myofibers and, therefore, this mechanism appears to unable to explain muscle's ability to take up foreign DNA. Denervated muscle (via unilateral dorsal root lesions) showed the same gene expression levels as innervated muscle suggesting that DNA uptake by muscle cells is not facilitated by the nervous system. Newborn and young adult rat muscle were both able to take up and express implanted DNA pellets. This suggests that uptake of DNA is still possible even though various anatomical and physiological aspects of newborn rat muscle, such as the T and sarcoplasmic reticulum systems, are not fully developed at one day of age (Schiaffino and Margreth, 1969; Edge, 1970; Wirtz et al., 1983).

It may be that a unique cytoarchitectural feature of striated muscle is responsible for the uptake of polynucleotides since skeletal and cardiac muscle appear to be better suited to take up and express injected foreign DNA vectors relative to other types of tissue (Wolff et al., 1990; Jiao et al., 1992b; Acsadi et al., 1991a;

Kitsis et al., 1991; Buttrick et al., 1992). There have been recent reports that other tissues, such as liver and thyroid, are in fact able to take up and express DNA after direct injection. However, it is unclear whether the efficiency of gene expresion is as high in these tissues as that in striated muscle (Sikes et al., 1993; Malone et al., 1993).

EXPRESSION OF NAKED PLASMID DNA BY CULTURED CELLS

In vitro results with various cell cultures also suggest that skeletal muscle cells are better able to take up DNA relative to other cell types (Wolff et al., 1992b). When primary rat muscle cell cultures, in various states of differentiation, were exposed to naked pRSVLux (de Wet et al., 1987) or pCMVLux (Acsadi et al., 1991), significant luciferase expression levels resulted, which were independent of the state of cell differentiation (Table 1). The fact that cell age did not affect expression suggests that muscle contractions, which are absent in myoblasts and which have been suggested to cause transient membrane disruptions in vivo (McNeil and Khakee, 1992), are not important in the uptake of foreign DNA. Some of the muscle

TABLE 1. Comparison of luciferase expression after exposure of primary rat muscle cells in various states of differentiation to plasmid pRSVLux and pCMVLux either as naked DNA or complexed with cationic lipids (Wolff et al., 1992b). Muscle cells were grown on gelatin-coated culture plates.

Day DNA Added[a]	Day Lux Assayed[a]	Mean Luciferase Activity (l.u. X 10^3)[b]			
		pRSVLux		pCMVLux	
		Naked DNA[c]	Cationic Lipid[d]	Naked DNA[c]	Cationic Lipid[d]
Day 2 myoblasts	Day 4 fusing myoblasts	98 ± 17 n=13 (26-207)	$1,299 \pm 285$ n=16 (131-2,970)	97 ± 13 n=12 (22-202)	$1,903 \pm 427$ n=12 (145-4,065)
Day 2 myoblasts	Day 8 large myotubes	129 ± 63 n=14 (8-822)	$4,016 \pm 448$ n=13 (2,176-7,538)	83 ± 49 n=10 (6-497)	$4,389 \pm 1,171$ n=11 (840-13,104)
Day 4 fusing myoblasts	Day 6 small myotubes	154 ± 39 n=15 (12-605)	$11,612 \pm 1,611$ n=13 (232-16,572)	274 ± 127 n=10 (34-451)	$11,160 \pm 1,832$ n=11 (5,280-21,355)
Day 8 large myotubes	Day 10 large myotubes	161 ± 65 n=12 (26-751)	$14,565 \pm 2,483$ n=10 (5,694-29,618)	45 ± 17 n=11 (1-117)	$15,810 \pm 5,109$ n=12 (1,310-60,401)

[a] Days post-plating.

[b] Luciferase activity in relative light units (l.u.) assayed in 20μl of the 200μl cell extract prepared from each of the plates 35mm in diameter containing approximately one million cells. The mean values, standard errors (+), number of plates (n), and ranges of values (in parentheses) are shown from three separate batches of muscle cells. Background luciferase levels were $\leq 0.5 \times 10^3$ l.u.

[c] Each culture plate was exposed to 200μg of naked plasmid DNA for 4 hours.

[d] Each culture plate was exposed to 10μg of plasmid DNA complexed with 30μg of Lipofectin®. Similar results were obtained with TransfectACE, another cationic lipid formulation.

TABLE 2. Comparison of luciferase expression after exposure of various cultured cells to naked plasmid pRSVLux or cationic lipid-pRSVLux complexes (Wolff et al., 1992b).

Type of Cell	Mean Luciferase Activity (l.u. X 10^3)[a]	
	Naked DNA[b]	Cationic Lipid[c]
immortalized mouse 3T3 fibroblasts	0.5 ± 0.1 n=12 (0.3-1.5)	733 ± 101 n=7 (315-1,158)
dividing rat primary fibroblasts	4.0 ± 1.3 n=9 (0.8-10.1)	$1,441 \pm 330$ n=8 (145-2,513)
confluent rat primary fibroblasts	9.2 ± 4.9 n=7 (0.5-29.8)	$1,682 \pm 167$ n=5 (1,289-2,135)
undifferentiated mouse C2-C12 myoblasts	1.6 ± 0.8 n=8 (0.3-7.3)	378 ± 120 n=7 (95-993)
differentiated mouse C2-C12 myotubes	25 ± 5 n=7 (8-42)	274 ± 108 n=7 (8-714)
rat primary fetal brain cells	12 ± 4 n=13 (0.8-50)	109 ± 37 n=12 (28-511)
dog primary smooth muscle cells	4 ± 1 n=7 (0.6-11)	446 ± 414 n=8 (13-3,346)

[a] Luciferase activity in relative light units (l.u.) assayed in 20μl of the 200μl cell extract prepared from each of the plates 35mm in diameter containing approximately one million cells. The mean values, standard errors (+), number of plates (n), and ranges of values (in parentheses) are shown from three separate batches of muscle cells. Background luciferase levels were $0.3–0.5 \times 10^3$ l.u.

[b] Each culture plate exposed to 200μg of naked plasmid DNA for 4 hours.

[c] Each culture plate exposed to 10μg of plasmid DNA complexed with 30μg of Lipofectin®. Similar results were obtained with TransfectACE, another cationic lipid formulation.

cell cultures contained luciferase expression levels which approached that observed after intramuscular injections of plasmid DNA in vivo. Luciferase expression obtained in muscle cells were greater than those obtained in other cell types (Table 2) suggesting that these cells are indeed unique relative to other cell types. All cell cultures expressed substantial luciferase activity with the either the RSV or CMV promoter in combination with or without lipofection (Tables 1 and 2) which suggests that all cell types were healthy and the promoter is able to function in each cell type. When the primary muscle cell cultures were lipofected with pRSVLux and pCMVLux, the luciferase activity of 8 day old cultures was greater than that

TABLE 3. Luciferase expression after exposure of primary rat muscle cells in various states of differentiation to plasmid pRSVLux alone or complexed with Lipofectin®. Muscle cells were grown on 1:100 Matrigel® matrix-coated culture dishes. Data is unpublished from our laboratory.

		Mean Luciferase Activity (l.u. X 10^3)[b]	
Day DNA added[a]	Day Lux assayed[a]	Naked DNA[c]	Cationic Lipid[d]
Day 2 myoblasts	Day 4 small myotubes	29 ± 53 n = 7 (0.4-147)	810 ± 1135 n = 2 (8-1613)
Day 2 myoblasts	Day 8 large myotubes	86 ± 112 n = 8 (1-288)	1325 ± 495 n = 2 (975-1675)
Day 4 small myotubes	Day 6 large myotubes	129 ± 153 n = 8 (2-381)	6 ± 2 n = 2 (5-8)
Day 8 large myotubes	Day 10 large myotubes	1357 ± 305 n = 8 (905-1736)	105 ± 55 n = 2 (66-144)

[a] Days post-plating.

[b] Luciferase activity in relative light units (l.u.) assayed in 40µl of the 400µl cell extract prepared from each of the plates 35mm in diameter containing approximately one million cells. The mean values, standard errors (+), number of plates (n), and ranges of values (in parentheses) are shown. Background luciferase levels were approximately $\leq 0.7 \times 10^3$ l.u.

[c] Each culture plate was exposed to 200µg of naked plasmid DNA for 4 hours.

[d] Each culture plate was exposed to 10µg of plasmid DNA complexed with 30µg of Lipofectin®.

of 2 day old muscle cells as well as other cell types (Tables 1 and 2), suggesting that the transcription and translation machinery may be more efficient in the older myotubes relative to younger myoblasts and other cell types.

The substrate on which muscle cells are grown appears to affect their ability to take up and express foreign DNA depending on whether the substrate promotes proliferation or differentiation of the cells. The data of Table 1 were obtained from muscle cells cultured on gelatin-coated culture plates. Conversely, if muscle cells are grown on Matrigel® basement membrane matrix (Collaborative Biomedical Products, Bedford, MA), the amount of protein expression resulting from application of naked pRSVLux increases with increasing age (Table 3). The levels of luciferase expression achieved in the myotubes with naked DNA was similar to the levels achieved in optimally transfected 3T3 fibroblasts. In addition, myoblasts that were transfected with cationic lipid complexed to plasmid DNA resulted in similar levels of expression as seen in Table 1, while myotubes transfected with cationic lipid resulted in approximately two orders of magnitude less protein expression (Table 3). Muscle cells grown on Matrigel® differentiate and begin to contract much faster than those grown on gelatin (our unpublished observation). It appears that the state of differentiation of a muscle cell appears to play a role in both the uptake of plasmid DNA into the cell and the ability of the cell to be transfected, which, in turn, is dependent on the substrate on which the cells are grown. This observation also suggests that other cell types may be better able to take up and express plasmid DNA depending on the conditions in which the cells are grown. In summary, the ability of muscle cells to take up and express foreign DNA is an exciting and interesting phenomena. The ability for cultured muscle cells to express naked plasmid DNA should be a valuable system for elucidating the mechanism of uptake.

LOCALIZATION OF THE PLASMID DNA AFTER INTRAMUSCULAR INJECTION

Although plasmid DNA can be taken up by muscle cells both in vivo and in vitro, it is less clear how the polynucleotide traverses the numerous barriers, such as extracellular matrix and plasma membrane, to eventually gain access to the sarcoplasm. Injected or implanted plasmid DNA in mouse muscle in vivo has been shown to distribute throughout the extracellular matrix, caveolae, and T tubules (Fig. 1 and 2) which suggests that the external lamina is not the rate-limiting step for protein expression (Wolff et al., 1992b). However, positively charged macromolecules, i.e. polyethylene glycol, polylysine, and lipofectin-plasmid DNA complexes, though seen in the external lamina, were only rarely found to have crossed the external lamina to gain access to the caveolae and T-tubules (Fig. 3) (Wolff et al., 1992b). In addition, polyglutamic acid, which has a net negative charge, also rarely crossed the external lamina (Wolff et al., 1992b). In effect, these data suggest that other properties of plasmid DNA, besides its negative charge, are involved in its ability to access myofibers. The study by Wolff et al. (1992b) also showed that there was a restriction of high molecular weight DNA by the external lamina suggesting that size also played a role in the transport of the plasmid DNA into the muscle cells (Fig. 4).

In primate muscle, the injected plasmid DNA was shown to be more restricted in its distribution in the muscle relative to mouse muscle (Wolff et al., 1992b). The efficiency of expression was less in primate muscle compared to mouse muscle which may be explained by this difference in distribution (Jiao et al., 1992b). It is possible that since the primate perimysium is thicker than the mouse perimysium (Jiao et al., 1992b), this property acted as a barrier to the entry of the plasmid into the endomysial space. However, the injection needle should have given DNA access to the endomysium in both species. Hence, it might be that the primate per-

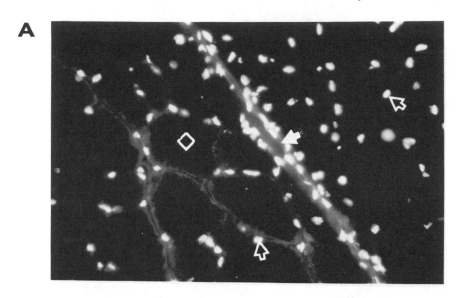

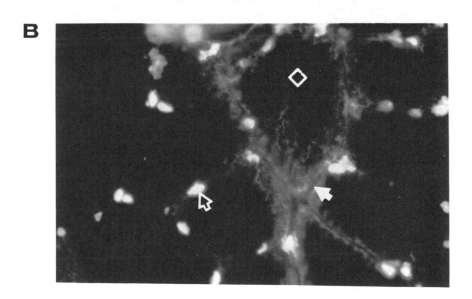

FIGURE 1. (A and B) The distribution of plasmid DNA after IM injection into mouse quadriceps seen with a fluoresence light microscope (Wolff et al., 1992b). Cross-sections of muscle samples. Stained with Hoechst 33258 (Molecular Probes) which stains DNA with AT selectivity. Diamond: a myofiber; open arrow, nucleus; closed arrow: extramyofiberal space. A. x250. B. x500.

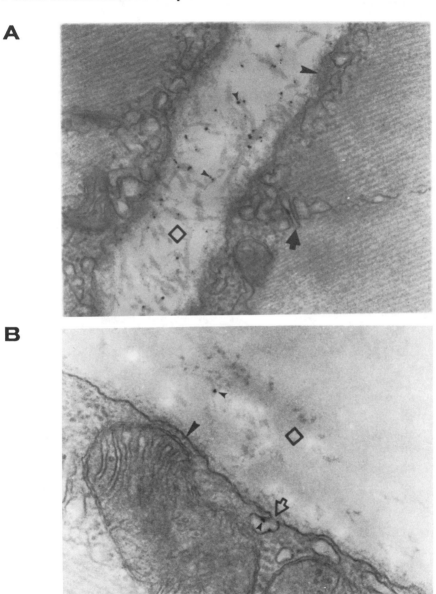

FIGURE 2. Electron microscopy after room temperature fixation of unstained sections from mouse quadriceps injected with 5 nm (average size) gold-conjugated DNA (Au₅-DNA) 15 min previously (Wolff et al., 1992b). (A) Longitudinal section showing Au₅-DNA (small arrowheads) present in the endomysium (diamond) between two myofibers and in a T tubule (filled arrow). (B) Longitudinal section showing Au₅-DNA (small arrowheads) present in a caveolae (open arrow) and perimysium (diamond). Large arrowhead points to the sarcolemma. A and B, x60,000.

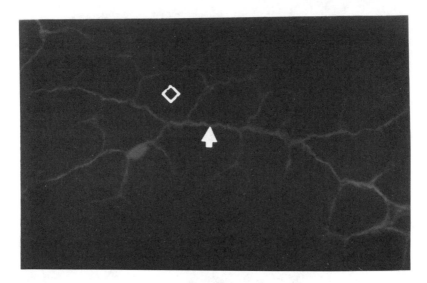

FIGURE 3. Cross sectional view of the distribution of polylysine-Texas Red after IM injection into mouse quadriceps (Wolff et al., 1992b). Note that the polycation is more limited to the extracellular space relative to DNA (Fig. 1). Diamond: a myofiber; filled arrow: extracellular space. x250.

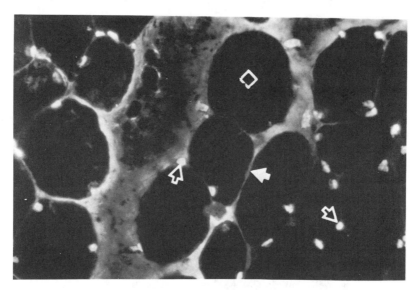

FIGURE 4. The distribution of high molecular weight (genomic) DNA after IM injection into mouse quadriceps stained with Hoechst 33258 (Wolff et al., 1992b). Note the restriction of entry of the DNA into myofibers (compare to Fig. 1). Cross-section of the muscle. Diamond: a myofiber; filled arrow: extracellular space; open arrow: nucleus. x500.

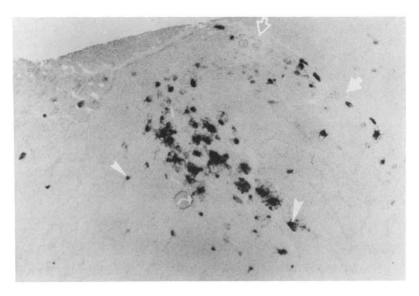

FIGURE 5. A cross-section of a muscle stained for ß-galactosidase expression one week after pRSVlacZ injection (Wolff et al., 1992b). Note the number of blue myofibers distant from the injection site. Open arrow: injection site, closed arrow: epimysium, arrowhead: ß-galactosidase positive cell.

imysium acts as a larger reservoir for the plasmid DNA and, therefore, limits the amount of DNA which is available for contact with the myofibers.

IS PLASMID DNA TAKEN UP BY MUSCLE CELLS VIA MEMBRANE DISRUPTIONS?

Electron microscope data with gold-labeled probes showed that gross membrane disruptions occurred at the site of injection only (Wolff et al., 1992b). However, β-galactosidase-positive myofibers were found distant from the injection site with both injected and implanted plasmid DNA (Fig. 5) (Wolff et al., 1992b). This information is not consistent with the hypothesis that DNA enters myofibers through irreversible membrane disruptions. The ability of cultured myotubes to express naked plasmid DNA in vitro also suggests that irreversible membrane damage is not responsible for the uptake of DNA in muscle cells. Each cell type was treated exactly in the same manner and, therefore, the cell membranes of myotubes would not be subjected to more physical stress relative to the other cultured cells. This data is consistent with the results reported by Wolff et al. (1991).

McNeil and co-authors have hypothesized that the plasma membrane of various cells can open and close after being wounded (McNeil and Ito, 1989; McNeil,

1991; McNeil and Kahkee, 1992). They have demonstrated that gastric epithelial and skin epidermis in situ will take up fluorescent dextran or horseradish peroxidase into their cytoplasm. They also suggested that these probes (McNeil and Kahkee, 1992) as well as serum albumin (McNeil, 1991) are able to enter the sarcoplasm of myofibers. These probes may indeed be taken up by cells through transient breaks in their plasma membrane. However, the pattern of fluorescence or diaminobenzidine staining in muscle was similar to that seen with plasmid DNA at the light microscope level (Fig. 1). Therefore, it is not clear where these probes may be since light microscope analysis does not allow the distinction between extracellular and intracellular compartments in muscle. Electron microscope data (Wolff et al., 1992b) showed that, for DNA, this type of light microscope staining pattern was consistent with localization in the extracellular compartments of the myofibers, i.e. T system and caveolae (Fig. 2). In addition, the ability for muscles in culture to take up and express naked plasmid DNA is also not easily explained by transient membrane disruptions. Myotubes may be able to take up naked DNA because they are contracting which may cause transient membrane disruptions. Furthermore, the inhibition of plasmid DNA uptake at 4°C could be the result of decrease transient membrane disruptions secondary to decreased muscle contractions or decreased membrane fluidity (Table 4) (Wolff et al., 1992b). However, this hypothesis would not explain why (under some culture conditions) myoblasts can take up naked plasmid DNA just as well as myotubes even though they are not contracting. Moreover, gold-labeled DNA, polyethylene glycol, polylysine, and polyglutamic acid (Wolff et al., 1992b) as well as ferritin (Wolff et al., 1992b; Huxley, 1964), analyzed with the electron microscope, were limited to T tubules and caveolae after intramuscular injection and were not found in the cytoplasm of intact myofibers, which does not support a transient membrane disruption hypothesis.

TABLE 4. Exposure of myotubes in 8 day old cultures of primary rat muscle cells to naked pRSVLux DNA at 37° and 4°C (Wolff et al., 1992b).

Condition	Mean Luciferase Activity (l.u. x 10^3) (n=7)[c]	
	1 hr exposure	4 hr exposure
control[a]	52.5 ± 19.4	41.9 ± 11.9
experimental[b]	14.0 ± 9.8	3.0 ± 1.5

[a] Control plates were first exposed to 100µg of naked pRSVLux at 37°C for 1 or 4 fours. After washing and adding media with serum, they were placed at 4°C for 1 or 4 hours, then returned to a 37°C incubator.

[b] Experimental plates were first exposed to 100µg of naked pRSVLux at 4°C for 1 or 4 hours before being washed and returned to the 37°C incubator with media containing serum.

[c] Luciferase was measured as in Table 1.

IS PLASMID DNA TAKEN UP BY MUSCLE CELLS BY ACTIVE TRANSPORT PROCESSES?

Cold treatment has been shown to inhibit endocytosis in cultured myotubes (Janeczko et al., 1985), which may account for the effect of cold on plasmid expression in cultured myotubes (Table 4) (Wolff et al., 1992b). However, electron microscope data did not show any evidence that DNA was taken up by receptor-mediated endocytosis or pinocytosis (Wolff et al., 1992b). In addition, no evidence for the endocytosis of polylysine, which is a marker for endocytosis, was seen (Wolff et al., 1992b). Nevertheless, it is possible that an endocytotic mechanism of DNA uptake exists, but that it is a rare event. Some authors have suggested that the mechanism of uptake of oligonucleotides in various cell types is consistent with an endocytotic process (Loke et al., 1989; Shoji et al., 1991). Further investigation is necessary to determine definitively whether or not foreign DNA is taken up by muscle cells via endocytosis.

Plasmid DNA was found to a great extent in T tubules and caveolae suggesting that these structures may play a role in the uptake of foreign DNA (Fig. 2B) (Wolff et al., 1992b). The ability of DNA to enter these regions at 4°C in vivo suggests that this distribution was energy-independent (Wolff et al., 1992b). Gold-labeled polyethylene glycol, polylysine, and polyglutamate were found in T tubules and caveolae, but to a much less extent than gold-labeled DNA (Wolff et al., 1992b). This suggests that a distinctive property of DNA may be responsible for its localization within these structures. It was not possible to wash out injected plasmid DNA, which appeared to have entered T tubules and caveolae, from unfixed sections suggesting that specific interactions may exist between DNA and these structures (Wolff et al., 1992b). Conversely, intramuscularly injected dextran, which appeared to have a similar distribution to DNA, was removed with multiple washings (Wolff et al., 1992b). Oligonucleotides have been shown to bind to specific membrane receptors (Loke et al., 1989; Yakubov et al., 1989; Wu-Pong et al., 1992) and, hence, it is possible that DNA also binds to some receptor on the cell membrane. Further studies will be required to test this hypothesis. DNA receptors have already been identified in human leukocytes where DNA is taken up by phagocytosis (Bennett et al., 1985; Bennett et al., 1988).

Caveolae have been postulated to play a role in transcytosis either by endocytosis or by the formation of transient channels in endothelial cells (Anderson, 1981). They have also been proposed to be associated with pinocytosis in muscle (Horwitz and Schotland, 1986), but other researchers have disagreed with this possibility (Franzini-Armstrong, 1986). In addition, caveolae have been shown to be involved in potocytosis, a recently proposed mechanism for folate uptake (Anderson et al., 1992). Even though potocytosis has been proposed as a mechanism for cellular uptake for molecules with molecular weights less than 1-2 kD, it is possible that DNA, with a diameter of 2 nm, could string itself through a small transporter pore. However, no gold-labeled DNA found its way into the cytoplasm of myofibers , which may have been due to the inability of the gold-labeled DNA to pass through the putative pores (Wolff et al., 1992b). If potocytosis of DNA exists in myofibers, it may occur via a general potocytotic pathway for polynucleotides or, for that matter, another molecule. It may also be specific to striated muscle which would explain the unique ability of muscle cells to take up DNA. The uptake of naked plasmid DNA by mammalian cells has never been described. However, the transformation of Gram positive bacteria occurs via the transport of single-stranded DNA though a protein pore in the bacterial membrane (Lacks and Greenberg, 1976). In addition, Gram negative bacteria, such as *Haemophilus influenzae*, have specific membrane receptors that enable double-stranded DNA to enter small surface vesicles, i.e. transformasomes, which resembles mammalian potocytosis (Biswas et al., 1989; Concino and Goodgal, 1981; Danner et al., 1982; Dorward et al., 1989; Kahn et al., 1982). Although, the uptake of DNA through caveolae is an interesting possibility, more study is required to test this hypothesis.

ENTRY OF PLASMID DNA INTO THE NUCLEUS

In addition to the necessary requirement of DNA to be transported across the plasma membrane, it must also cross the nuclear membrane and enter the nucleus. The nuclear uptake of DNA is currently being investigated in our laboratory. We have shown that approximately 50% of primary rat myotubes, which were cytoplasmically microinjected with plasmid DNA, will take up the foreign DNA into their nuclei and express the protein encoded by the vector (manuscript in preparation). This appears to be a unique property of the myotubes in that all other cell types which have been cytoplasmically microinjected with DNA showed negligible expression (Capecchi, 1980; Brinster et al., 1985; Mirzayans et al., 1992; Thorburn and Alberts, 1993). The absence of expression cannot be explained by a technical problem of the injection technique because if the same cells were injected directly into their nuclei, 50 to 100% of the cells showed protein expression. It is not completely clear why myotubes express cytoplasmically injected DNA better than other cell types for which there may be, at this time, a plethora of possible explanations. It is not an issue of cell survival because all cell types showed similar viability postinjection. The postmitotic state of myotubes may be an important factor. There may be greater nucleocytoplasmic transport in this cell state. The presence of multiple nuclei in myotubes may provide a greater target for nuclear transport of DNA. Regardless of the reasons for plasmid DNA uptake into the nuclei of myotubes, this observation provides indisuptable evidence that cytoplasmic plasmid DNA can traverse a postmitotic and intact nuclear membrane. This muscle/microinjection system will be invaluable in elucidating the mechanism of plasmid transport into the nucleus.

CONCLUSIONS

It is clear that more research is necessary before the exact mechanism of DNA uptake by muscle cells through the plasma membrane can be defined. Certainly, it does not appear to be a trivial disruption of the plasma membrane through which DNA may enter the myofiber. Defining the mechanism is complicated by the fact that not all muscle cells take up and express DNA and the amount taken up is apparently small, which leads to technical difficulties of quantification. On the other hand, cultured muscle cell systems are available and are constantly being improved to better define both the plasma membrane and nuclear uptake processes. Any information related to the transport mechanisms of foreign DNA into cells may be useful in increasing the efficiency of this process. The ability of muscle cells to take up and express foreign DNA has exciting applications for the treatment of many different types of acquired and genetic diseases (Acsadi et al., 1991; Jiao et al., 1993).

REFERENCES

Acsadi G, Jiao S, Jani A, Duke D, Williams P, Wang C, Wolff JA (1991a): Direct gene transfer and expression into rat heart in vivo. *The New Biologist* 3:71-81

Acsadi G, Dickson G, Love DR, Jani A, Walsh FS, Gurusinghe A, Wolff JA, Davies KE (1991b): Human dystrophin expression in mdx mice after intramuscular injection of DNA constructs. *Nature* 352:815-818

Anderson R (1981): Cell surface membrane structure and the function of endothelial cells. In *Structure and Function of the Circulation*, vol. 3 (ed. CJ Schwartz, N Werthessen, and S Wolf), pp. 239-86. New York: Plenum Press

Anderson RGW, Kamen BA, Rothberg KG, Lacey SW (1992): Potocytosis: sequestration and transport of small molecules by caveolae. *Science* 255:410-411

Bennet RM, Gabor GT, Merritt MM (1985): DNA binding to human leukocytes; evidence for a receptor-mediated association, internalization, and degradation of DNA. *J Clin Invest* 76:2182-2190

Bennet RM, Hefeneider SH, Bakke A, Merritt M, Smith CA, Mourich D, Heinrich MC (1988): The production and characterization of murine monoclonal antibodies to a DNA receptor on human leukocytes. *J Immunology* 140:2937-2942

Benvenisty N, Reshef L (1986): Direct introduction of genes into rats and expression of the genes. *Proc Natl Acad Sci USA* 83:9551-9555

Biswas GD, Lacks SA, Sparling PF (1989): Transformation-deficient mutants of piliated Neisseria gonorrhoeae. *J Bacteriology* 171:657-664

Brinster RL, Chen HY, Trumbauer ME, Yagle MK, Palmiter RD (1985): Factors affecting the efficiency of introducing foreign DNA into mice by microinjecting eggs. *Proc Natl Acad Sci USA* 82:4438-4442

Buttrick PM, Kass A, Kitsis RN, Kaplan ML, Leinwand LA (1992): Behavior of genes directly injected into the rat heart in vivo. *Circulation Research* 70:193-198

Capecchi MR (1980): High efficiency transformation by direct microinjection of DNA into cultured mammalian cells. *Cell* 22:479-488

Chin DJ, Green GA, Zon G, Szoka Jr FC, Straubinger RM (1990): Rapid nuclear accumulation of injected oligodeoxyribonucleotides. *The New Biologist*

2:1091-1100

Chu G, Hayakawa H, Berg P (1987): Electroporation for the efficient transfection of mammalian cells with DNA. *Nucleic Acids Res* 15:1311-1326

Concino MF, Goodgal SH (1981): Haemophilus influenzae polypeptides involved in deoxyribonucleic acid uptake detected by cellular surface protein iodination. *J Bacteriology* 148:220-231

Danner DB, Smith HO, Narang SA (1982): Construct of DNA recognition sites active in Haemophilus transformation. *Proc Natl Acad Sci USA* 79:2393-2397

de Wet JR, Wood KV, DeLuca M, Helinski DR, Subramani S (1987): Firefly luciferase gene; structure and expression in mammalian cells. *Mol Cell Biol* 7:725

Dorward DW, Garon CF, Judd RC (1989): Export and intercellular transfer of DNA via membrane blebs of Neisseria gonorrhoeae. *J Bacteriology* 171:2399-2505

Edge M (1970): Development of apposed sarcoplasmic reticulum at the T system and sarcolemma and the change in orientation of triads in rat skeletal muscle. *Dev Biol* 23:634-650

Felgner PL, Gadek TR, Holm M, Roman R, Chan HW, Wenz M, Northrop JP, Ringold GM, Danielsen M (1987): Lipofection: a highly efficient, lipid-mediated DNA-transfection procedure. *Proc Natl Acad Sci USA* 84:7413-7417

Felgner PL, Ringold GM (1989): Cationic liposome-mediated transfection. *Nature* 337:387-388

Franzini-Armstrong C (1986) The sarcoplasmic reticulum and the transverse tubules. In: *Myology.* (ed. AG Engel and BQ Banker) pp. 125-153. New York: McGraw-Hill

Horwitz AF, Schotland DL (1986): The plasma membrane of the muscle fiber. In: *Myology.* (ed. AG Engel and BQ Banker) pp. 177-207. New York: McGraw-Hill

Huxley HE (1964): Evidence for continuity between the central elements of the triads and extracellular space in frog sartorius muscle. *Nature* 202:1067-1071

Janeczko RA, Carriere RM, Etlinger JD (1985): Endocytosis, proteolysis, and exocytosis of exogenous proteins by cultured myotubes. *J Biol Chem* 260:7051-7058

Jiao S, Acsadi G, Jani A, Felgner P, Wolff JA (1992a): Persistence of plasmid DNA and expression in rat brain cells in vivo. *Exp Neuro* 115:400-413

Jiao S, Williams P, Berg RK, Hodgeman BA, Liu L, Repetto G, Wolff JA (1992b): Direct gene transfer into non-human primate myofibers in vivo. *Human Gene Therapy* 3:21-33

Jiao S, Gurevich V, Wolff JA (1993) Long-term correction of rat model of Parkinson's disease by gene therapy. *Nature* 362:450-453

Kahn ME, Maul G, Goodgal SH (1982): Possible mechanism for donor DNA binding and transport in Haemophilus. *Proc Natl Acad Sci USA* 79:6370-6374

Kaneda A, Iwai K, Uchida T (1989): Increased expression of DNA cointroduced with nuclear protein in adult rat liver. *Science* 243:375-378

Kitsis RN, Buttrick PM, McNally EM, Kaplan ML, Leinwand LA (1991) Hormonal modulation of a gene injected into rat heart in vivo. *Proc Natl Acad Sci*

USA 88:4138-4142

Lacks S, Greenberg B (1976): Single-strand breakage on binding of DNA to cells in the genetic transformation of Diplococcus pneumoniae. *J Mol Biol* 101:255-175

Lin SS, Levitan IB (1991): Concanavalin A: a tool to investigate neuronal plasticity.*Trends in Neuroscience* 14:273-277

Loke S, Stein C, Zhang X, Mori K, Nakanishi M, Subasinghe C, Cohen J (1989): Characterization of oligonucleotides transport into living cells. *Proc Natl Acad Sci USA* 86:3474-3478

Malone RW, Hickman MA, Lehmann K, Walzem R, Bassiri M, Powell JS (1993) Hepatic gene transfer following direct in vivo injection. *J Cell Biochem* 17E:239

McNeil PL (1991): Cell wounding and healing. *American Scientist* 79:222-235

McNeil PL, Ito S (1989): Gastrointestinal cell membrane wounding and resealing in vivo. *Gastroenterology* 96:1238-1248

McNeil PL, Kahkee R (1992) Disruptions of muscle fiber plasma membranes: role in exercise-induced damage. *Am J Path* 140:1097-1109

Miller AD (1990): Retrovirus packaging cells. *Hum Gene Ther* 1:5-14

Mirzayans R, Aubin RA, Paterson MC (1992): Differential expression and stability of foreign genes introduced into human fibroblasts by nuclear versus cytoplasmic microinjection. *Mutation Res* 281:115-122

Ralston E, Hall Z (1989): Transfer of protein encoded by a single nucleus to nearby nuclei in multinucleated myotubes. *Science* 244:1066-1069

Schiaffino S, Margreth A (1969): Coordinated development of the sarcoplasmic reticulum and T system during postnatal differentiation of rat skeletal muscle. *J Cell Biol* 41:855-875

Sikes ML, O'Malley Jr BW, Ledley FD (1993) In vivo gene transfer into rabbit thyroid by direct DNA injection: a novel strategy for gene therapy. *J Cell Biochem* 17E:208

Shoji Y, Akhtar S, Periasamy A, Herman B, Juliano RL (1991): Mechanism of cellular uptake of modified oligodeozynucleotides containing methylphosphonate linkages. *Nucl Acid Res* 19:5543-5550

Thorburn AM, Alberts AS (1993): Efficient expression of miniprep plasmid DNA after needle microinjection into somatic cells. *BioTechniques* 14:356-358

Wirtz P, Loermans H, Peer P, Reintjes A (1983): Postnatal growth and differentiation of muscle fibers in the mouse. I. a histochemical and morphometrical investigation of normal muscle. *J Anat* 137:109-126

Wolff JA, Ludtke JJ, Acsadi G, Williams P, Agnes J (1992a): Long-term persistence of plasmid DNA and foreign gene expression in mouse muscle. *Human Molecular Genetics* 1:363-369

Wolff JA, Dowty ME, Jiao S, Repetto G, Berg RK, Ludtke JJ, Williams P (1992b): Expression of naked plasmids by cultured myotubes and entry of plasmids into T tubules and caveolae of mammalian skeletal muscle. *J Cell Sci* 103:1249-1259

Wolff JA, Malone RW, Williams P, Chong W, Acsadi G, Jani A, Felgner PL (1990): Direct gene transfer into mouse muscle in vivo. *Science* 247:1465-1468

Wolff JA, Williams P, Acsadi G, Jiao S, Jani A, Wang C (1991): Conditions affecting direct gene transfer into rodent muscle in vivo. *BioTechniques* 11:474-485

Wu GY, Wu CH (1988): Receptor-mediated gene delivery and expression in vivo. *J Biol Chem* 263:14621-14624

Wu-Pong S, Weiss TL, Hunt CA (1992): Antisense c-myc oligodeoxyribo-nucleotide cellular uptake. *Pharm Res* 9:1010-1017

Yakubov L, Deeva E, Zarytova V, Ivanova E, Ryte A, Yurchenko L, Vlassov V (1989): Mechanism of oligonucleotides uptake by cells: involvement of specific receptors. *Proc Natl Acad Sci USA* 86:6454-6458

Yang NS, Burkholder J, Roberts B, Martinell B, McCabe D (1990): In vivo and in vitro gene transfer to mammalian somatic cells by particle bombardment. *Proc Natl Acad Sci USA* 87:9568-9572

RECEPTOR-MEDIATED GENE DELIVERY EMPLOYING ADENOVIRUS-POLYLYSINE-DNA COMPLEXES

David T. Curiel

GENE DELIVERY VIA THE RECEPTOR-MEDIATED PATHWAY

Gene transfer to eucaryotic cells may be accomplished by capitalizing on endogenous cellular pathways of macromolecular transport. In this regard, gene transfer has been accomplished via the receptor-mediated endocytosis pathway employing molecular conjugate vectors (Wu and Wu, 1987; Wu et al., 1989; Wagner et al., 1990; Wagner et al., 1991b; Cotten et al., 1990; Curiel et al., 1992a; Huckett et al., 1990; Rosenkranz et al., 1992). The molecular conjugate is a synthetic bifunctional agent employed to serve two functions: binding of the heterologous DNA to form a conjugate-DNA complex, and attachment of the conjugate-DNA complex to the target cell to facilitate internalization. The initial step of binding the heterologous DNA to form a conjugate-DNA complex is mediated through a domain of the conjugate comprised by a polycation amine, such as polylysine. This electrostatic interaction between the negatively charged DNA and the positively charged DNA-binding domain serves not only to bind the DNA, but also to condense it into a compact toroid structure (Wagner et al., 1991a). As the ligand is covalently linked to the polylysine DNA-binding domain, after binding of the DNA, at least a portion of the ligand is presented on the surface of the complex, free to interact with its cognate receptor. The attachment of the conjugate-DNA complex to the target cell is then mediated through the specificity of the ligand domain for its corresponding receptor. Thus, after the conjugate-DNA complex accomplishes attachment, it is internalized through the corresponding cellular transport pathway.

There are several potential advantages deriving from this strategy of gene delivery. Many cellular internalization pathways are highly efficient. For example, the transport protein transferrin may be internalized in selected cell populations at rates on the order of thousands of molecules per second (Testa, 1985; Newman et al., 1982). Thus, this methodology possesses the capacity to achieve highly efficient gene delivery. In addition, as the DNA entry occurs via a physiologic internalization pathway, vector-associated toxicity consequent to membrane perturbation is circumvented. This minimization of toxicity thus offers the poten-

Gene Therapeutics: Methods and Applications of Direct Gene Transfer
Jon A. Wolff, Editor • ©1994 *Birkhäuser Boston*

tial to deliver the DNA on a continuous or repetitive basis (Zenke et al., 1990). The design of the conjugate also provides the basis to achieve cell-specific delivery of nucleic acids. Since delivery is dictated by the specificity of the ligand for its receptor, it should be possible to design a vector specifically targetable through a receptor of interest.

Various strategies to accomplish receptor-mediated gene delivery have been developed (Wu and Wu, 1987; Wu et al., 1989; Wagner et al., 1990; Wagner et al., 1991b; Cotten et al., 1990; Curiel et al., 1992a; Huckett et al., 1990; Rosenkranz et al., 1992). Targeting of cells of hepatocyte derivation has been shown in both in vitro and in vivo contexts (Wu and Wu, 1987; Wu et al., 1989; Plank et al., 1992; Wu and Wu, 1988). These studies have capitalized on the unique localization of the asialoglycoprotein receptor on hepatocytes to allow conjugate internalization by this route. In this regard, Wu et al. have convincingly shown cell-specific delivery through the asialoglycoprotein receptor in vitro. In addition, asialoglycoprotein-polylysine-DNA complexes delivered systemically have been shown to achieve delivery to hepatocytes in vivo (Wu et al., 1989; Wu and Wu, 1988; Wu et al., 1991; Wilson et al., 1992b; Wilson et al., 1992a). Gene transfer has also been documented via the transferrin pathway (Figure 1) (Zatloukal et al., 1992; Zenke et al., 1990; Cotten et al., 1990; Cotten et al., 1991; Zatloukal et al., 1992; Wagner et al., 1991b; Curiel et al., 1992a). Transferrin-polylysine conjugates were shown by Birnstiel et al. to mediate in vitro delivery to a variety of cell lines. Strategies to target specific airway epithelial subsets have also been proposed utilizing internalization pathways for polymerized IgA (Ferkol et al., 1992) and surfactant protein C (Baatz et al., 1992). Thus, extensive work has demonstrated the potential application of gene delivery by the receptor-mediated endocytosis pathway to accomplish in vitro and in vivo gene delivery.

Despite these many potential advantages, in practice, the realization of strategies to accomplish gene delivery by the receptor-mediated pathway has been limited. This has largely been a consequence of the fact that effective gene transfer by this route is often idiosyncratic, despite the presence of an appropriate receptor on the target cell. Thus, target cells known to be characterized by the presence of a specific internalization pathway may nonetheless show limited, or absent, gene transfer by this pathway using molecular conjugate vectors. This observation reflects the fact that the conjugate-DNA complex lacks a specific mechanism to escape the cell vesicle system once internalized by the receptor-mediated pathway. Thus, endosome internalized DNA may be largely targeted for lysosomal pathways eventuating in destruction of the delivered material. This concept has been corroborated in studies that show that selected lysosomotropic substances can enhance overall gene transfer efficiency, presumably by mitigating lysosomal destruction of conjugate-delivered DNA (Cotten et al., 1990). Thus, despite the fact that molecular conjugate vectors possess the means to achieve high efficiency cellular delivery through endogenous internalization pathways, the fact that they lack a specific mechanism to allow escape of the internalized DNA from the cell vesicle system severely limits their overall utility.

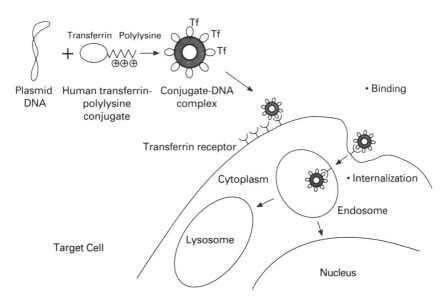

FIGURE 1. Gene transfer via the receptor-mediated endocytosis pathway. A bifunctional molecular conjugate is employed to bind DNA and transport it via cellular macromolecular transport mechanisms. The conjugate consists of a DNA-binding domain, comprised by a cationic polylysine moiety, which is covalently linked to a ligand for a cell surface receptor, in this case transferrin. Plasmid DNA bound to the polylysine moiety of the conjugate undergoes marked condensation to yield an 80- to 100-nm toroid with surface localized transferrin molecules. When the transferrin ligand domain is bound by its corresponding cell surface receptor, the conjugate is internalized by the receptor-mediated endocytosis pathway, co-transporting bound DNA. Escape from the cell vesicle system is achieved by a fraction of the internalized conjugate-DNA complex to achieve nuclear localization where heterologous gene expression is effected.

ADENOVIRUS-FACILIATED GENE DELIVERY VIA THE RECEPTOR-MEDIATED PATHWAY

With the recognition that gene transfer via the receptor-mediated endocytosis pathway was limited due to endosome entrapment of the conjugate-DNA complex, it was hypothesized that maneuvers to facilitate exit of the delivered DNA from the cell vesicle system might overcome this limitation. In this regard, a variety of viruses are known to enter cells via the receptor-mediated pathway. Unlike conjugate vectors, however, many of these viral agents possess specific mechanisms to accomplish cell vesicle escape after entry, thereby allowing an infectious cycle to be completed in the target cell cytoplasm or nucleus. One virus with a well-characterized receptor-mediated entry mechanism is the adenovirus [(Pastan et al., 1986), Figure 2]. The adenovirus is a double-strand DNA virus with a naked protein capsid (Philipson, 1983). The entry pathway of the adenovirus involves an initial

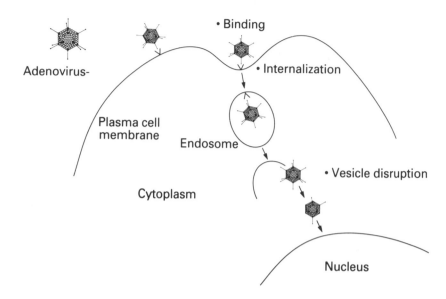

FIGURE 2. Pathway of adenoviral entry. Adenoviral attachment to target cells is accomplished by binding of the adenoviral fiber protein to an uncharacterized membrane surface receptor. Specific internalization of the receptor-bound virion is via the receptor-mediated endocytosis pathway. After internalization, the adenovirus is localized within the endocytotic vesicles. Endosome acidification induces hydrophobic alterations in the capsid proteins, allowing interaction with the vesicle membranes. This interaction results in vesicle disruption. The virion thereby achieves escape from the cell vesicle system and localizes to the nucleus, where viral DNA is translocated, likely through target cell nuclear pores.

binding to an uncharacterized cell surface receptor followed by cellular internalization; initially in clathrin-coated pits and then within cellular endosomes. Acidification of the endosome allows the virus to disrupt the cell vesicle to achieve escape to the cell cytoplasm. After ingress into the cytoplasm, the virus localizes to the host nucleus in order to translocate its DNA. Thus, the entry pathway of adenovirus is analogous to that of the conjugate vector in certain respects. Like the molecular conjugate vector, the adenovirus has an efficient internalization mechanism via a cellular internalization pathway. Unlike the molecular conjugate vector, however, after entry the adenovirus possesses a specific mechanism to achieve escape from the cell vesicle system and thus avoid lysosomal degradation.

Several lines of evidence suggested the feasibility of exploiting the entry mechanism of adenovirus to facilitate conjugate-mediated gene delivery. First, early work by Carrasco et al. showed that a variety of viruses could facilitate cellular uptake of macromolecules (Fernandez-Puentes and Carrasco, 1980). These studies did not discriminate between facilitation by receptor-mediated and other pathways, or delineate the mechanistic basis for the effect; however, this work did establish the concept that viral entry could be linked to the entry of other macro-

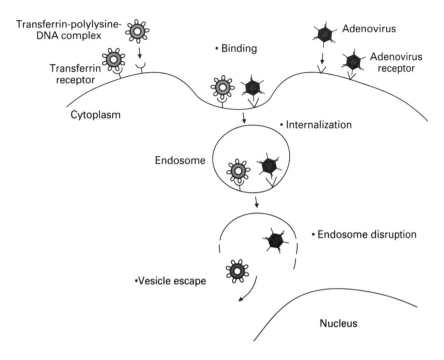

FIGURE 3. Mechanism of adenoviral facilitation of molecular conjugate-mediated gene transfer. After binding to their respective cell surface receptors, cointernalization of the transferrin-polylysine conjugate and the adenovirus is within the same endocytotic vesicle. Adenovirus-mediated endosome disruption allows vesicle escape for both the virion and the conjugate-DNA complex.

molecules. Later work by Pastan et al. showed that adenoviruses could specifically facilitate entry of macromolecules through the receptor-mediated pathway (FitzGerald et al., 1983). These studies established that heterogeneous receptor-bound ligands could be co-internalized within the same endosome and that co-delivery of adenovirus could facilitate the cytoplasmic delivery of the ligands. On the basis of these studies, it was demonstrated that adenovirus could dramatically facilitate the efficacy of protein conjugate cytotoxins delivered by the receptor mediated pathway. This effect derived specifically from the ability of the adenovirus to disrupt cellular endosomes and thus allow ingress of the conjugates into the target cell cytosol.

To test the hypothesis that adenovirus-mediated vesicle disruption could facilitate DNA delivery by molecular conjugate vectors, we co-delivered transferrin-polylysine-DNA complexes in combination with adenovirus to HeLa cells (Figure 3). This cell line possesses cellular receptors for both transferrin and adenovirus. The delivery of increasing amounts of adenovirus resulted in a dose-dependent augmentation of conjugate-mediated gene transfer (Figure 4). Peak

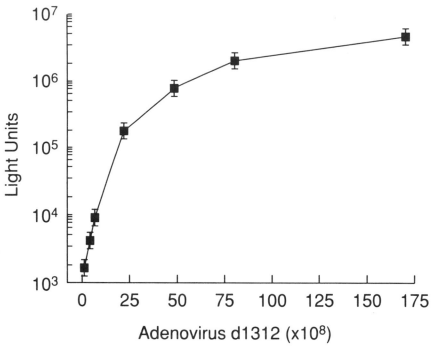

FIGURE 4. Effect of adenoviral infection on gene transfer by transferrin-polylysine conjugates. For complex formation 6 μg of luciferase-encoding plasmid DNA (pRSVL) was
mixed with 12 μg of human transferrin-polylysine conjugate (hTfpL). Conjugate-DNA
complex plus variable amounts of the replication-defective adenovirus dl312 (0.05 - 3.2 x
10^4 viral particles per cell) were added to HeLa cells. Cell lysates were standardized for
total protein content and analyzed for luciferase enzyme activity. Results are expressed as
"light units" per 50 μg of total cellular protein. Data are the mean of two to four separate
experiments; error bars represent SEM.

levels of heterologous gene expression achieved with the adenovirus augmentation were at least three orders of magnitude greater than levels achieved with transferrin-polylysine conjugates alone (Curiel et al., 1991). In this analysis, it was
observed that the amount of adenovirus required to achieve these peak levels of
augmented gene expression corresponded to the number of receptors for adenovirus on the target cell (Svensson, 1985; Defer et al., 1990). This is consistent with
the concept that the observed effect of the adenovirus is mediated through receptor
binding as a limiting factor of its augmentation capacity. To determine the specific
mechanism whereby the adenovirus augmented conjugate-mediated gene transfer,
experiments were repeated utilizing virus that had been heat-inactivated. This
treatment ablates the capacity of the virus to mediate vesicle disruption without
perturbing the structural integrity of the viral gene elements (Defer et al., 1990).
Heat treatment resulted in the complete abrogation of the virus's ability to facilitate conjugate-mediated gene transfer (data not shown). This finding establishes

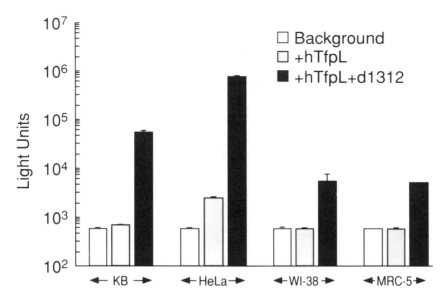

FIGURE 5. Effect of adenoviral infection on gene transfer by transferrin-polylysine conjugates in selected cell lines. Conjugate-DNA complexes (6 μg of pRSVL plus 12 μg of hTfpL) were added to KB, HeLa, WI-38, and MRC-5 cells with or without adenovirus dl312 (1.0 x 10⁴ viral particles per cell).

that it is the capacity of the virus to mediate endosome disruption that is specifically responsible for its observed effect on augmenting molecular conjugate vector-mediated gene transfer. This is also consistent with the concept that it is the lack of an endosome escape mechanism that is the principal factor limiting the gene transfer efficiency of molecular conjugate vectors.

The capacity of the adenovirus to disrupt the cell vesicle overcomes the principal factor limiting the overall efficiency of conjugate vectors. This is observed not only in terms of net levels of gene expression achieved but also in terms of transduction frequency. Transduction of HeLa cells with transferrin-polylysine conjugates utilizing a ß-galactosidase reporter gene achieves transduction of less than 1% of the target cells. With the addition of adenovirus as a facilitator, the percent transduction achieved is greater than 90% (data not shown). The ability of adenovirus to augment molecular conjugate-mediated gene transfer may be observed for a variety of immortalized and primary cells in vitro (Figure 5). It can be seen that for a variety of cellular targets putatively showing very limited or absent susceptibility to transferrin-polylysine, appreciable levels of heterologous gene expression can be achieved when adenovirus is employed to facilitate cellular entry. In those instances where the cells appeared refractory to transferrin-polylysine-mediated gene transfer without adenovirus facilitation, it is clear that the requisite receptors were present and conjugate internalization achieved; however

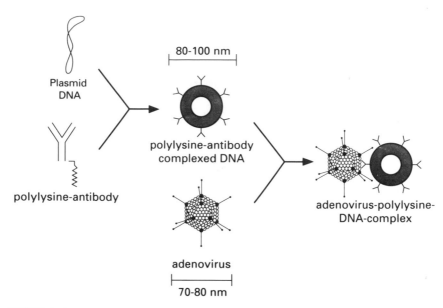

FIGURE 6. Schematic of approach to derive adenovirus-polylysine-DNA complexes containing heterologous DNA attached to exterior of adenovirus capsid. To accomplish linkage of an adenoviral cognate domain and a polycationic DNA-binding domain, the chimeric adenovirus P202-Ad5 containing a heterologous epitope in the exterior domain of its hexon protein was employed in conjunction with a monoclonal antibody specific for this epitope. Control experiments demonstrated that attachment of the monoclonal antibody was non-neutralizing for adenovirus P202-Ad5. The monoclonal antibody was rendered competent to carry foreign DNA sequences by attaching a polylysine moiety. Interaction of the polylysine-antibody complexed DNA with adenovirus P202-Ad5 occurs via the specificity of the conjugated antibody.

processing of the internalized conjugate-DNA complex via degradative pathways was more complete. Thus, the employment of adenovirus to provide endosome disruption capacity expands the range of applications of molecular conjugate-mediated gene transfer.

ADENOVIRUS-COMPONENT MOLECULAR CONJUGATE VECTORS

As conjugate efficacy is limited by the lack of an endosome escape mechanism, it was hypothesized that the incorporation of such a mechanism into the conjugate design could overcome this limitation, with a favorable outcome on overall gene transfer efficacy (Curiel et al., 1992b; Wagner et al., 1992). Since adenovirus can provide endosome disruption function, a strategy to incorporate the adenovirus into conjugate design was derived (Figure 6). In developing a means to link the virus to the conjugate structure, consideration was given to the fact that attach-

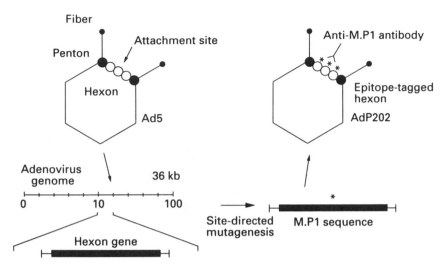

FIGURE 7. Construction of chimeric adenovirus containing heterologous epitope in surface region of hexon capsid protein. Since the adenoviral capsid proteins fiber and penton are important mediators of the adenoviral entry mechanism, attachment of capsid-bound DNA was targeted to the hexon protein. A specific attachment site for an immunologic linkage was created by introducing a heterologous epitope into the surface region of the hexon protein by site-directed mutagenesis of the corresponding region of the adenoviral hexon gene. The introduced foreign epitope is a portion of Mycoplasma pneumoniae P1 protein.

ment via the viral capsid proteins might perturb the same viral functions that were being exploited. In this regard, the adenovirus binds to target cells by virtue of its fiber protein, and accomplishes cell vesicle disruption by means of capsid proteins in the peri-pentonal region (Pastan et al., 1986; Seth et al., 1984; Seth et al., 1985). Both of these functions are important to the adenoviral entry capacity. In contrast, the major capsid protein, hexon, is less important in this regard. Thus, it was deemed desirable to link polylysine-condensed DNA to the exterior aspect of the adenoviral hexon protein. To achieve this, a heterologous epitope was introduced into the surface region of the hexon capsid protein by site-directed mutagenesis of the adenoviral hexon gene. Utilizing a monoclonal antibody against this epitope, a method of linkage to the exterior of the virus could be derived whereby no perturbation of capsid proteins involved in cellular entry occurred (Figure 7). In this schema, conjugating the polylysine to the monoclonal antibody allows DNA binding directly to the exterior of the virus with the interposition of the antibody to provide the linkage. To test the feasibility of this approach, adenovirus-polylysine-DNA complexes were derived by serial addition of the epitope-tagged virus, the antibody-polylysine, and reporter plasmid DNA. It could be demonstrated that all of these specific components were required to allow effective gene transfer (Figure 8). The various control studies emphasize the crucial nature of the linkage

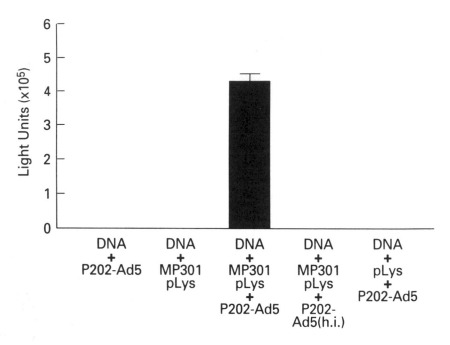

FIGURE 8. Gene transfer mediated by adenovirus-polylysine-DNA complexes. Various combinations of specific and nonspecific complex components were combined and evaluated for the capacity to mediate gene transfer to HeLa cells. DNA is the reporter plasmid pRSVL. The specific virus P202-Ad5 contains an epitope recognized by the polylysine monoclonal antibody MP301pL. This was employed as viable virus or heat-inactivated (h.i.). Non-antibody-conjugated polylysine (pL) was also evaluated.

between the DNA and the virus. Thus, by including an endosome escape mechanism within the conjugate design, it was possible to overcome cell vesicle entrapment. The resulting molecular conjugate vector thus possessed the capacity to accomplish high efficiency gene transfer.

The adenovirus-polylysine-DNA complexes contain specific mechanisms to accomplish cellular internalization and escape from entrapment in the cell vesicle system. By virtue of cellular entry via the receptor-mediated pathway, the adenovirus-polylysine-DNA complexes possess the advantages described for molecular conjugate vectors. The inclusion of the capacity to achieve endosome disruption confers the additional property of high efficiency gene delivery. To determine the level of efficiency of gene delivery, serial dilutions of the complexes were delivered to HeLa cells. It could be seen that as few as 10 DNA molecules delivered per cell resulted in detectable levels of reporter gene expression (data not shown). This compares favorably to the requirement of approximately 500,000 DNA molecules per cell required for reporter gene expression employing other DNA-mediated gene transfer techniques. Peak levels of heterologous gene expression achieved by adenovirus-polylysine-DNA complexes were several orders of magnitude higher than peak levels observed when free adenovirus was used to facilitate transferrin-polylysine-mediated gene transfer. This difference likely reflects the fact that in the linked configuration the adenovirus provides additional functions facilitating gene transfer besides its ability to disrupt the endosome. In this regard, morphometric analysis of adenovirus entry has shown that the capsid retains its overall integrity at the level of the nuclear membrane of the target cell (Chardonnet and Dales, 1970). The adenovirus in the adenovirus-polylysine-DNA configuration could thus possess the capacity to transport the heterologous DNA to this region of the cell. In contrast, free virus can only facilitate transferrin-polylysine conjugate ingress into the target cell cytosol. After localization in the cytoplasm the transferrin-polylysine conjugate does not possess a specific mechanism to facilitate transport to the nucleus. This observation has important consequences with regard to strategies to utilize subparticles of the virus in the conjugate design. Capsid components mediating only endosomolysis will thus not provide all of the functions of the intact virus necessary to benefit overall gene transfer efficiency. In this regard, the use of synthetic fusogenic peptides to provide endosome disruption capacity to molecular conjugates has not allowed the same high efficiency gene transfer characteristics as noted with the adenovirus-polylysine-DNA complexes (Plank et al., 1992). It is thus clear that it is both the endosome disruption capacity and the nuclear localization characteristics of the adenovirus that contribute to its facilitation of gene delivery in the adenovirus-polylysine configuration.

The transport of heterologous DNA in the configuration of adenovirus-polylysine-DNA complexes is within the conceptual framework of recombinant virion-mediated gene transfer. The transport of heterologous DNA via recombinant virions has heretofore involved integration of the foreign DNA into the genome of the virion. In this fashion, this strategy capitalizes on the efficient mechanisms of delivery of the viral genome to target cells. However, this strategy suffers from several disadvantages. The size of the foreign DNA that can be transported is limited by packaging constraints of the virus. In addition, because the heterologous DNA is expressed in the context of viral gene elements, the possibility of cis-acting effects deriving from the viral gene elements may confound efforts to achieve specific regulation by heterologous promoter elements. Over and above these practical constraints, the obligatory co-delivery of viral gene elements presents potential safety hazards. The carrying of DNA on the exterior of the virion represents a radical conceptual departure from these recombinant virion strategies. Because DNA is carried on the exterior of the virion, the size that can be transported is not limited by packaging constraints of the virus. As the polylysine DNA-binding domain of the conjugate interacts with nucleic acids in a sequence-independent manner, DNA of any design may be incorporated into the complexes. Thus, cis-acting interactions with viral genes are obviated. Of more fundamental importance, this strategy exploits viral entry features in a selective manner. Since for the adenovirus the entry properties derive from capsid proteins (Pastan et al., 1986), the integrity of viral genes is not an essential feature. In fact, steps may be

FIGURE 9. Effect of replication capacity on ability of adenovirus to function as an endosomolysis agent. Adenovirus-polylysine-DNA complexes were formed as before containing epitope-marked adenovirus that was replication-competent (P202) or replication-incompetent (P259A). The adenovirus strain P259A is derived from P202 by completely deleting the E1A/E1B gene regions. The deletion of these gene regions renders the adenovirus replication-incompetent. Complexes were delivered to HeLa cells and reporter gene expression assayed as before.

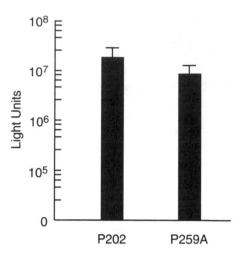

taken to inactivate the viral genes without impairing the capacity of the adenovirus moiety to facilitate the entry of the complexes (Figure 9) (Cotten et al., 1992). Thus, by the simple expedient of transporting DNA on the viral exterior rather than integrated into the virion's genome, important benefits accrue.

ADENOVIRUS-COMPONENT MOLECULAR CONJUGATE VECTORS CONTAINING AN ALTERNATE LIGAND DOMAIN

In the adenovirus-polylysine configuration, the adenovirus functions not only as an endosomolysis agent but also as the ligand domain of the conjugate. Thus, the susceptibility of cellular targets to this vector would be expected to reflect the range of tropism of the virus. When a variety of cellular targets were examined, this was found to be the case; cell types characterized by a high number of adenoviral receptors were highly susceptible to the adenovirus-polylysine complexes, whereas cell types characterized by a low number of the receptors were much less transducible by this vector (Figure 10). Since the adenovirus was incorporated for the specific purpose of accomplishing cell vesicle escape, we wondered whether the virus could accomplish this in the context of an alternate ligand. To derive combination complexes that contained distinct endosomolysis and ligand domains, sequential addition of adenovirus and antibody polylysine was followed by plasmid DNA plus a secondary ligand-polylysine, in this case transferrin-polylysine (Figure 11). These complexes were delivered to HeLa cells, which possess receptors for both adenovirus and transferrin. It could be shown that the "combination complexes" carried out a significantly augmented level of gene transfer compared to the transferrin-polylysine or the adenovirus-polylysine complexes (Figure 12). As this level of gene transfer exceeded any possible additive effect of transferrin-polylysine and adenovirus-polylysine complexes, it suggested some element of cooperativity. This result implied that the combination complexes could internal-

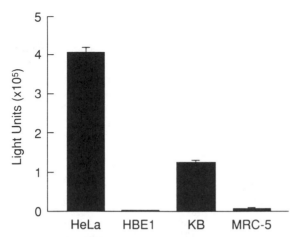

FIGURE 10. Gene transfer to various cell lines mediated by adenoviral-polylysine-DNA complexes. Complexes were evaluated for the capacity to mediate gene transfer to cell lines with a high number of adenovirus cell surface receptors (HeLa and KB) or a low number of such receptors (HBE1 and MRC-5).

ize by either of two entry pathways. Furthermore, entry by either pathway was associated with adenoviral-mediated endosomolysis facilitating gene delivery. Thus, it appeared that the virus did not need to bind to its native receptor in order to mediate the subsequent steps of viral entry, including vesicle disruption. To prove this concept, we delivered the combination complexes to a cell line that was

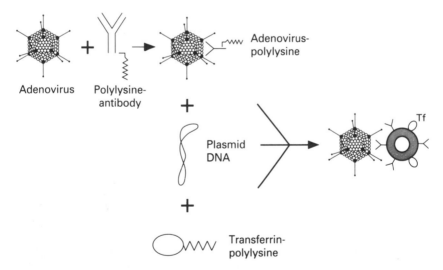

FIGURE 11. Strategy for the employment of chimeric conjugates containing adenovirus and transferrin. Complexes were derived that contain transferrin as the ligand domain and adenovirus as an endosomolysis domain. These chimeric complexes possess the potential to enter cells via the transferrin or adenovirus pathway. In the former instance, after entry via the transferrin pathway the adenovirus would function exclusively in the capacity of an endosomolysis agent. Such conjugates thus possess both specific internalization and endosome escape mechanisms.

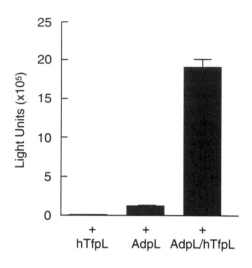

FIGURE 12. Gene transfer mediated by chimeric conjugates. Reporter gene expression mediated by human transferrin-polylysine conjugates (hTfpL) and adenoviral-polylysine-DNA complexes (AdpL) was compared to gene transfer mediated by chimeric conjugates containing human transferrin and adenovirus ligands in HeLa cells. The chimeric conjugates were formed by combination of epitope-tagged adenovirus P202-Ad5 (0.25×10^{11} particles) plus monoclonal antibody polylysine MP301pL (2 μg). Reporter plasmid DNA pRSVL (6 μg) was added to the resulting adenovirus polylysine to form adenoviral-polylysine-DNA complexes. Complete condensation of the DNA was achieved by addition of human transferrin polylysine conjugate hTfpL (9 μg). The resulting complexes were added to HeLa cells and evaluation of reporter gene expression accomplished as before.

not susceptible to adenovirus-polylysine complexes, as it lacked adenoviral receptors. This cell line was nonetheless highly susceptible to transduction utilizing combination complexes, thereby establishing that adenovirus could function exclusively in the capacity of an endosomolysis agent (Figure 13). Furthermore, these results established that, within the context of the adenoviral entry pathway, virion binding and viral-mediated vesicle disruption are not functionally linked.

FIGURE 13. Gene transfer to various cell lines mediated by ternary conjugates. The ternary conjugates containing adenovirus and human transferrin (AdpL/hTfpL) were delivered to a cell line possessing receptors for both conjugate ligands (HeLa) and a cell line possessing receptors uniquely for the transferrin ligand (HBE1). The HBE1 cell line was shown to lack susceptibility to gene transfer by adenovirus-polylysine-DNA complexes (AdpL) in FIGURE 10 based on a paucity of adenoviral receptors.

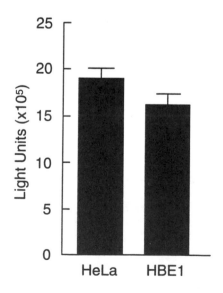

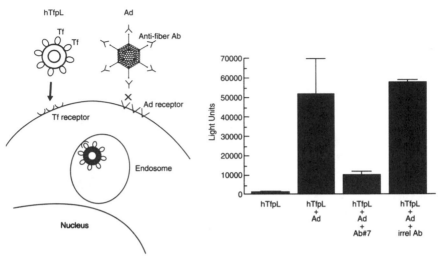

FIGURE 14. Effect of anti-fiber antibody on ability of free adenovirus to facilitate molecular conjugate-mediated gene transfer. Cells were treated with human transferrin-polylysine-DNA complexes plus free adenovirus dβ12. Adenovirus was used to facilitate gene transfer through its ability to disrupt cellular endosomes, thus allowing conjugate-DNA-complex ingress into the target cell cytosol. The adenovirus had been pretreated with either an antifiber antibody (αfiberAb#7) or an irrelevant antibody (PY203). Cell lysates were evaluated for reporter gene expression as before.

The derivation of combination complexes possessing separate domains mediating binding and vesicle disruption suggests the possibility of deriving conjugates with independent functional units acting in a concerted manner to effect gene delivery.

Whereas the adenovirus moiety can function as an endosomolysis agent in the context of an alternate ligand, in the combination complex configuration it could also function as a competitor ligand. Thus, the potential to achieve cell-specific targeting would potentially be undermined. This is especially relevant as adenoviral receptors are rather ubiquitously expressed. Since it was established that adenoviral binding and endosomolysis are not functionally linked, we wondered whether we could block adenoviral binding while retaining the adenovirus-mediated endosome disruption capacity as a functional component of the complex. To accomplish blockade of adenoviral binding to its receptor, monoclonal antibody was prepared to purified adenoviral fiber protein. Antifiber antibodies possessing the capacity to block viral entry were thus derived. It could be shown that the antibody could effectively block the ability of free adenovirus to facilitate transferrin-polylysine conjugate-mediated gene transfer, confirming that blockade of viral entry ablated any possible vesicle disruption (Figure 14). When the antibody was then applied to combination complexes, there was no appreciable effect on overall gene transfer efficiency (Figure 15). Since the entry via the viral pathway was effectively blocked by this maneuver, the non-binding virus was nonetheless able

D. T. Curiel

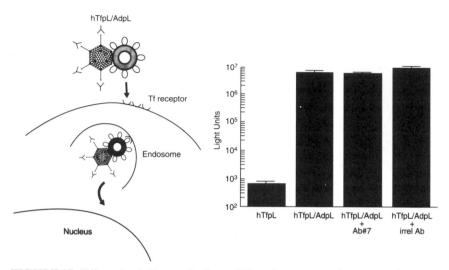

FIGURE 15. Effect of anti-fiber antibody on ability of ternary complexes to mediate gene transfer. Ternary complexes were prepared containing human transferrin and adenovirus (hTfpL/AdpL) as before. The incorporated adenovirus had been pre-treated with either an anti-fiber antibody (αfiberAb#7) or an irrelevant antibody (PY203). Cell lysates were evaluated for reporter gene expression as before.

to accomplish cell vesicle disruption. The incorporation of the non-binding virions into the linked configuration of the combination complexes allowed the retention of high level gene transfer deriving from effective cell vesicle disruption, but without the potentially confounding variable of the adenovirus functioning as a competitor ligand. This employment of the adenovirus exploits not only its entry feature for conjugate facilitation, but, by ablation of adenoviral binding, exploits only a selective aspect of the entry pathway.

ACKNOWLEDGEMENTS

The author would like to acknowledge his collaborators Ping-chuan Hu at the University of North Carolina at Chapel Hill and Ernst Wagner and Matt Cotten at the Research Institute for Molecular Pathology in Vienna, Austria.

REFERENCES

Baatz JF, Ciraolo P, Bruno M, Glasser S, Stripp B, Korfhagen TR (1992): Utilization of modified surfactant-associated protein B for delivery of DNA to airway cells in culture. *Pediatr Pulmonol Suppl* 8:263

Chardonnet, Dales S (1970): Early events in the interaction of adenoviruses with HeLa cells. 1. Penetration of Type 5 and intracellular release of the DNA genome. *Virology* 40:462-477

Cotten M, Langle-Rouault F, Kirlappos H, Wagner E, Mechtler K, Zenke M, Beug H, Birnstiel ML (1990): Transferrin-polycation-mediated introduction of DNA into human leukemic cells: Stimulation by agents that affect the survival of transfected DNA or modulate transferrin receptor levels. *Proc Natl Acad Sci USA* 87:4033-4037

Cotten M, Wagner E, Birnstiel ML (1991): Receptor mediated transport of DNA into eukaryotic cells. *Methods Enzymol* (In Press)

Cotten M, Wagner E, Zatloukal K, Phillips S, Curiel DT, Birnstiel ML (1992): High-efficiency receptor-mediated delivery of small and large (48 kilobase) gene constructs using the endosome-disruption activity of defective or chemically inactivated adenovirus particles. *Proc Natl Acad Sci USA* 89:6094-6098

Curiel DT, Agarwal S, Wagner E, Cotten M (1991): Adenovirus enhancement of transferrin-polylysine-mediated gene delivery. *Proc Natl Acad Sci USA* 88:8850-8854

Curiel DT, Agarwal S, Romer N, Wagner E, Cotten M, Birnstiel ML, Boucher RC (1992a): Gene transfer to respiratory epithelial cells via the receptor-mediated endocytosis pathway. *Am J Respir Cell Mol Biol* 6:247-252

Curiel DT, Wagner E, Cotten M, Birnstiel ML, Li C-m, Loechel S, Agarwal S, Hu P-C (1992b): High efficiency gene transfer mediated by adenovirus coupled to DNA-polylysine complexes. *Hum Gene Ther* 3:147-154

Defer C, Belin M-T, Caillet-Boudin M-L, Boulanger P (1990): Human adenovirus-host cell interactions: Comparative study with members of subgroups B and C. *J. Virol* 64:3661-3673

Ferkol T, Davis P, Kaetzel C, Hanson R (1992): Targeted gene delivery to respiratory epithelial cells. *Pediatr Pulmonol* (Abstract)

Fernandez-Puentes C, Carrasco L (1980): Viral infection permeabilizes mammalian cells to protein toxins. *Cell* 20:769-775

FitzGerald DJP, Padmanabhan R, Pastan I, Willingham MC (1983): Adenovirus-induced release of epidermal growth factor and Pseudomonas toxin into the cytosol of KB cells during receptor-mediated endocytosis. *Cell* 32:607-617

Huckett B, Ariatti M, Hawtrey AO (1990): Evidence for targeted gene transfer by receptor-mediated endocytosis. *Biochem Pharmacol* 40:253-263

Newman R, Schneider C, Sutherland R, Vodinelich L, Greaves M (1982): The transferrin receptor. *Trends Biochem Sci* 7:397-400

Pastan I, Seth P, FitzGerald D, Willingham M (1986): Adenovirus entry into cells: Some new observations on an old problem. In: *Virus attachment and entry into cells.* edited by R.L. Crowell, K. Lonberg-Holm. Washington, DC, American Society for Microbiology, pp. 141-146

Philipson L (1983): Structure and assembly of adenoviruses. *Curr Top Microbiol Immunol* 109:2-52

Plank C, Zatloukal K, Cotten M, Mechtler K, Wagner E (1992): Gene transfer into hepatocytes using asialoglycoprotein receptor mediated endocytosis of DNA complexed with an artificial tetra-antennary galactose ligand. *Bioconjugate Chem* (In Press)

Rosenkranz AA, Yachmenev SV, Jans DA, Serebryakova NV, Murav'ev VI, Peters R, Sobolev AS (1992): Receptor-mediated endocytosis and nuclear transport of a transfecting DNA construct. *Exp Cell Res* 199:323-329

Seth P, FitzGerald D, Ginsberg H, Willingham M, Pastan I (1984): Evidence that the penton base of adenovirus is involved in potentiation of toxicity of Pseudomonas exotoxin conjugated to epidermal growth factor. *Mol Cell Biol* 4:1528-1533

Seth P, Willingham MC, Pastan I (1985): Binding of adenovirus and its external proteins to Triton X-114. Dependence on pH. *J Biol Chem* 260:14431-14434

Svensson U (1985): Role of vesicles during adenovirus 2 internalization into HeLa cells. *J Virol* 55:442-449

Testa U (1985): Transferrin receptors: Structure and function. *Curr Top Hematol* 5:127-161

Wagner E, Zenke M, Cotten M, Beug H, Birnstiel ML (1990): Transferrin-polycation conjugates as carriers for DNA uptake into cells. *Proc Natl Acad Sci USA* 87:3410-3414

Wagner E, Cotten M, Foisner R, Birnstiel ML (1991a): Transferrin-polycation-DNA complexes: The effect of polycations on the structure of the complex and DNA delivery to cells. *Proc Natl Acad Sci USA* 88:4255-4259

Wagner E, Cotten M, Mechtler K, Kirlappos H, Birnstiel ML (1991b): DNA-binding transferrin conjugates as functional gene delivery agents: synthesis by linkage of polylysine or ethidium homodimer to the transferrin carbohydrate moiety. *Bioconjugate Chem* 2:226-231

Wagner E, Zatloukal K, Cotten M, Kirlappos H, Mechtler K, Curiel DT, Birnstiel ML (1992): Coupling of adenovirus to transferrin-polylysine/DNA complexes greatly enhances receptor-mediated gene delivery and expression of transfected genes. *Proc Natl Acad Sci USA* 89:6099-6103

Wilson JM, Grossman M, Cabrera JA, Wu CH, Wu GY (1992a): A novel mechanism for achieving transgene persistence in vivo after somatic gene transfer into hepatocytes. *J Biol Chem* 267:11483-11489

Wilson JM, Grossman M, Wu CH, Chowdhury NR, Wu GY, Chowdhury JR (1992b): Hepatocyte-directed gene transfer in vivo leads to transient improvement of hypercholesterolemia in low density lipoprotein receptor-deficient rabbits. *J Biol Chem* 267:963-967

Wu C, Wilson J, Wu G (1989): Targeting genes: delivery and persistent expression of a foreign gene driven by mammalian regulatory elements in vivo. *J Biol Chem* 264:16985-16987

Wu GY, Wilson JM, Shalaby F, Grossman M, Shafritz DA, Wu CH (1991): Receptor-mediated gene delivery in vivo. Partial correction of genetic analbuminemia in nagase rats. *J Biol Chem* 266:14338-14342

Wu GY, Wu CH (1987): Receptor-mediated in vitro gene transformation by a soluble DNA carrier system. *J Biol Chem* 262:4429-4432

Wu GY, Wu CH (1988): Receptor-mediated gene delivery and expression in vivo. *J Biol Chem* 263:14621-14624

Zatloukal K, Wagner E, Cotten M, Phillips S, Plank C, Steinlein P, Curiel DT, Birnstiel ML (1992): Transferrinfection: A highly efficient way to express gene constructs in eukaryotic cells. NYAcademy of Sciences Antisense strategies conference (In Press)

Zenke M, Steinlein P, Wagner E, Cotten M, Beug H, Birnstiel ML (1990): Receptor-mediated endocytosis of transferrin-polycation conjugates: An efficient way to introduce DNA into hematopoietic cells. *Proc Natl Acad Sci USA* 87:3655-3659

GENE TRANSFER IN MAMMALIAN CELLS USING LIPOSOMES AS CARRIERS

Arun Singhal and Leaf Huang

INTRODUCTION

After understanding the molecular genetic cause(s) for human diseases, gene therapy is a method of treatment under active research. As the name implies, gene therapy involves treatment of diseases by product(s) of foreign gene which return(s) affected cells or tissues to normal status. The successful application of this approach begins with the development of a suitable carrier for the target specific delivery of genetic material followed by expression of DNA at that site. This carrier should also be able to protect the DNA from surrounding environment, e.g., from plasma for in vivo delivery. Under ideal conditions this expression should be controlled by using inducible or tissue specific promoters. Different kinds of systems are being used to effectively transfer and express the foreign DNA in various types of mammalian cells. These are classified below:

(i) agents which deliver DNA by physical means: e.g. microinjection (Capecchi, 1980), electroporation (Paquereau and Cam, 1992), biobalistic or particle bombardment (Yang et al., 1990) and jet injection (Furth et al., 1992).

(ii) agents which deliver DNA by chemical means: e.g. calcium phosphate (Wigler et al., 1977), DEAE dextran (Ishikawa and Homcy, 1992), polylysine conjugates (Wu and Wu, 1987; Wagner et al., 1990), polybrene-dimethyl sulfoxide (Kawai and Nishizawa, 1984) and liposomes (Felgner et al., 1987; Gao and Huang, 1991)

(iii) agents which deliver DNA by biological means: e.g. virus derived vectors (Ferry et al., 1991; Culver et al., 1992).

These reagents have been used in vitro as well as in vivo studies with varying efficiency but none of the methods described so far meet all the requirements of an "ideal" drug/DNA carrier. Although the physical methods such as microinjection and electroporation and chemical methods e.g. calcium phosphate and DEAE dextran can transfer DNA to a wide variety of cells, their efficiency is relatively low. Moreover, physical methods such as microinjection and electroporation often need special and sophisticated instruments and are not suitable for in vivo gene delivery for practical reasons.

Gene Therapeutics: Methods and Applications of Direct Gene Transfer
Jon A. Wolff, Editor • ©1994 *Birkhäuser Boston*

Viral vectors, which often give high level of transfection have received considerable amount of interest as gene carriers. They are replication defective retroviruses (Gilboa et al., 1986) or adenoviruses (Rosenfeld et al., 1991), which are defective in producing some of their own proteins without affecting their ability to express the foreign genes inserted into the viral genome. Thus, the only viral elements that are required in these vectors are the long terminal repeat (LTR), the packaging signal, Psi, and both the primer binding sites. The remaining space can be filled with the exogenous DNA sequence. These viral vectors offer many advantages including the efficient and stable integration of foreign DNA into a wide variety of host genomes as well as the ability to infect a large population of cells (Verma, 1985). On the other hand they also exhibit several disadvantages, e.g.(i) they can not be used for non dividing cells (Miller et al., 1990), (ii) the replication defective virus can be converted to infectious form by possible recombination, (iii) they have a size limit for foreign DNA which can be inserted into the viral genome, and (iv) viruses can cause random integration of genes into the host chromosomes (Temin, 1990). However, retroviral vectors have been recently developed for delivery of DNA to hepatocytes in vivo (Ferry et al., 1991) and treatment of experimental brain tumors (Culver et al., 1992).

After carefully considering various factors for gene transfer to mammalian cells, liposomes have emerged with great promises. Since 1965, when liposomes were first introduced as a model cellular membrane (Bangham et al., 1965), they have been widely used as carriers for various kinds of substances for delivery to cells both in vitro and in vivo.

Liposomes offer several advantages for their use in the delivery of drugs or DNA, e.g., (i) both hydrophobic and hydrophilic materials can be accommodated into liposomes, (ii) liposomes can protect DNA (or RNA) from inactivation or degradation, and (iii) can be targeted to specific cells or tissues. Moreover, liposomes can potentially overcome the problems associated with viral vectors. For example, the absence of viral DNA and their inability for self replication in vivo completely eliminate the possibility of obtaining dangerous recombinants. Furthermore, liposomes can carry large pieces of DNA, potentially up to chromosomal size. Many studies have been done to discover and improve the different aspects of liposome mediated DNA transfer (for a review see, Hug and Sleight, 1991). Recently, a direct gene transfer protocol using a liposome-DNA complex has been approved for injection into the solid tumors of the patients (Nabel et al., 1992a). This phase I/II clinical trial is currently now underway at the University of Michigan. In this present review, we will discuss the ability of liposomes to mediate transfection both in vitro and in vivo with the specific focus on cationic liposomes.

LIPOSOME-DNA COMPLEX

The first step in the delivery of DNA with the help of liposomes is making a stable complex of DNA and liposomes of sufficiently small size so that it can enter into

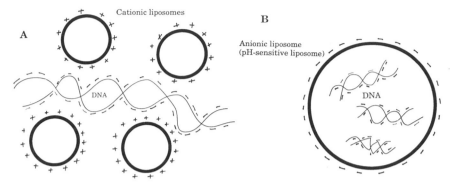

FIGURE 1. Schematic representation of liposome-DNA complex. DNA is held by charge interactions and remain outside to the positively charged liposomes (A), whereas in negatively charged liposomes (B) it is entrapped.

the cells. Since DNA is a highly negatively charged molecule it can be held with positively charged liposomes to make a complex (Figure 1A). The other way of loading the liposomes with DNA is to entrap the DNA in the aqueous interior of liposome (Figure 1B). These liposomes are generally made from negatively charged lipids which, in some cases have a property to destabilize the liposomal membrane at the low pH. Because of their sensitivity to pH, these liposomes are also known as pH-sensitive liposomes. This is an important property for the purpose of delivering DNA, as will be discussed in a later section. On the basis of the mode of entrapment of DNA, the liposomes can be grouped in two categories:

(A) positively charged or cationic liposomes and
(B) negatively charged or pH-sensitive liposomes.

Cationic liposomes

As shown in Figure 1A, DNA, when mixed with positively charged liposomes, make a complex with liposomes because of charge interactions. These liposomes mainly consist of a positively charged lipid and a co-lipid (also termed as helper lipid), e.g. dioleoyl phosphatidylethanolamine (DOPE) or dioleoyl phosphatidylcholine (DOPC). In some cases, the addition of a helper lipid is necessary for making stable liposomes, although DOPE also helps in the cytoplasmic delivery of the DNA, as will be discussed in a later section. Several different kinds of cationic lipids have been developed including lipofectin, quaternary ammonium detergents, cationic derivatives of cholesterol-diacyl glycerol and lipid derivative of polyamines. In the following paragraphs each of them is discussed separately:

i. Lipofectin
The commercially available lipofectin is a mixture of cationic lipid, N-[1-(2,3-dioleyloxy)propyl]-N,N,N,-trimethylammonium chloride (DOTMA, Figure

2A), and DOPE and was first reported by Felgner and co-workers (1987) to transfect cells in culture. DOTMA, either by itself or in combination with other neutral phospholipids, spontaneously forms multilamellar vesicles (MLV) which can be converted to small unilamellar vesicles (SUV) by sonication. DNA interacts spontaneously with lipofectin, to form lipid-DNA complexes with 100% loading efficiency. This association was supported by sucrose density gradient centrifugation (Felgner et al., 1987; Felgner and Holm,1989). When DNA was mixed with lipid (1:5 wt/wt) and loaded on a sucrose gradient, all of the DNA remained associated with lipid and floated to top of the gradient, whereas in absence of lipid, the DNA migrates to the bottom of the gradient. It is presumed that complex formation results from ionic interactions between the positively charged head group of DOTMA and the negatively charged phosphate groups of DNA. Both the lipid-DNA ratio as well as the overall lipid concentration are critical for efficient transfection. It was suggested (Felgner and Ringold, 1989) that a liposome of size of 250 nm made from equal amount of DOPE/DOTMA will have 2500 total lipid molecules or 1250 positively charged DOTMA molecules. Approximately four of these liposomes will be necessary to neutralize 5000 negative charges present in a standard 2.5 kb plasmid. Since there is only a slight variation in size of the complex from original liposome size of about 250 nm, it is assumed that each complex contains few or only one plasmid. This is an idealized calculation and does not include any changes which arise when the complex is mixed with serum or other body fluids resulting in more extensive aggregation.

The liposome-DNA complex has been used for both transient and stable transfection of various cell lines including T lymphoblastoid and macrophage cell lines in suspension cultures (Dorman and Yong, 1989; Belkowski et al., 1989), primary cultures of rat pituitary cells (Maurer, 1989), pancreatic islet cells (Welsh et al., 1990), fibroblasts and hepatocytes (Legendre and Szoka,1992), and hybridomas (Felgner and Ringold, 1989). Lipofectin has also been used to deliver RNA (Malone et al., 1989) and proteins to cells (Debs et al., 1990). The transfection efficiency of lipofectin-DNA complex was from 5 to 100 fold more effective than Ca phosphate or DEAE-dextran methods. However, significant toxicities (Felgner et al., 1987) for various cells limit its use as a general DNA carrier in vivo and lead other efforts to develop new agents for transfection.

ii. Cationic derivatives of cholesterol and diacyl glycerol
Leventis and Silvius (1990) have synthesized other cationic lipids, e.g. 1,2-bis(oleoyloxy)-3-(trimethylammonio) propane (DOTAP), 1,2-dioleoyl-3-(4'-trimethyl ammonio) butanoyl-sn-glycerol (DOTB), 1,2-dioleoyl-3-succinyl-sn-glycerol choline ester (DOSC) and cholesteryl (4'-trimethylammonio) butanoate (ChoTB), (see Figure 2B for structures). These derivatives when combined with DOPE mediated transfection of CV-1 and NIH3T3 cells more efficiently than DEAE dextran. Use of fluorescent coumarin-labeled analogs of DOTB and DOSC also indicated that these lipids undergo degradation, suggesting reduced toxicities of these compounds. In fact, DOTAP has been found to be less toxic than lipofectin

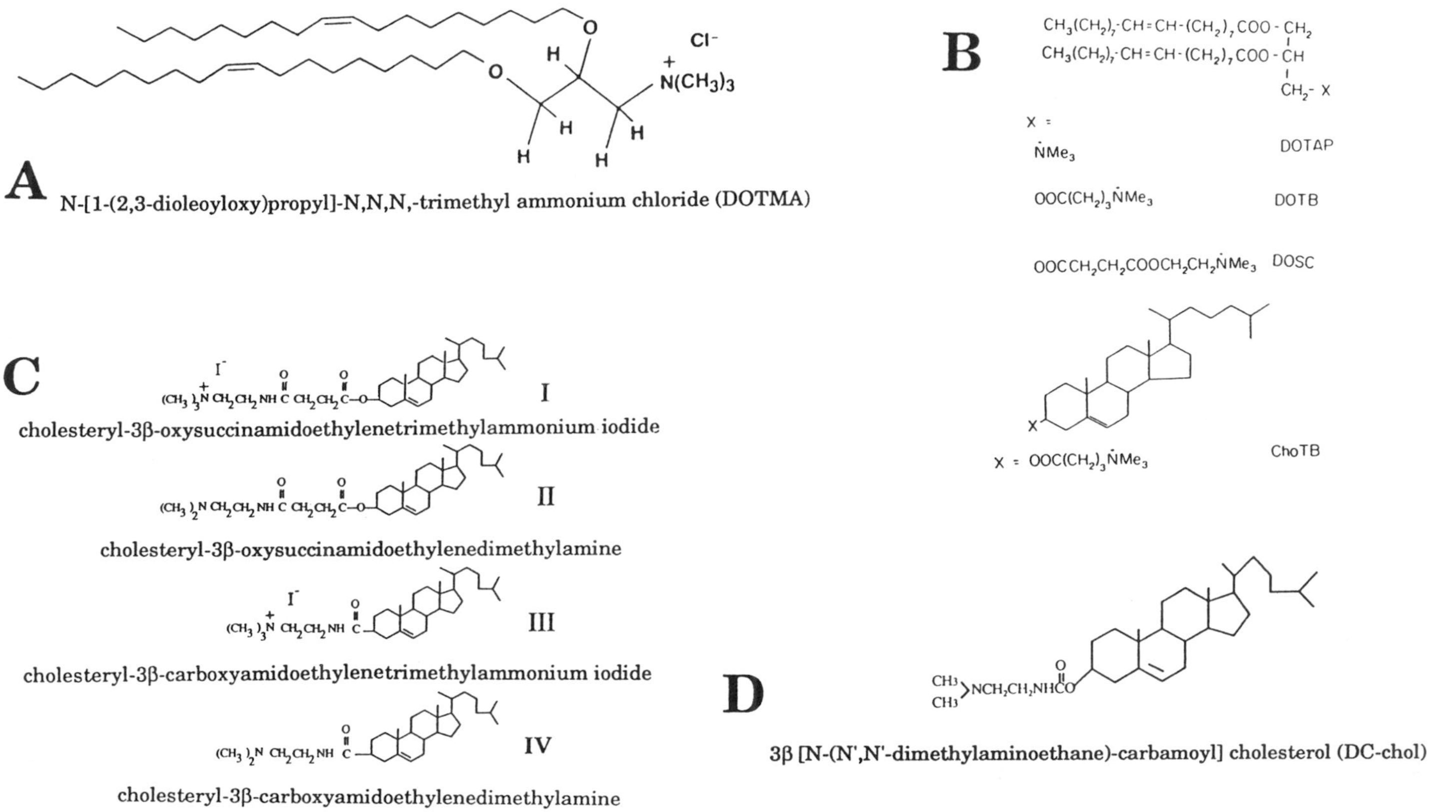

FIGURE 2. Structures of different cationic lipid derivatives used for transfection. See text for complete names for lipids of B.

(unpublished data). However, continous search is being made to develop more active and less toxic agents for DNA delivery. A detailed study on the structural and functional aspects of cationic liposomes has been done by our laboratory along with the development of more efficient systems for DNA delivery. These studies will be presented in a separate section.

iii. Lipopolyamines

A new type of lipophilic molecule has been reported as an efficient transfection reagent, i.e. lipopolyamine (Behr et al., 1989). This reagent mediates the transfection by itself and does not require any co-lipid for activity. In other words, a micellar complex of lipopolyamine and DNA is sufficient for transfection. The cationic polyamine is the essential part of the reagent since it complexes with the anionic DNA. However, there are only four primary amino groups on the polyamine and if any one of these is used to conjugate with the lipid, the net charge for DNA binding will be reduced. Therefore, a larger polycation, poly-L-lysine (PLL) was employed, which is advantageous as different ligands can be coupled with its primary amino groups. Receptor mediated, target specific delivery of DNA has been shown for asialooromucoid (Wu and Wu, 1988), transferrin (Wagner, 1990) and antibody (Trubetskoy et al., 1992a,b) conjugated with PLL. The PLL has also been conjugated with N-glutaryl-phosphatidylethanolamine (NGPE) to make a phospholipid derivative, which is known as lipopoly-L-lysine (LPLL) (Zhou et al., 1991). Mouse L929 cells were efficiently transfected with DNA/LPLL complexes. It was about threefold more effective than lipofectin and the activity was more compatible with the presence of serum than lipofectin. It can tolerate up to 30%-40% serum before losing the transfection activity completely. However, in order to obtain gene expression cells have to be mechanically scrapped. This obstacle was eliminated by adding a colipid, DOPE, along with lipopolylylysine (Zhou,1992). The optimal molar ratio LPLL and DOPE was 1:8 for transfection. The optimal liposome-DNA complex had a positive to negative charge ratio of about 9. This high level of net positive charge of the complex facilitates a high affinity binding of the complex to the negatively charged cell surface, resulting in an efficient uptake into the cells. The effect of poly-D-lysine (PDL) was also studied by making its phospholipid derivative (LPDL) (Zhou, 1992). The same level of transfection was achieved by using LPDL/DOPE liposomes, suggesting that degradation of the polylysine chain, which likely takes place in the lysosomes is not necessary for the cytoplasmic delivery of the DNA. A detailed mechanism of transfection mediated by these complexes will be discussed in a later section.

iv. Other cationic lipids

Other than lipids described above, liposomes composed of cationic amphiphiles such as a quaternary ammonium detergent and DOPE have been used as a carrier for DNA delivery to the cells (for a review see Zhou and Huang 1992). Various detergents, including cetyltrimethylammonium bromide (CTAB), didecyltrimethylammonium bromide (DTAB) and tetradecyl trimethylammonium bromide (TTAB) form liposomes in the presence of DOPE. These liposomes show various levels of toxicities with CTAB being the least toxic. The transfection efficiency has been demonstrated by the expression of a chloramphenicol acetyl transferase (CAT) reporter gene in mouse L 929 fibroblasts (Pinnaduwage et al., 1989). However, lipofectin was less toxic to the mouse L929 cells than the DOPE/CTAB liposomes, and transfected these cells with a slightly greater efficiency.

The single chain amphiphile, stearylamine (SA), has been used to form positively charged liposomes with phosphatidylcholine (Martin and McDonald 1976). However, SA is cytotoxic to mammalian cells (Hannun and Bell, 1989) and SA/DOPE liposomes are completely inactive for DNA delivery (Felgner and Ringold, 1989). Another type of cationic lipid, dimethyldioctadecyl-ammonium bromide (DDAB), which is now commercially available, has been reported to deliver DNA in different cell lines (Rose et al., 1991).

pH-sensitive liposomes

pH-sensitive or negatively charged liposomes carry DNA in a totally different way than the cationic liposomes (Figure 1B). Since both DNA and liposomes exhibit the same type of charge, there is a repulsion rather than complex formation between the two. However, some DNA can be entrapped in the aqueous interior of the liposomes. These liposomes were developed as a efficient system for cytoplasmic delivery, since they are destabilized in response to low pH in the endocytic vacuoles and release the contents into the cytoplasm. However, the cationic liposomes have been reported to be more efficient for gene transfer, probably because of their stronger adherence to the negatively charged cell membrane, resulting in a higher level of uptake (Legendre and Szoka, 1992).

Liposomes composed of DOPE and palmitoylhomocysteine (Connor et al., 1984), free fatty acids (Huang et al., 1987; Collins and Huang, 1987), or diacyl succinyl glycerol (Liu and Huang, 1990; Collins et al., 1990) fuse spontaneously with other lipid bilayers at low pH. Because liposomes enter the cells mainly via the endocytic pathway, this type of liposomes have the potential for efficient intracellular delivery of various entrapped substances. Successful delivery of a fluorescent dye calcein (Connor and Huang, 1985), FITC dextran (Straubinger et al., 1985), diphtheria toxin A (Collins and Huang, 1987), various drugs (Connor and Huang, 1986) and DNA has been shown by using these liposomes. Delivery of DNA has been shown both in vitro (Wang and Huang, 1989; Wang et al., 1986; Legendre and Szoka,1992) and in vivo (Wang and Huang, 1987). The ability of DOPE to form nonbilayer structures under appropriate physiological conditions is essential for the design of pH-sensitive liposomes.

pH-sensitive liposomes can also be prepared to contain specific ligand molecules for target specific delivery, both in cultured cells (Wang and Huang, 1989) and in a mouse model (Wang and Huang, 1987). However, due to the low entrapment of DNA into liposomes, the therapeutic application of the system was not fully developed. Recently, the entrapment of DNA by these liposomes has been

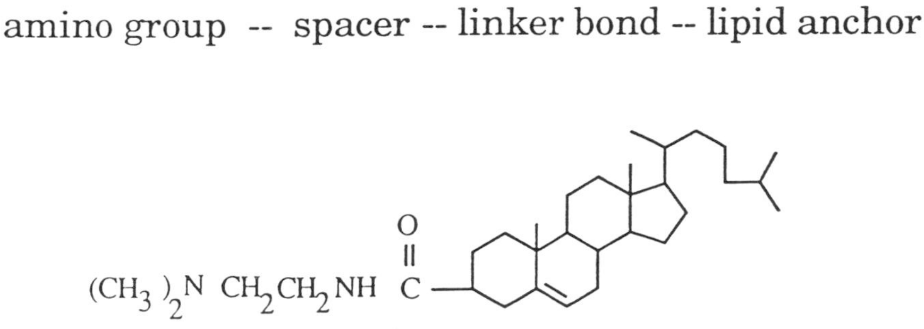

amino group -- spacer -- linker bond -- lipid anchor

$(CH_3)_2N\ CH_2CH_2\ NH\ C$ —

FIGURE 3. General structure of cationic derivatives of cholesterol.

improved by employing a freeze and thaw method (Zhou et al., 1992). Using this method the degree of DNA entrapment which is dependent on the size of DNA and lipid composition and concentration, has been increased up to 43%. It is suggested that freeze and thaw cycles cause destabilization of the membrane bilayer and generate transient "holes" in the membrane which in turn allow the DNA to penetrate into the liposomes. Very little damage to DNA was seen as the result of these mild freeze and thaw cycles.

STRUCTURAL AND FUNCTIONAL STUDIES OF CATIONIC LIPOSOMES

The general structure of a cationic lipid is shown in Figure 3. It consist of a cationic moiety containing an amino group (primary, secondary, tertiary or quaternary), a spacer arm which links the amino group with the lipid anchor and the lipid anchor itself. The transfection efficiency and toxicity depend mainly on the type of amino group, spacer arm, lipid anchor and the linker bond between the spacer arm and lipid anchor. As a lipid anchor, cholesterol was chosen because of its lipid bilayer stabilizing activity and minimal toxic effects to the treated cells. A series of compounds were synthesized either by us or in collaboration of Epand and Bottega. The following discussions are focused on the studies using these compounds.

As it is well known that protein kinase C (PKC) is vital to normal cellular functions including the regulation of gene expression and probably the uptake of liposome-DNA complex (Stabel and Parker, 1991). Certain cationic amphiphiles e.g. sphingosine, a naturally occuring cationic lipid, can inhibit PKC activity (Hannun et al., 1986; Bottega and Epand, 1992). Activators of PKC can increase the transfection efficiency by Ca phosphate method (Reston et al., 1991). It is, therefore, speculated that inhibition of PKC by cationic liposomes could be a critical factor which determines the transfection efficiency and cytotoxicity.

To evaluate the effect of spacer arm, linker bond and type of amino group on the transfection and PKC activity, several cationic derivatives of cholesterol (Figure 2C, I to IV), in which the cationic moiety containing quaternary (derivatives I

and III) or tertiary (derivatives II and IV) amino headgroup was linked to cholesterol with a ester or amide bond were studied (Farhood et al., 1992). Derivatives I
and II have succinyl spacer arm between the substituted ethylenediamine and cholesterol whereas compounds III and IV have a shorter spacer arm. The results
showed that tertiary amine derivatives were weak inhibitors of PKC (Ki > 100
mM) whereas quaternary amine derivatives were stronger PKC inhibitors with Ki
values about 4 to 20-fold lower than those of corresponding tertiary amine derivatives. The cytotoxicity of cationic liposomes prepared with these derivatives and
DOPE correlated well to the PKC inhibitory activity, i.e. the tertiary amine derivatives were less toxic than the quaternary amine derivatives.

When tested for transfection activity in tissue culture cells, quaternary amine
derivatives were found to have very little or no activity whereas derivative II,
cholesteroyl-3β-oxysuccinamidoethylenedimethylamine, which has a succinyl
spacer arm and a tertiary amino group, resulted about 3 fold higher transfection
activity than lipofectin with less toxicity in murine L929 cells (derivative IV which
also has tertiary amino group but shorter spacer arm is much less efficient). However, like lipofectin, the transfection efficiency of derivative II was also inhibited
by serum (Farhood et al., 1992). Large amounts of negatively charged serum
proteins probably complex with the liposomes and interfere with the binding with
the cells. In this regard, the behavior of derivative II is similar to lipofectin.
Moreover, it is relatively unstable because of the labile ester bond which are not
expected to be stable due to the ammonium group catalyzed reaction.

The following conclusions were drawn based upon work done on transfection
of cells by cationic liposomes containing cationic cholesterol derivatives:
(i).   Cationic lipids containing nondegradable ether linker bonds such as DOTMA
in the lipofectin formulation are generally more toxic than those containing biodegradable linker bonds such as ester, amide and carboamyl bonds.
(ii).   Toxicity is also dependent on the activity of cationic lipid to inhibit protein
kinase C. Relatively strong inhibitors (Ki= 1-10 mM) are more toxic to the treated
cells than the weak inhibitors (Ki>100 mM).
(iii). Cationic lipids containing a tertiary amino group are generally more efficient
in transfection than those containing a quaternary amino group.
(iv). A spacer arm of about 3-6 atoms between the amino group and the linker
bond is necessary for activity.
(v). Liposomes formulated with cationic lipids containing an ester linker bond
are not stable for storage (4°C, pH 7.4). It shows half-life of only 1-2 days,
whereas cationic lipids containing ether, amide and carbamoyl linker bonds are
stable for at least 3-4 weeks.
(vi). The other active ingredient termed "co-lipid" or "helper lipid" of cationic
liposomes is a phospholipid (Table 1 summarizes different lipids used for this
purposes). Those phospholipid having a strong tendency to form the inverted
hexagonal structures (H_{II} phase), such as DOPE, are best co-lipids. DOPC, which
does not form H_{II} phase under physiological conditions has little or no activity.

Based on the above empirical rules, a derivative of cholesterol, 3b[N-(N',N'-dimethylaminoethane)-carbamoyl] cholesterol (DC-chol) has been developed (Gao and Huang, 1991) in our lab. This novel lipid (Figure 2D) has a carbamoyl bond, a spacer arm of 3 atoms and a tertiary amino group. The carbamoyl bond was chosen because it is easily hydrolyzed by cellular esterases (unlike DOTMA which has nondegradable ether bonds). Liposomes prepared with DC-chol and DOPE by sonication retain their full transfection activity after storage at 4°C for 4 months (Gao and Huang, unpublished data). The transfection of different cell lines in vitro including human epidermoid carcinoma cells (A431), human lung epithelial carcinoma cells (A549), murine fibroblasts (L929), minipig primary endothelial cells (YPT) (Gao and Huang, 1991), human embryonal kidney cells (293), HeLa, rabbit synoviocytes,Vero,IB3-1 cells from airway epithelium of a cystic fibrosis patient (Gao and Huang, unpublished results) has been done successfully with these liposomes. The transfection activity of DC-chol liposomes varies among cell lines with a maximum of about 4-5 fold over that of lipofectin. In general, epithelial cells and fibroblasts are easier to transfect wheareas these liposomes do not or very poorly transfect cells like lymphocytes, macrophages and endothelial cells. Using β-galactosidase gene as a histochemical marker, it was observed (Singhal and Huang, unpublished data) that the degree of transfection varies among cells of the same type in a homogenous culture. The cause of this heterogeneity is still unknown, however the transfection does not seem to be dependent on cell division as nondividing cells can be efficiently transfected (Gao and Huang, unpublished data). The transfection also depends on the density of the culture. In A431 cells, cultures of 60% to 80% confluency are optimal. Transfection with lower confluency usually leads to lower efficiency, probably due to the fact that cells take up excess cationic liposomes and their growth is inhibited. Although the carbamoyl bond in DC-chol is designed to be biodegradable, these liposomes can still cause acute toxicities, if used in overdose and may kill the cells. The toxicity varies among cell types and dependent on the confluency of the cell culture. Confluent cells are more resistant to toxicity. For a given confluency, DC-chol liposomes have been found to be at least fivefold less toxic than that of lipofectin (Gao and Huang, 1991).

These liposomes are prepared as 3:2 molar ratio of DC-chol and DOPE. The addition of a co-lipid such as DOPE or DOPC is required because DC-chol does not form stable dispersion by itself at physiological pH. It is necessary to add at least 10% co-lipid to obtain a stable liposome dispersion. However, addition of DOPE also increases the transfection efficiency significantly, as will be discussed in the following sections. The mixture of lipid is dispersed in 20mM Hepes buffer, pH 7.8 and converted into SUV by sonication. DNA in Tris-EDTA buffer (Tris 10 mM, EDTA 1mM, pH 8.0) is then mixed with liposomes at different ratios (1:1 to 1:10 wt/wt, liposomes:DNA). This complex formation is typically performed in 0.1ml of serum free media for 1mg of DNA which is sufficient for 4×10^4 cells. DNA being negatively charged interact immediately with DC-chol liposomes and form a complex. This complex is added to tissue culture cells and incubated at

TABLE 1. Phospholipids used as "co-lipid" in the formation of liposomes for transfection.

Co-lipid[a]	Cationic or pH-sensitive lipid[b]	Target cell[c]	Transfection efficiency[d]	Ref.[e]
	Cationic liposomes			
DOPE	DOTMA	CV-1; COS-7	+	1
	DOTAP[f]	CV-1; 3T3	+	2
	Derivative II	L929	+	3
	DC-chol	A431	+	4
	LPLL	L929	+	5
DOPC	Derivative II	L929	-	3
	LPLL	L929	-	5
DEPE	LPLL	L929	+/-	5
MMDOPE	LPLL	L929	+/-	5
DMDOPE	LPLL	L929	-	5
DOPS	LPLL	L929	-	5
DPSG	LPLL	L929	-	5
MGDG	LPLL	L929	-	5
Cholesterol	LPLL	L929	-	5
	pH-sensitive liposomes			
DOPE	DOSG	L929	+	6
	CHEMS	CV-1	+	7
DOPC	DOSG	L929	-	6
	CHEMS	CV-1	-	7
Cholesterol/DOPE	Oleic acid	RDM-4	+	8
Cholesterol/DOPE	Oleic acid	Pancreatic Islet cells	+	9
Cholesterol/DOPC	Oleic acid	RDM-4	-	8

Codes for table are on the next page.

37°C in serum free media for 5 hours. The cells are then washed and incubated in regular media containing a normal amount of fetal bovine serum. Cells are harvested 2 days later and the transfection efficiency is estimated by enzymatic assays for the reporter gene product, e.g. CAT, luciferase or β-galactosidase in cell extracts.

DC-chol/DOPE liposomes have also been extensively studied for their suitability in vivo using mouse, rabbit and pig as models (Stewart et al., 1992; Nabel et al., 1992b). The biodistribution of liposome-DNA complex administered by intravenous (i.v.) injection or direct intratumor injection in mouse was monitored by the polymerase chain reaction (PCR) method and possible toxic effects were evaluated by pathological, electrocardiographic and clinical biochemical studies. The results showed that 20 days after i.v. injection, exogenous DNA mainly localized in the lung and the heart, and occasionally in the kidney. After intratumor injection, DNA was consistently detectable in the tumor and occasionally in tissues outside the injected tumor. These animals showed neither any sign of inflammatory response nor any major abnormality. No significant changes were found in liver functions or blood concentration of tissue specific enzymes. Since there was exogenous DNA accumulated in the heart of i.v. injected mice, acute cardiac toxicity of the heart was studied by measurement of total creatine phosphokinase activity and electrocardiography, which were found to be normal. Cardiac rhythm was found to be normal and no acute ichemic changes were observed. The long term effects on autoimmunity and gonadal localization were also studied (Nabel et al., 1992b). In rabbits and pigs, these liposomes containing class I MHC gene were given by i.v. injection, or direct transfection of arteries was conducted using a catheter (Nabel et al., 1990). Histological examination of different organs showed no clinically significant immunopathology or organ damage. These studies suggest that uptake of foreign DNA following gene transfer through DC-chol liposomes in major organs is not associated with autoimmunity, toxicity or gonadal localization. Based on this safety and toxicity data, a phase I/II protocol for

---

a.   DOPE, dioleoylphosphatidylethanolamine; DOPC, dioleoylphosphatidylcholine; DEPE, dielaidoylphatidylethanolamine; MMDOPE, N-monomethyldioleoylphosphatidylethanolamine; DMDOPE, N-dimethyldioleoylphosphatidylethanolamine; DOPS, dioleoylphosphatidylserine; DPSG, dipalmitoylsuccinylglycerol; DOSG, dioloelsuccinylglycerol; MGDG, monogalactosyldiglyceride.

b.   See text for complete names of DOTMA, DOTAP, DC-chol and LPLL. Derivative II, Cholesteroyl-3β-oxysuccinamidoethylenedimethylamine; CHEMS, Cholesterol hemisuccinate morpholine salt.

c.   CV-1, African green monkey kidney cell; COS-7, Monkey kidney cell expressing T antigen of simian virus (SV 40); 3T3, Murine fibroblast cell line; L929, Murine fibroblast cell line; A431, Human epidermoid carcinoma cell line; RDM-4, Murine lymphoma cells.

d.   Transfection efficiencies are not related to each other. Significant transfection activity is shown as (+), whereas little or no activity is shown as (+/-) or (-), respectively.

e.   1. Felgner et al., 1987; 2. Leventis and Silvius, 1990; 3. Farhood et al., 1992; 4. Gao and Huang, 1991; 5. Zhou, 1992; 6. Zhou et al., 1992; 7, Legendre and Szoka, 1992; 8, Wang and Huang, 1987; 9, Welsh et al., 1990.

f.   Some other cationic lipids were are also used in the same study with similar results.

human melanoma gene therapy by using HLA B7 gene complexed with DC-chol/ DOPE liposomes has been approved and is currently under investigation at the University of Michigan (Nabel et al., 1992a).

SITE SPECIFIC DELIVERY OF LIPOSOMES TO CELLS AND TISSUES

Delivery of nucleic acids to desired sites in the body is a major goal for liposomes as carriers. In fact, liposomes show considerable promise as carriers for the delivery of therapeutic agents in vivo. However, a major obstacle in their wide spread utilization in medicine is that the injected liposomes are rapidly removed from the blood by the cells of reticuloendothelial system (RES), primarily the liver Kupffer cells and splenic macrophages (Hwang, 1987; Senior, 1987). The RES uptake of liposomes depends upon the lipid composition and size of liposomes as well as on the route of injection (Senior, 1987). Efforts have been made to divert the liposomes from being taken by RES. The specificity of liposomes towards a target site has been attempted by using different approaches which are mainly based upon the following principles:

(A) effect of route of injection in vivo,

(B) effect of liposomal composition/size, and

(C) effect of attaching site specific ligands to liposomes.

Effect of route of injection of liposomes in vivo

Intravenous injection is the most common way of introducing liposomes into the body. The injected liposomes are sequestered in the liver and spleen (Hwang, 1987). Injection of liposomes other than intravenously can provide some degree of reduced uptake by RES. For example, liposomes when injected into the peritoneal cavity of mice and rats, enter the lymphatics and then into the circulation (Ellens et al., 1981; Parker et al., 1981) causing a delay in the uptake by RES. Intramuscular (i.m.) and subcutaneous (s.c.) injections of liposomes also show similar effects (Poste et al., 1984; Tuner et al., 1983). Therefore, if liposomes are to be targeted to a cell type within or accessible from the lymphatic system, they may be able to reach the target by i.m. or s.c. injection routes.

Administration of liposomes to the lung has been reported by intratracheal instillation. This pathway has been used to administer both liposomally encapsulated drugs (Fielding and Abra, 1992) and lipofectin-DNA complexes (Brigham et al., 1989). In one study, Yoshimura et al. (1992) showed the presence of mRNA of human cystic fibrosis transmembrane conductance (CFTR) regulator gene in mouse lungs after intratracheal administration of the corresponding plasmid with lipofectin. Reporter gene activity for luciferase and b-galactosidase was also shown in the lungs, suggesting that most of the airway epithelial cells were transfected. Brigham et al. (1989) also used lipofectin-DNA complexes to transfect mouse lungs by intratracheal instillation as well as intravenous and intraperitoneal injections. Recently, the expression of CAT gene has been reported in mouse lung after administration of liposome-DNA complexes in an aerosol form (Stribling et al., 1992). DC-chol liposome-DNA complexes have been directly injected into the tumor (Stewart et al, 1992) and also administered into arterial endothelial cells by catheters (Nabel et al., 1992b).

Effect of liposome composition and size

Irrespective of the site of injection of liposomes in the body, liposomes come in the blood circulation after certain time and taken up by the RES. Liposomes composed of DC-chol/DOPE also found to be sequestered in the RES within 30 minutes of i.v. injection (Singhal and Huang, unpublished data). Therefore, it is necessary to develop methods which increase the survival time of liposomes in circulation. This way, liposomes will stay in circulation for a longer period of time which, in turn, will give more chance for liposomes to interact with the target cells.

The survival time of liposomes in circulation can be increased by changing the lipid composition and size. Addition of ganglioside GM_1 (Liu et al., 1992; Allen et al., 1987), hydrogenated phosphatidylionisitol (PI)(Gabizon and Papahadjopolous, 1988) or N-(polyethyleneglycol) phosphatidylethanolamine (PEG-PE) (Klibanov et al., 1990; Mori et al., 1991; Blume and Cevc, 1990: Allen et al., 1991) to egg PC/cholesterol liposomes has been shown to increase the circulation time in blood. It has been suggested that the effect of these agents to prolong the circulation time is dependent on the co-lipid (Litzinger and Huang, 1992b) and works only with properly sized (diameter between 80-300 nm) liposomes (Liu et al., 1991,1992; Klibanov et al., 1991). As discussed in the following section, these liposomes with additionally attached site specific ligands may serve as efficient DNA carriers.

Effect of attaching ligands on the liposome surface

Among the different methods of targeting of liposomes, attachment of ligands on the surface of liposomes is the most efficient way for their delivery to the selective sites. Both antibodies and ligands to cell surface receptors have been used.

i. Antibodies

Antibodies and other site specific proteins can be attached to the liposomes on their surface (Heath, 1987) or be incorporated in their membrane as the liposomes are formed (Huang et al., 1984; Holmberg et al., 1989). When these liposomes are injected, they bind specifically and efficiently to the target site, if the liposomes are prepared with a lipid formulation which confers low RES uptake of liposomes (Maruyama et al., 1990). Because the lipids used in these liposomes forms stable bilayers, the liposomes remain intact after the binding of the antibody to the target cells. A monoclonal antibody against an epitope expressed on the lung endothelial cells was covalently attached to the negatively charged liposome surface and effective lung targeting of these immunoliposomes was observed (Litzinger and Huang, 1992c). However, this approach does not work for the cationic liposomes (Zhou and Huang, unpublished data), probably because of the strong RES uptake of the cationic liposomes. Therefore, a novel approach using these antibodies as a recognition molecule, has recently been developed in our laboratory (Trubetskoy et al., 1992 a,b). In this, the antibodies were covalently linked to positively charged polylysine chains (mean molecular weight 3000) and a ternary complex with positively charged liposomes and DNA (Figure 4) was formed. The DNA, used in this study was a expression vector containing CAT as reporter gene under control of SV40 promoter. When this ternary complex was added to lung endothelial cells in culture, the CAT activity was increased 10-20 fold over the complex containing non-specific antibodies. This increase in transfection activity was suggested as a result of two reasons. Firstly, the antibodies help the complex in binding to the surface of the target cells and secondly, the liposomal lipid destabilize the endosomes releasing the DNA into the cytoplasm (Trubetskoy et al., 1992b). The action of cationic liposomes is evidenced by the finding that complex containing only DNA and antibody-polylysine conjugates showed low transfection efficiency while retaining specific binding activity to cells (Trubetskoy et al., 1992b). Thus, this new ternary complex has promising activity and specificity to be used as an injectable and targetable transfection agent. The in vivo transfection activity of these liposomes might be further increased by using long circulating liposomes to avoid rapid uptake of liposomes by the RES.

Attachment of antibodies to the surface of pH sensitive liposomes is another way of using antibody directed approach. These immunoliposomes have been shown to transfect different cell types in vitro (Wang and Huang, 1989; Zhou et al., 1992). Tumors cells grown in peritoneal cavity of mice were transfected by intraperitoneal injection of immunoliposomes (Wang and Huang, 1987). Thus, these liposomes offer a working model for targeted DNA delivery in vivo.

ii. Other ligands

In another approach to targeted delivery of DNA, ligands to different cell surface receptors can be incorporated into the surface of liposomes by covalently modifying the ligand with a lipid group and adding it during the formation of liposomes. Stavridis et al.(1986) have complexed transferrin with stearylamine present in the liposomal membrane and targeted these liposomes to erythroid precursor cells in the bone marrow. Since the capillaries of the bone marrow are fenestrated, all classes of the bone marrow cells may be potentially transfected in vivo by using suitable receptor-ligand combinations.

Some degree of target selectivity can also be achieved by using a target specific promoter and/or enhancer for expression of the exogenous gene. Thus, specific gene expression occurs only at the desired cells (Wang and Huang, 1987; Stripp et al., 1990).

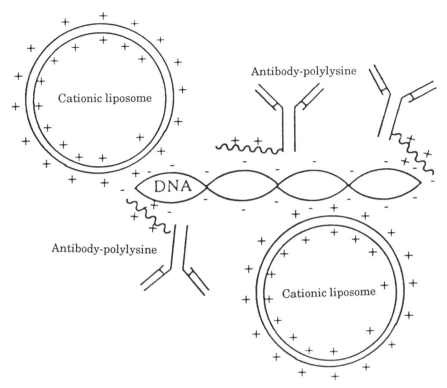

FIGURE 4. Schematic representation of ternary antibody-polylysine/DNA-cationic liposome complex.

MECHANISM OF LIPOSOME-CELL INTERACTION

The efficiency of liposomal delivery of genetic material depends on the understanding of liposome-cell interactions. Both cationic and pH-sensitive liposomes apparently share the same mechanism of interaction which can be divided in three steps:
(A) internalization of liposome-DNA complex,
(B) delivery of DNA into the cytosol, and
(C) entry of DNA into the nucleus.

Internalization of liposome-DNA complex

Endocytosis is the major mechanism by which pH-sensitive liposomes are internalized into the cells (Litzinger and Huang,1992a) (Figure 5). Nonspecific binding of pH-sensitive liposomes without an attached ligand is usually low. On the other hand, cationic liposome-DNA complex binds strongly to the cells due to favorable charge interactions. Therefore, cationic liposomes have been found to be more efficient in interaction than the ligand-free, pH-sensitive liposomes (Legendre and Szoka, 1992). However, cellular binding of pH-sensitive liposomes can be significantly enhanced if an appropriate ligand, such as an antibody is attached to the liposome surface. The actual mechanism of internalization of the cationic liposomes is not fully elucidated. However, fusion of the cationic liposome membrane with the cell membrane has been suggested for the interaction of lipofectin with mouse L cells (Felgner et al., 1987). Rhodamine fluorescence was observed throughout the surface of the these cells, when transfection was performed using a lipofectin-DNA complex containing trace amount of rhodamine-labelled DOPE. Substitution of DOPE with DOPC in the lipofectin liposomes resulted in only puntate fluorescence suggesting the absence of fusion. A classical fusion process, however, is not sufficient to explain the intracellular delivery of DNA which is tightly bound to the external surface of liposomes. Free quaternary ammonium detergent complexed with DNA mediates weak but detectable transfection (Pinnaduwage et al., 1989), where fusion of free detergent micelles with the plasma membrane is very unlikely. Thus, existing evidence does not support a classical fusion mechanism as the major entry pathway of DNA-liposome complex. However, electron microscopic studies using LPLL/DOPE liposomes indicate that a small (less than 1%) fraction of the complex causes a localized destabilization at the plasma membrane, resulting in direct penetration of the complex into the cytosol (Zhou, 1992). The major internalization mechanism of the cationic liposome-DNA complex is still via the pathway of adsorptive endocytosis (Figure 5).

Delivery of DNA into cytosol

The release of the DNA from endosomes containing DNA-liposome complex is dependent upon several factors; (i) low pH in the endosome vacuoles, (ii) the appropriate liposomal lipid, i.e. pH-sensitive or cationic lipid, and (iii) the co-lipid. The acidic pH (pH 5-6.5) of endosomes is mainly responsible for the release of DNA along with other factors. A diagramatic representation of the *proposed* mechanism of delivery of DNA is shown in Figure 5.

It is well known that endosomes fuse with lysosomes and the contents of endosomes are degraded by lysosomal enzymes (Figure 5, steps a and b). However, the contents of an endosome can escape degradation and be released into the cytosol, if the endosome membrane is destabilized before it fuses with the lysosome (steps c to e). The acidic pH in the endosome triggers fusion of the pH-sensitive liposome membrane with the endosome membrane which results in release of the DNA both in the cytosol and within the endosome (step c). Subsequently or simultaneously, the co-lipid (DOPE) of the liposomes induces a destabilization of the endosome membrane which releases more DNA into the cytosol (step d). In the case of cationic liposomes, no fusion between liposome and endosome occurs, but destabilization of the endosome membrane causes the release of the intact

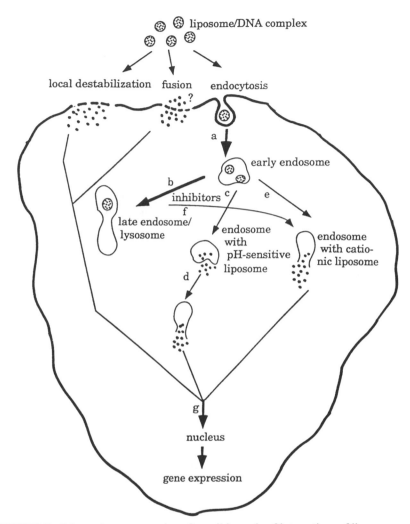

FIGURE 5. Schematic representation of possible mode of interactions of liposomes with cells which lead to intracellular delivery of DNA. Liposomes can enter the cells by local destabilization of plasma membrane, fusion or endocytosis. The release of DNA by fusion is not very clear. In endocytosis, early endosomes are formed containing liposome-DNA complex (step a). These can either be degraded in lysosomes (step b) or enter into different steps for release of the DNA. It is proposed that in early endosomes (containing pH-sensitive liposome complex), fusion of endosome and liposome membrane occurs (step c) followed by rupture of the endosome membrane (step d), releasing the DNA into the cytoplasm. Other early endosomes, containing cationic liposome-DNA complex, rupture due to membrane destabilization (step e), releasing the liposome-DNA complex into the cytoplasm. The lysosomotropic drugs inhibit the fusion of endosomes with lysosomes which, in some cases, results in greater release of DNA into the cytoplasm (step f). The released DNA or cationic liposome-DNA complex reach into the nucleus (step g), and gene expression occurs. Major events are shown by thick arrows. See text for more details.

liposome-DNA complex into the cytosol (step e). Since only a small fraction (about 15%) of endosomes undergo the destabilization process (Zhou, 1992), the majority of the liposome-DNA complexes are still delivered to the lysosomes for degradation (step b). Thus, it has been suggested that the transfection efficiency could be enhanced if the cells are treated with various lysosomotropic drugs e.g. chloroquine, ammonium chloride or cytochalasin B (step f). It was observed that these drugs indeed increase the transfection activity, when used with lipofectin-DNA (Legendre and Szoka, 1992) or LPLL/DOPE/DNA complexes (Zhou, 1992). However, transfection mediated by DC-chol liposomes is inhibited by chloroquine (Gao and Huang, unpublished data), suggesting that the site of entry into the cytosol is the late endosome-lysosome.

The different steps described above have been supported by a number of experiments. The role of acidic pH in the endosomes has been shown by using pH-sensitive lipids with different pKa's. Liposomes composed of palmitoyl homocysteine/DOPE, which destabilize in less acidic conditions (found in the early stages of endosomes or early endosomes), the site of delivery was the early endosomes (Collins et al., 1989,1990). Liposomes containing 1,2-dioleoyl-sn-3-succinylglycerol or 1,3-dipalmitoyl-2-succinylglycerol, which destabilize only in a more acidic condition (found in the late stages of endosomes), the site of delivery was the late endosomes (Collins et al., 1989,1990). The efficiency of transfection by using transferrin-polylysine/DNA complex was greatly enhanced by co-delivery of adenovirus (Wagner et al., 1992), as adenovirus causes endosome destabilization (Seth et al., 1984). The function of the co-lipid is similar to that of the adenovirus, because liposomes containing DOPE also cause destabilization. This activity of DOPE is probably related to its ability to resume nonbilayer structures, such as the H_{II} phase. When DOPC replaces DOPE as the co-lipid, liposomes do not make transition into non-bilayer phases and exhibit little, if any, transfection activity. The role of the co-lipid is summarized in Table 1.

Entry of DNA into the nucleus

Very little is known about the mechanism by which DNA moves from the cytosol into the nucleus, except that this process is likely very inefficient. DNA microinjected into the cytosol induces much less gene expression than if the same DNA is directly injected into the nucleus (Capecchi, 1980). The cationic liposome-DNA complex may enter into the nucleus as intact complexes (Friend et al., 1990).

CONCLUSION

We have summarized various factors involved in the use of liposomes as carriers for DNA delivery. Several parameters need to be better understood and improved before liposomes can be used as a general carrier for genetic material. These include the improvement in the targetbility and transfection efficiency, especially in vivo. Moreover, the DNA carrying capacity also need to be improved. It is generally realized that liposome mediated transfection is only transient; long-term transfection efficiency is very low. Therefore, methods must be developed for stable integration of the foreign gene at the desired site for long term gene expression. Furthermore, since different cell types behave differently towards a given type of liposome in terms of transfection, efficiency and toxicity, the molecular and cellular basis of this variability needs to be studied. Experiments are in progress at our laboratory to investigate these problems.

In spite of the needed research work, liposomal vectors offer unique advantages over other vectors, e.g., retrovirus vectors. Preparation and packaging of the exogenous gene can be easily done with liposomes. It is possible to deliver the liposomal genes to the desired sites, at least to those sites where a targeting system has been developed. Furthermore, liposomal vectors are relatively nontoxic and can be prepared in large quantities. It was with these advantages in mind that the first in vivo human gene therapy trial was carried out using liposomes as a vector (Nabel et al., 1992a). It is likely that many more applications will be performed in the future.

ACKNOWLEDGMENT

The original work from this laboratory was supported by NIH grants AI 29893, CA 59327, and HL 50256.

REFERENCES

Allen TM, Hansen C, Martin F, Redemann C, Yau-Young A (1991): Liposomes containing synthetic lipid derivatives of poly (ethylene glycol) show prolonged circulation half-lives in vivo. *Biochim Biophys Acta* 1066:29-36

Allen TM , Chonn A (1987): Large unilamellar liposomes with low uptake into the reticuloendothelial system. *FEBS Lett* 223:42-46

Bangham AD, Standish MM, Watkins JC (1965): Diffusion of univalent ions across the lamellae of swollen phospholipids. *J Mol Biol* 13:238-252

Behr JP, Demeneix B, Loeffler J-P, Perez-Mutul J (1989): Efficient gene transfer into mammalian priamry endocrine cells with lipopolyamine-coated DNA. *Proc Natl Acad Sci USA* 86:6982-6986

Belkowski LS, Fan X, Bloom BR (1989): Transfection of murine and human macrophage-like cell lines by cationic liposomes. *Focus* 11:35-36

Blume G, Gregor C (1990): Liposomes for the sustained drug release in vivo. *Biochim Biophys Acta* 1029:91-97

Bottega R, Epand RM (1992): Inhibition of protein kinase C by cationic amphiphiles. *Biochemistry* 31:9025-9030

Brigham KL, Meyrick B, Christian B, Magnuson M, King G, Berry L (1989): In vivo transfection of murine lungs with a functioning prokaryotic gene using a liposomes vehicle. *Am J Med Sci* 298: 278-281

Capecchi MR (1980): High efficiency transformation by direct microinjection of

DNA into cultured mammalian cells. *Cell* 22:479-485

Collins D, Litzinger DC, Huang L (1990): Structural and functional comparisons of pH-sensitive liposomes composed of phosphatidylethanolamine and three different diacylsuccinylglycerols. *Biochim Biophys Acta* 1025:234-242

Collins D, Maxfield F, Huang L (1989): Immunoliposomes with different acid sensitives as probes for the cellular endocytic pathway. *Biochim Biophys Acta* 987:47-55

Collins D, Huang L (1987): Cytotoxicity of diphtheria toxin A fragment to toxin-resisted murine cells delivery by pH-sensitive immunoliposomes. *Cancer Res* 47:735-739

Connor J, Huang L (1986): pH-sensitive immunoliposomes as an efficient and target-specific carrier for antitumor drugs. *Cancer Res* 46:3431-3435

Connor J, Huang L (1985): Efficient cytoplasmic delivery of a fluorescent dye by pH-sensitive immunoliposomes. *J Cell Biol* 101:582-589

Culver KW, Ram Z, Wallbridge S, Ishii H, Oldfield EH, Blaese RM (1992): In vivo gene transfer with retroviral vector-producer cells for treatment of experimental brain tumors. *Science* 256:1550-1552

Debs RJ, Freedman LP, Edmunds S, Gaensler KL, Duzgunes N, Yamamoto KR (1990): Regulation of gene expression in vivo by liposome-mediated delivery of a purified transition factor. *J Biol Chem* 265:10189-10192

Dorman L, Yong H (1989): Cationic liposomes-mediated transfection of suspension cultures. *Focus* 11:37

Ellens H, Morselt H, Scherphof G (1981): In vivo fate of large unilamellar sphingomylein-cholesterol liposomes after intraperitoneal and intravenous injection into rats. *Biochim Biophys Acta* 674:10-18

Farhood H, Bottega R, Epand RM, Huang L (1992): Effect of cationic cholesterol derivatives on gene transfer and protein kinase C activity. *Biochim Biophys Acta* 1111:239-246

Felgner PL, Gadek YR, Holm M, Roman R, Chan HW, Wenz M, Northop JP, Ringold GM, Danielson M (1987): Lipofection: A highly efficient, lipid-mediated DNA-transfection procedure. *Proc Natl Acad Sci USA* 84:7413-7417

Felgner PL, Holm M (1989): Cationic liposome-mediated transfection. *Focus* 11:21-25

Felgner PL, Ringold GM (1989): Cationic liposome-mediated transfection. *Nature* 337:387-388

Ferry N, Duplessis O, Hopussin D, Danos O, Heard J-M (1991): Retroviral-mediated gene transfer into hepatocytes in vivo. *Proc Natl Acad Sci USA* 88:8377-8381

Fielding RM, Abra RM (1992): Factors affecting the release rate of terbutaline from liposome formulations after intratracheal instillation in the guinea pig. *Pharm Res* 9:220-223

Friend DS, Debs RJ, Duzunes N (1990): Interactions between DOTMA liposomes, CV-1 and U937 cells and their isolated nuclei. 30th annual meeting of the American Society for Cell Biology, San Diego. *J Cell Biol* 111:663

Furth PA, Shamay A, Wall RJ, Hennighausen L (1992): Gene transfer into somatic tissues by jet injection. *Anal Biochem* 205:365-368

Gabizon A, Papahadjopoulos D (1988): Liposome formulation with prolonged circulation time in blood and enhanced uptake by tumors. *Proc Natl Acad Sci USA* 85:6949-6953

Gao X, Huang L (1991): A novel cationic liposome reagent for efficient transfection of mammalian cells. *Biochem Biophys Res Commun* 179:280-285

Gilboa E, Eglitis MA, Kantoff PW, French Anderson W (1986): Transfer and expression of cloned genes using retroviral vectors. *Biotechniques* 4:504-512

Hannun YA, Bell RM (1989): Functions of sphingolipids and sphingolipid breakdown products in cellular regulation. *Science* 243:500-507

Hannun YA, Loomis CR, Merrill Jr AH, Bell RM (1986): Sphingosine inhibition of protein kinase C activity and phorbol diburate binding in vitro and in human platelets. *J Biol Chem* 261:12604-12609

Heath TD (1987): Covalent attachment of proteins to liposomes. *Meth Enzymol* 149:111-119

Holmberg E, Maruyama K, Litzinger DC, Wright S, Davis M, Kabalka GW, Kennel SJ, Huang L (1989): Highly efficient immunoliposomes prepared with a method which is compatible with various lipid compositions. *Biochem Biophys Res Commun* 165:1272-1278

Huang L, Connor J, Wang C-Y (1987): pH-sensitive immunoliposomes. *Meth Enzymol* 149:88-99

Huang L, Huang A, Kennel S (1984): Coupling of antibodies with liposomes. In: *Liposome Technology* (Gregoriadis G; ed.) , volume 3, CRC press, Boca Raton, pp. 51-62

Hug P, Sleight RG (1991): Liposomes for the transformation of eukaryotic cells. *Biochim Biophys Acta* 1097:1-17

Hwang KJ (1987): Liposome pharmacokinetics. In: *Liposomes: From biophysics to therapeutics*, (Ostro MJ ed.), Marcel Dekker, New York, pp. 109-156

Ishikawa Y, Homcy CJ (1992): High efficiency gene transfer into mammalian cells by a double trasnfection protocol. *Nuc Acids Res* 20:4367

Kawai S, Nishizawa M (1984): New procedure for DNA transfection with polycation and dimethyl sulphoxide. *Mol Cell Biol* 4:1172-1174

Klibanov AL, Maruyama K, Beckerleg AM, Torchilin VP, Huang L (1991): Acitivity of amphipathic poly (ethylene glycol) 5000 to prolong the circulation time of liposomes depends on the liposome size and is unfavorable for immunoliposomes binding to target. *Biochim Biophys Acta* 1062:142-148

Klibanov AL, Maruyama K, Torchilin VP, Huang L (1990): Amphipathic polyethyleneglycols effectively prolong the circulation time of liposomes. *FEBS Lett* 268:235-237

Legendre J-Y, Szoka FC (1992): Delivery of plasmid DNA into mammalian cell lines using pH-sensitive liposomes: Comparison with cationic liposomes. *Pharm Res* 9:1235-1242

Leventis R, Silvius JR (1990): Interaction of mammalian cells with lipid dispersions containing novel metabolizable cationic amphiphiles. *Biochim Biophys Acta* 1023:124-132

Litzinger D, Huang L (1992a): Phosphatidylethanolamine liposomes: drug delivery, gene transfer and immunodiagnostic applications. *Biochim Biophys Acta* 1113:201-227

Litzinger D, Huang L (1992b): Amphipathic poly(ethylene glycol) 5000-stabilized dioleoylphosphatidylethanolamine liposomes accumulate in spleen. *Biochim Biophys Acta* 1127:249-254

Litzinger D, Huang L (1992c): Biodistribution and immunotargetability of ganglioside-stabilized dioleoylphosphatidylethanolamine liposomes. *Biochim Biophys Acta* 1104:179-187

Liu D, Mori A, Huang L (1992): Role of liposome size and RES blockade in controlling biodistribution and tumor uptake of GM_1 containing liposomes. *Biochim Biophys Acta* 1104:95-101

Liu D, Mori A, Huang L (1991): Large liposomes containing ganglioside GM_1 accumulate effectively in spleen. *Biochim Biophys Acta* 1066:159-165

Liu D, Huang L (1990): pH-sensitive, plasma-stable liposomes with relatively prolonged residence in circulation. *Biochim Biophys Acta* 1022:348-354

Malone RW, Felgner PL, Verma IM (1989): Cationic liposome-mediated RNA transfection. *Proc Natl Acad Sci USA* 86:6077-6081

Martin FG, MacDonald RC (1976): Lipid vesicle-cell interactions. III. Introduction of a new antigenic determinant into erythrocyte membranes. *J Cell Biol* 70:515-526

Maruyama K, Kennel SJ, Huang L (1990): Lipid composition is important for highly efficient target binding and retention of immunoliposomes. *Proc Natl Acad Sci USA* 87:5744-5748

Maurer RA (1989): Cation liposome-mediated transfection of primary cultures of rat pituitary cells. *Focus* 11:25-27

Miller DG, Adam MA, Miller AD (1990): Gene transfer by retrovirus vectors occurs only in cells that are actively replicating at the time of infection. *Mol Cell Biol* 10:4239-4242

Mori A, Klibanov AL, Torchilin VP, Huang L (1991): Influence of the steric barrier activity of amphipathic poly (ethylene glycol) and ganglioside GM_1 on the circulation time of liposomes and on the target binding of immunoliposomes in vivo. *FEBS Lett* 284:263-266

Nabel GJ, Chang A, Nabel EG, Plautz G, Fox BA, Huang L, Shu S (1992a): Clinical protocol: Immunotherapy of malignancy by in vivo gene transfer into tumors. *Human Gene Therapy* 3:399-410

Nabel EG, Gordon D, Yang Z-Y, Xu L, San H, Plautz GE, Wu B-Y, Gao X, Huang L, Nabel GJ (1992b): Gene transfer in vivo with DNA-liposome complexes: Lack of autoimmunity and gonadal localization. *Human Gene Therapy* 3:649-656

Nabel EG, Plautz G, Nabel GJ (1990): Site-specific gene expression in vivo by direct gene transfer into arterial wall. *Science* 249:1285-1288

Paquereau L, Cam AL (1992): Electroporation-mediated gene transfer into hepatocytes: preservation of a growth hormone response. *Anal Biochem* 204:147-151

Parker RJ, Sieber SM, Weinstein JN (1981): Effect of liposome encapsulation of a fluorescent dye on its uptake by the lymphatics of the rat. *Pharmacol* 23:128-136

Pinnaduwage P, Schmitt L, Huang L (1989): Use of a quaternary ammonium detergent in liposome mediated DNA transfection of mouse L-cells. *Biochim Biophys Acta* 985:33-37

Poste G, Kirsh R, Koestler T (1984): The challenge of liposome targeting in vivo. In: *Liposome Technology* (Gregoriadis G; ed.), volume 3, CRC press, Boca Raton, pp. 1-28

Reston JT, Gould-Fogerite S, Mannino RJ (1991): Potentiation of DNA mediated gene transfer in NIH3T3 cells by activators of protein kinase C. *Biochim Biophys Acta* 1088:270-276

Rose JK, Buonocore L, Whitt MA (1991): A new cationic liposome reagent mediating nearly quantitative transfection of animal cells. *Biotechniques* 10:520-525

Rosenfeld MA, Siegfried W, Yoshimura K, Yoneyama K, Fukayama M, Stier LE, Pakko PK, Gilardi P, Straford-Perricaudet LD, Perricaudet M, Jallat S, Pavirani A, Lecocq JP, Crystal RG (1991): Adenovirus-mediated transfer of a recombinant alpha 1-antitrypsin gene to the lung epithelium in vivo. *Science* 252:431-434

Satbel S, Parker PJ (1991): Protein Kinase C. *Pharmac Ther* 51:71-95

Senior JR (1987): Fate and behavior of liposomes in vivo: a review of controlling factors. *CRC Cri Rev Therp Drug Carr Sys* 3:123-193

Seth P, Fitzgerald DJP, Willingham MC, Pastan I (1984): Role of a low-pH environment in adenovirus enhancement of the toxicity of a *Pseudomonas* exotoxin-epidermal growth factor conjugate. *J Virol* 51:650-655

Stavridis JC, Deliconstantinos G, Psallidopoulos MC, Armenakas NA, Hadjiminas DJ, Hadjiminas J (1986): Construction of transferrin-coated liposomes for in vivo transport of exogenous DNA to bone marrow erythroblasts in rabbits. *Exp Cell Res* 164:568-572

Stewart MJ, Plautz GE, Buono LD, Yang ZY, Xu L, Gao X, Huang L, Nabel EG, Nabel GJ (1992): Gene transfer in vivo with DNA-liposome complexes: safety and acute toxicity in mice. *Human Gene Therapy* 3:267-275

Straubinger RM, Duzgunes N, Papahadjopoulos D (1985): pH-sensitive liposomes mediate cytoplasmic delivery of encapsulated macromolecules. *FEBS Lett* 179:148-154

Stribling R, Brunette E, Liggitt D, Gaensler K, Debs R (1992): Aerosol gene delivery in vivo. *Proc Natl Acad Sci USA* 89:11277-11281

Stripp BR, Whitsett JA, Lattier DL (1990): Strategies for analysis of gene expression: pulmonary surfactant proteins. *American J Physol* 259:185-197

Temin HM (1990): Safety considerations in somatic gene therapy of human disease with retrovirus vectors. *Human Gene Therapy* 1:111-123

Trubetskoy VS, Torchilin VP, Kennel S, Huang L (1992a): Use of N-terminal modified poly-L-lysine-antibody conjugate as a carrier for targeted gene delivery in mouse lung endothelial cells. *Bioconjugate Chem* 3:323-327

Trubetskoy VS, Torchilin VP, Kennel S, Huang L (1992b): Cationic liposomes enhance targeted delivery and expression of exogenous DNA mediated by N-terminal modified poly-L-lysine-antibody conjugate in mouse lung endothelial cells. *Biochim Biophys Acta* 1131:311-313

Tuner A, Kirby C, Senior J, Gregoriadis G (1983): Fate of cholesterol-rich liposomes after subcutaneous injection into rats. *Biochim Biophys Acta* 760:119-125

Verma IM (1985): Retroviral vectors for gene transfer. In: *Microbiology* (Leive L et al., eds.) American Society of Microbiology, Washington, DC, p. 229

Wagner E, Zatloukal K, Cotten M, Kirlappos H, Mechtrler K, Curiel DT, Birnstiel ML (1992): Coupling of adenovirus to transferrin-polylysine/DNA complexes greatly enhances receptor-mediated gene delivery and expression of trans-fected genes. *Proc Natl Acad Sci USA* 89:6099-6103

Wagner E, Zenk M, Cotten M, Beug H, Birnsteil ML (1990): Transferrin-polycation conjugates as carriers for DNA uptake into the cells. *Proc Natl Acad Sci USA* 87:3410-3414

Wang C-Y, Huang L (1989): Highly efficient DNA delivery mediated by pH-sensitive immunoliposomes. *Biochemistry* 28:9508-9514

Wang C-Y, Huang L (1987): pH-sensitive immunoliposomes mediate target-cell-specific delivery and controlled expression of a foreign gene in mouse. *Proc Natl Acad Sci USA* 84:7851-7855

Wang C-Y, Hughes K, Huang L (1986): Improved cytoplasmic delivery to plant protoplasts via pH-sensitive liposomes. *Plant Physiology* 82:179-184

Welsh N, Oberg C, Hellerstrom C, Welsh M (1990): Liposome mediated in vivo transfection of pancreatic islet cells. *Biomed Biochim Acta* 49:1157-1164

Wigler M, Silverstein S, Lee L-S, Pellicer A, Cheng Y-C, Axel R (1977): Transfer of purified herpes virus thymidine kinase gene to cultured mouse cells. *Cell* 11:223-232

Wu GY, Wu CH (1988): Receptor-mediated gene delivery and expression in vivo. *J Biol Chem* 263:14621-14624

Wu GY, Wu CH (1987): Receptor-mediated in vitro gene transformation by a soluble DNA carrier system. *J Biol Chem* 262:4429-4432

Yang N-S, Burkholder J, Roberts B, Martinell B, McCabe D (1990): *Proc Natl Acad Sci USA* 87:9568-9572

Yoshimura K, Rosenfeld M, Nakamura H, Scherer MM, Pavirani A, Lecocq J-P, Crystal RG (1992): Expression of the human cystic fibrosis transmembrane conductance regulator gene in the mouse lung after in vivo intracheal plas-mid-mediated gene transfer. *Nuc Acid Res* 20:3233-3240

Zhou X (1992): Liposome mediated gene transfer in mammalian cells. PhD thesis, University of Tennessee, Knoxville, USA

Zhou X, Huang L (1992): Targeted delivery of DNA by liposomes and polymers. *J Controlled Release* 19:269-274

Zhou X, Klibanov AL, Huang L (1992): Improved encapsulation of DNA in pH-sensitive liposomes for transfection. *J Liposome Res* 2:125-139

Zhou X, Klibanov AL, Huang L (1991): Lipophilic polylysine mediates efficient DNA transfection in mammalian cells. *Biochim Biophys Acta* 1065:8-14

IN VIVO GENE THERAPY VIA RECEPTOR-MEDIATED DNA DELIVERY

Henry C. Chiou, George L. Spitalny, June R. Merwin, and Mark A. Findeis

Human gene therapy has advanced during the past ten years from a theoretical concept to a rapidly emerging technology. Tremendous technological strides in recombinant DNA methodologies have fostered molecular studies in such fields as regulation of gene expression, human genetics and disease states, and gene transfer techniques. The confluence of these fields has led to the emergence of gene therapy as a reality, albeit limited at present to a small number of clinical studies (Anderson, 1992; Miller, 1992). As practiced today most gene therapy protocols lie within the realm of high-cost, technology-intensive, individualized treatments, akin to such procedures as organ and bone marrow transplantation (Mulligan, 1991). This type of procedure, though beneficial, is limited in usefulness since it is not readily accessible to much of the population. Even for those to whom this type of gene therapy strategy would be available, the current inability to achieve permanent transgene expression necessitates periodic retreatments, making these procedures highly cost-ineffective over the long term.

To realize the full potential of gene therapy, gene-based therapeutics will need to evolve in the direction of traditional drug-based therapies. As such, current and developing gene therapy strategies should be assessed with respect to the issues normally considered in the development of pharmaceuticals. For example, emphasis should be placed upon the implementation of gene transfer strategies that deliver therapeutic transgenes into selected target cells in vivo with minimal manipulation or intervention. Ideally, the "gene-drug" would be introduced into the body by some form of parenteral injection or oral ingestion. These forms of administration would allow for more practical re-administrations of the gene formulation to maintain sufficient long-term expression of the therapeutic gene. Like other pharmaceuticals, gene-based drugs will need to demonstrate in vivo specificity; in this case by expressing their protein products only in the target tissues. Such specificity could be achieved by delivering genes solely to target tissue, or by construction of tissue-specific expression vectors. Other important issues to be considered involve the physicochemical aspects of the gene-based therapeutic and its manufacture. These issues include the relative costs and availability of the components that make up the gene-drug, efficiency and yield of production, ease of storage, the shelf-life of the gene formulation, the maximum DNA capacity of the gene transfer system, lack of immunogenicity or toxicity, and pharmacokinetic properties.

Gene Therapeutics: Methods and Applications of Direct Gene Transfer
Jon A. Wolff, Editor • ©1994 *Birkhäuser Boston*

DIRECT GENE TRANSFER BY TARGETED DELIVERY
TO HEPATOCYTES

Most of the points discussed above coalesce around the fundamental question of developing a practical and effective method of gene transfer in vivo, and, concomitantly, the formulation for the gene delivery vehicle. Selective, targeted delivery for in vivo gene transfer is one strategy for bringing gene therapy into the realm of accessible, easy to administer pharmaceuticals. The concept of targeted delivery of therapeutic agents was initially proposed by Paul Ehrlich over eighty years ago (Baümler, 1984). In its essence, targeted delivery utilizes specific receptor-ligand interactions to selectively deliver therapeutic agents. This concept has been applied to cancer therapy, autoimmune diseases, and infectious diseases, mainly by covalent coupling of antibody or growth factor ligands to cytotoxic agents (Arnon and Sela, 1982; Freeman and Mayhew, 1986; Braslawsky et al., 1990; Vitetta, 1990; Pastan et al., 1992). For gene therapy, the use of recombinant viruses to deliver genetic material to cells can be considered a form of targeted delivery. The viruses attach to and enter cells via receptor-ligand binding. However, receptors for the more common viral vectors currently in use, retroviruses, herpesviruses, and adenovirus, are found on a broad range of cell types. Thus, although targeted, lack of cell or tissue specificity limits their usefulness in vivo.

Parenchymal hepatocytes display highly specific receptors that recognize and bind galactose-terminal glycoproteins, or asialoglycoproteins (ASGP) (Ashwell and Morell, 1974). The ASGP receptor (ASGPr) provides a housekeeping function, removing desialylated glycoproteins from the circulation by clathrin-coated pit endocytosis. The exclusive localization of the ASGPr on hepatocytes makes it a good candidate for targeted delivery. Between 100,000 and 500,000 ASGP binding sites are present per cell, randomly distributed over the sinusoidal, or blood-facing, domain of the plasma membrane (Spiess, 1990). A relatively constant number of receptors are always available on the cell surface. The ASGPr rapidly and constitutively recycles, and the receptor population is continually replenished from large intracellular reservoirs. Thus a tremendous number of ligands can be rapidly bound and internalized without an appreciable decrease in the capacity of the liver to take up more ligand shortly thereafter. These characteristics, in addition to tissue selectivity, are highly advantageous for targeted delivery since they suggest that large quantities of DNA-ASGP complexes could be rapidly delivered to hepatocytes, and therefore exhibit a favorable pharmacokinetic profile within the circulation.

Gene transfer to hepatocytes offers tremendous potential for a broad spectrum of gene therapies (Findeis et al., 1993). The liver is the largest gland in the body, accounting for one-fiftieth of total body weight (Schwartz, 1991). It produces 90-95% of all plasma proteins, including most of the factors involved in blood coagulation. The rate of plasma protein production can be as high as thirty to sixty grams per day (Guyton, 1981); suggesting that it is an ideal site for high level expression of therapeutic proteins. The liver is highly vascularized, with a fifth of the cardiac output flowing through each minute (Rappaport, 1987). This assures rapid delivery of intravenously injected gene complexes, and efficient systemic distribution of therapeutic proteins synthesized in the liver and secreted into the circulation. The liver is essential in the maintenance of homeostasis, and plays a central role in numerous processes such as the metabolism of lipids, carbohydrates, and proteins, and the detoxification of exogenous chemicals. As such, it is an excellent site for gene transfer and expression to treat numerous diseases which either affect liver function, or which may be ameliorated by modification of liver metabolism.

IN VIVO GENE TRANSFER USING ASIALOGLYCOPROTEIN-DNA COMPLEXES

The pioneering studies of Wu and Wu (1987; 1988a; 1988b) and their colleagues (Wu et al., 1989; Wu et al., 1991; Wilson et al., 1992; Furs and Wu, this volume) were the first to successfully implement gene transfer by targeted delivery, both in vivo and in vitro. The general strategy used involves covalent coupling of the polycationic polypeptide, poly-L-lysine (PL), to ASOR. The ASOR-PL conjugate binds and highly condenses DNA by electrostatic attraction between the negatively charged nucleic acid and the polycation (Figure 1). Our own electron microscopic studies, as well as those of others (Wagner et al., 1991) have shown that these DNA-PL-ligand complexes condense into rodlike and toroidal structures, 75 to 125 nm in size. We believe that this condensation helps to protect the DNA from degradation and facilitates its entry into cells. Once internalized, DNA is released from the ASOR-PL conjugate and is able to get into the nucleus, where it is expressed. Applying the same concept, Birnstiel and coworkers have used transferrin-polycation conjugates in vitro for receptor-mediated delivery of genes encoding luciferase and β-galactosidase (Zenke et al., 1990; Cotten et al., 1990; Wagner et al., 1990; Wagner et al., 1991; Wagner et al., 1992b). The transferrin receptor is highly represented on the surface of hematopoietic cells and rapidly proliferating cells, such as those found in neoplasms, but is also found on most other cell types. It thus does not offer the advantage of selectivity that is present in the ASOR-ASGPr system. Transferrin however, may be useful for applications where generalized gene delivery is desired, or where tissue-specific expression systems are employed. To date, in vivo gene transfer has yet to be reported using this system.

The soluble DNA-PL-ASOR complex appears to be quite stable and can be easily administered by intravenous injection (Figure 2). Anecdotal evidence suggests that the DNA-protein complex will retain full activity for several months when stored as a solution at 4°C. The efficiency and specificity of delivery is illustrated by in vivo experiments which have shown that 85% of ^{32}P-labeled DNA complexed with ASOR-PL was internalized into the liver ten minutes after injection (Wu and Wu, 1988a). No other tissue contained more than five percent of the total amount of label injected. Our own in vivo targeting and clearance studies have confirmed these findings. We have also observed by cryo-autoradiography that labeled complex is evenly, and selectively distributed to hepatocytes through-

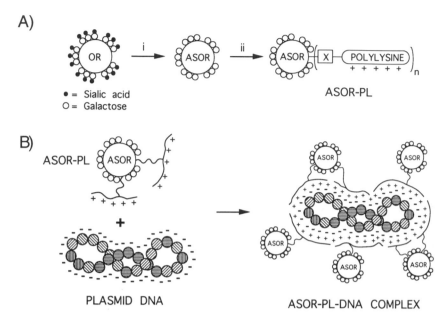

FIGURE 1. Preparation of asialoorosomucoid-polylysine (ASOR-PL) conjugates and ASOR-PL-DNA complexes. (A) Terminal sialic acid is removed from orosomucoid (OR) by treatment with acid or neuraminidase (i) to obtain asialoorosomucoid. ASOR is crosslinked with polylysine using carbodiimide or thiol chemistry (ii), in which the covalent coupling X is via amide or disulfide bonds, respectively. (B) ASOR-PL conjugates are combined in solution with plasmid DNA to form an electrostatic complex. The ASOR on the surface of the complex recognizes and binds to ASGPr on the surface of hepatocytes.

out the entire organ. The nonparenchymal vascular cells of the liver, namely endothelia and smooth muscle cells, did not exhibit any uptake of the complex, while a small portion was non-specifically phagocytosed into the Kupffer cells.

Intravenous injection satisfies the need for an undemanding method of administration, making periodic retreatment of patients a feasible, practical strategy. It is anticipated that ASOR-PL-DNA complexes will elicit little or no immune response in humans, even after multiple injections. Although clinical studies using the complete complex have not as yet been performed, each of the components have been clinically examined with no evidence of immunogenicity. It is well established that DNAs are rapidly destroyed in plasma by nucleases, and that none of the breakdown products are immunogenic. Asialoorosomucoid is a naturally occurring derivative of the plasma protein orosomucoid (OR), a nonpolymorphic protein. As such it should not be immunogenic. In addition, it has been observed that orosomucoid is a common and substantial contaminant found in human serum albumin preparations used as plasma extenders. Antibodies have not been detected in patients infused with albumin. Polylysine has been used to stabilize clinical

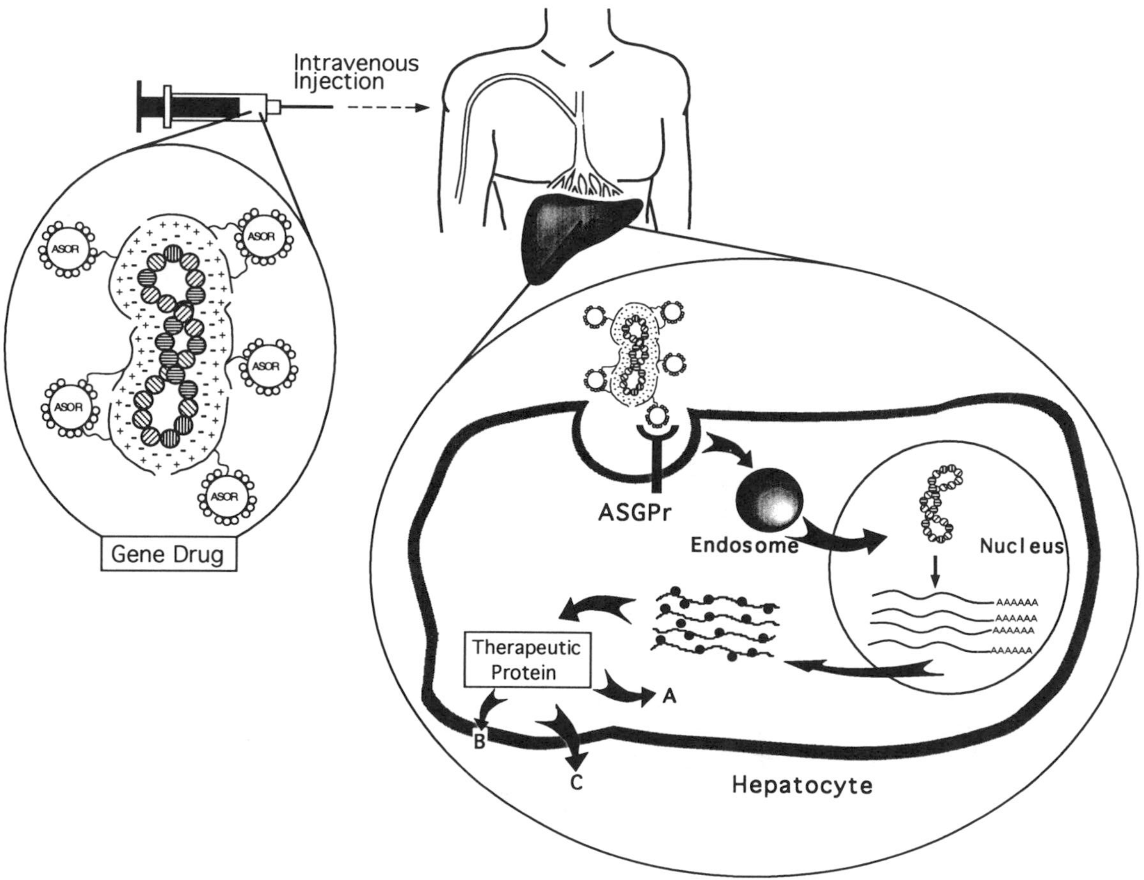

FIGURE 2. Strategy for direct in vivo gene transfer via receptor-mediated DNA delivery. Soluble ASOR-PL-DNA complex is administered by intravenous injection. The complex is taken up into hepatocytes from the circulation via asialoglycoprotein receptor-mediated endocytosis. DNA is released from the complex within the endosome and travels to the nucleus where it is transcribed into mRNA. The mRNA is translated to produce the therapeutic protein. Depending upon the application, the therapeutic protein may be (A) intracellular, (B) membrane bound, or (C) secreted.

preparations of the interferon inducer polyI-polyC (Lampkin et al., 1985; Hartmann et al., 1987; Ewel et al., 1992). Published clinical studies have not reported the development of antibodies against either the polypeptide, or the polynucleotide, though multiple doses of PL-polyI-polyC complex were administered (Lampkin et al., 1985; Ewel et al., 1992). With the exception of ASOR, this complex is similar to ASOR-PL-DNA complexes, which suggests a lack of immunogenicity for the latter protein-DNA formulation.

EXPRESSION OF GENES DELIVERED IN THE FORM OF DNA-PROTEIN COMPLEXES

The possibility of regular, periodic gene therapy treatments lessens the prevailing problem of transient expression. With a nonimmunogenic, easily administered therapeutic, expression can be manipulated not only at the level of the DNA sequence, but also by the amount of complex administered and the frequency of treatment. As in most other gene therapy strategies (Thompson, 1992; Felgner 1993; Mulligan, 1993), the efficiency of expression from ASOR-PL-DNA complexes is low to moderate, and declines over time. ASGPr-mediated endocytosis delivers large quantities of DNA very rapidly to hepatocytes in vivo. However, a large percentage of the DNA is destroyed intracellularly, within the endosomal-lysosomal compartment. It is at this stage of gene transfer that viral mechanisms have a distinct advantage. After viruses enter cells, many, such as adenoviruses, have the ability to disrupt endosomes, or neutralize cellular defense mechanisms in other ways, in order to safeguard their genetic payloads. This advantage, plus the ability of adenoviruses to express in nondividing cells, has stimulated much interest in their use for gene transfer.

Adenovirus have been used for in vivo delivery of the cystic fibrosis transmembrane conductance regulator (CFTR) gene to the lung epithelium of cotton rats (Rosenfeld et al., 1992). In these experiments, CFTR mRNA was observed for as long as 42 days after gene transfer. Lung epithelial cells are a natural target for adenovirus. However, the virus can infect most other cell types as well. For gene transfer in the lung, the pulmonary lining acts as a barrier against penetration of the adenovirus to other tissues. Other applications where the ability to physically restrict the infectivity of the virus is absent would be more problematic. The benefits of using viruses for in vivo gene transfer may be negated by their inherent immunogenicity, which will certainly limit repeated administrations. For viruses found in a large percentage of the population, such as adenovirus and herpesvirus, the initial treatments with these virus-based vectors may themselves induce undesirable side effects. Packaging of transgenes in viral capsids is also handicapped by limitations on the size of the transgene construct that can be accommodated within the viral genome. Adenoviruses can accommodate about seven to ten kilobase pairs (kbp) of foreign sequence, while retroviruses are limited to roughly five kilobases. Polylysine-protein conjugates have been shown to condense and deliver DNAs as small as 21 nucleotides (Wu and Wu, 1992), and as large as a 48 kbp double-stranded DNA (Cotten et al., 1992). Further work is required to take full advantage of the beneficial functions of viruses while minimizing their limitations.

To circumvent packaging constraints while harnessing their endosomal escape functions, adenovirus has been used to co-infect cultured cells treated with DNA-protein complexes. Co-infection greatly enhanced expression of the transgenes in these studies (Curiel et al., 1991, Cotten et al., 1992; Cristiano et al., 1993). Even more promising for in vivo delivery, however, has been gene delivery formulations where the endosomal disruption function of adenovirus was combined with selective tissue targeting by physical coupling of adenovirus to PL-ASOR or PL-transferrin conjugates (Wagner et al., 1992a; Wu et al., 1992; Michael et al., 1993). Optimal tissue selectivity however, required inactivation of viral binding to its receptor (Wu et al., 1992; Michael et al., 1993). A 25 to 1,000-fold enhancement of gene expression in vitro and 10-fold enhancement in vivo was observed in these experiments. In another adaptation of the membrane active properties of viruses, synthetic viral-sequence peptides from influenza virus hemagglutinin have been incorporated into DNA-binding conjugates to enhance DNA release from endosomes (Wagner, 1992b; Plank et al., 1992). The use of small peptides or fusion proteins may help to lessen the problem of virus protein induced immunogenicity.

Inhibition of the intracellular degradation of the transgene can also be accomplished by use of agents known to alter the endocytic-lysosomal pathway. For example, chloroquine, which has been shown to accumulate in and raise the pH of the endosomal-lysosomal compartment (Homewood et al., 1972), has been shown in vitro to enhance expression of DNA-PL-transferrin complexes (Cotten et al., 1990). The lysosomatropic agents are thought to act by inhibiting the pH sensitive degradative enzymes present in the lysosome. A second strategy for inhibition of endosomal/lysosomal destruction employs pharmacological agents that are known to disrupt microtubules and interfere with intracellular transport. This disruption potentially inhibits the transfer of lysosomal contents to endosomes. In this regard, studies have shown that a single dose (75 mg/kg) of colchicine 60 minutes prior to injection of a protein-DNA complex into rats induced prolonged intracellular expression for a minimum of six weeks (Chowdhury et al., 1993).

Fibric acid derivatives are another class of compounds being examined for their ability to enhance gene expression. These agents have multiple effects in stimulating liver cell physiology including activation of hepatocyte peroxisomes (Ochsner et al., 1990; Orton and Parker, 1982). Two drugs in this class, Clofibrate (2-(4-chlorophenoxy)-2-methyl propanoic acid ethyl ester) and Gemfibrizol (5-(2,5-dimethylphenoxy)-2,2-dimethyl pentanoic acid), are FDA approved for treatment of lipoprotein metabolism related to increased risk of coronary heart disease. Nafenopin ([2-methyl-2-p-(1,2,3,4-tetrahydro-1-napthly)phenoxy proprionic acid), a more potent chemical derivative, has been shown to both increase and prolong gene expression in vivo (Wu et al., 1990).

PRACTICAL ASPECTS OF CONJUGATE AND COMPLEX PREPARATION

Developing a targetable DNA complex for use as a traditional injectable pharmaceutical requires that several issues be considered. First, the targeting ligand, an appropriate polycation, and the DNA containing the therapeutic gene must be available in sufficient quantity, and at reasonable cost, for large scale production. Proteins such as orosomucoid and transferrin are readily available from human plasma and basic poly-amino acids such as polylysine are commercial reagents. Potentially useful targeting ligands such as vitamins, or other metabolites are also readily available. The gene to be delivered must be coupled with appropriate promoter sequences or other regulatory elements to obtain therapeutic levels of expression. Once engineered, plasmids can be produced through fermentation in lab-scale apparatus to yield tens to hundreds of milligrams at a time. Economical industrial production of plasmid DNA of high quality on the gram-scale or larger however, is a process that has yet to be reduced to practice.

Covalent coupling between the ligand and polycation ensures that the complexed DNA will be carried to the target cell. The chemistry of bioconjugate formation is diverse and well developed, although many of the available reagents are costly (Wong, 1993). The chemistry used for crosslinking ligand and polycation must be chosen to ensure that the receptor-binding ability of the ligand is not impaired. Crosslinking reactions between macromolecules invariably generate complex product mixtures. Fractionation of these mixtures to isolate the desired conjugate fraction can prove difficult. For some purposes, dialyzed crude product may be adequately functional. Generally, however, a more involved fractionation, in which unreacted starting materials are removed along with low molecular weight byproducts, is essential. Further fractionation of the partially purified conjugate may require one or more chromatographic or electrophoretic steps to obtain a fraction satisfactory for the preparation of functional DNA complexes.

In our experience, a hallmark of inadequate fractionation is that DNA complexes made with these materials will often have low solubilities. Based on anecdotal evidence, it appears that the difficulties encountered by some investigators who have attempted targeted delivery strategies may be due to incomplete appreciation of the need to better purify the conjugates. Attempts to prepare DNA complexes at higher concentrations (e.g. ~ 1 mg/ml of complexed DNA) will result in significant precipitation of the complex. After filtration, the recovery of the soluble complexed DNA will be quite low. Even with "better" conjugates the solubility of DNA complexes is finite and it appears to be difficult to achieve the formation of complexes at concentrations of DNA greater than about 1 mg/ml. In light of the nature of the ionic complex between DNA and a polycation this is not a surprising result. The energy of association of the polyphosphate backbone of DNA and a polycation such as polylysine, based on multiple noncovalent ionic bonds, can easily exceed that of a covalent bond. For a 5 kb plasmid, this energy of association will be the equivalent of several hundred covalent bonds. Even the association of a twenty-base oligonucleotide with a polycation under nondenaturing conditions can have an energy of association equal to roughly one covalent bond. A consequence of this tight association is that the net charge of the resulting complex is greatly reduced. As with a protein brought to the pH of its isoelectric point, the solubility of fully complexed DNA is reduced by its incorporation into a complex with low overall net charge. For most in vitro applications, preparation of complexes at lower concentrations ($\leq$ 100 μg/ml of complexed DNA) is quite acceptable and usually affords high recoveries of targetable complex. However, limited solubility may become a concern for in vivo applications, where the complex must be sufficiently concentrated to allow injection in a practical volume.

ASIALOOROSOMUCOID-POLYLYSINE CONJUGATES AND THEIR COMPLEXES

Orosomucoid (also referred to as α_1-acid glycoprotein or AAG) can be isolated from human plasma with a yield of about 450 mg per liter (Schmid, 1975), by simple ion-exchange chromatography and ammonium sulfate precipitation (Whitehead and Sammons, 1966). Desialylation generates galactose-terminal asialoorosomucoid, a high-affinity ligand for the ASGPr. The physical robustness of OR allows desialylation by acid hydrolysis at pH 1.5 for one hour at 80°C (Schmid et al., 1967). This procedure avoids the more cumbersome and expensive approach of an enzymic hydrolysis of sialic acids with neuraminidase, and the resulting ASOR is as effective a ligand. An added advantage of acid hydrolysis is that the procedure should effectively neutralize any blood-borne contaminants, such as viruses, which may have been carried over during plasma fractionation. In principle, OR is available in large quantities as a byproduct of the plasma fractionation industry, which processes several million liters of plasma a year in the US alone. After the isolation of albumin from fraction V of the classic Cohn process, the resulting supernatant contains OR as one of the main protein components. This OR-enriched fraction serves as a better starting material than whole plasma, and should be more economical.

The polycation of choice in the synthesis of protein ligand-polycation conjugates has been poly-L-lysine, which is commercially available in a range of molecular weights. Two primary strategies have been used for crosslinking ligand and PL: carbodiimide-mediated amide bond formation (Wu and Wu, 1992) and thiol chemistry-based crosslinking (Wu and Wu, 1988a; Wagner, et al., 1990). These conjugation chemistries are well-suited to glycoproteins such as OR since the carbohydrate groups involved in receptor binding are unreactive under these reactions. The resulting product mixtures are typically heterogeneous and require fractionation by one or more chromatographic techniques such as ion-exchange (Wu and Wu, 1992) or gel-filtration (Wu and Wu, 1987; Wagner, et al., 1990) to isolate the desired fraction, which is then used to prepare DNA complexes for functional gene transfer.

An agarose gel retardation assay is used to determine the quantity of purified conjugate required to fully complex a selected DNA plasmid (Wu and Wu, 1988b).

As cationic conjugate is added, the polyanionic phosphodiester backbone of the DNA is progressively neutralized and the DNA's electrophoretic mobility is reduced. The ratio of conjugate to DNA at which the DNA will not migrate in the gel is taken as full complexation, and is used to prepare DNA complex for gene transfer. An alternate approach is to test varying ratios of conjugate and DNA using an in vitro expression assay to select an optimal ratio for complex formation (Wagner, et al., 1990). This latter approach may be useful to probe variations in gene expression obtained in relation to the solubility of complexes observed at or near full retardation.

THE POTENTIAL OF SYNTHETIC LIGANDS IN TARGETED DELIVERY

A relatively undeveloped area is the use of synthetic ligands in targeted gene transfer. The ligand specificity of the ASGPr has been extensively studied, allowing the development of synthetic and semisynthetic ligands (Ashwell and Harford, 1982; Schwartz, 1984). Synthetic ligands of the ASGPr have been developed with binding constants in the subnanomolar range (Lee and Lee, 1987). These studies spurred the development of carbohydrate-modified recombinant murine leukemia virus carrying the gene for β-galactosidase. Expression was observed in ASGPr-positive cells, but not in ASGPr-negative cells, nor in ASGPr-positive cells in the presence of excess ASOR (Neda et al., 1991). In another development, a tetra-galactosyl peptide conjugated to polylysine was used to transfer DNA into hepatocyte-derived cells (Plank et al., 1992). This last result represents the use of a totally synthetic conjugate to carry DNA into receptor-positive cells. The utility of these materials for practical gene transfer will depend in part on the ability to prepare them readily, their targeting efficiency, and their immunogenicity in comparison with naturally derived proteins such as asialoorosomucoid.

Related to the synthetic ligands described above is the use of glycolipids incorporated into liposomes to effect targeted delivery. In one report, lactosyl ceramide containing liposomes were used to carry a plasmid into the liver after intravenous injection into rats (Soriano et al., 1983). In the absence of lactosyl ceramide less than 14% of the plasmid was delivered to the hepatocytes, with over 80% in the Kupffer cells, and 4% in liver endothelial cells. Even with glycolipid, only 19% of the plasmid was delivered to hepatocytes. No results were reported on gene expression. A limitation with this approach appears to be that even with the glycolipid present, inadequate specificity for hepatocytes is observed. Liposomes are by no means inappropriate vehicles for gene delivery, however. The recent report from Debs and coworkers on aerosol gene delivery to the lungs is promising in this regard (Stribling et al., 1992). The liposomes appeared to be effective at transferring their contents to the epithelial and alveolar cells, resulting in gene expression for weeks. Transfer of DNA from liposomes to cells may circumvent the endocytotic pathway, allowing a greater proportion of the DNA to reach the nucleus. Liposome-mediated gene transfer could be a promising technology if the problem of tissue specificity can be resolved.

CONCLUSIONS

Gene therapy can be a powerful strategy for the treatment of inherited or acquired diseases. Most current gene therapy protocols however, are technology-intensive, individualized treatments, putting them out of the reach of the general population. Implementation of gene transfer methods more like traditional drug-based therapies will broaden the scope and impact of this emerging technology. Direct in vivo gene transfer by targeted delivery is one approach to this problem. ASOR-PL-DNA complexes specifically target hepatocytes in vivo and have been shown to effect transgene expression. This DNA formulation exhibits many pharmacologically advantageous characteristics. Further refinement of this strategy involves improving the amount and persistence of gene expression achieved. Using this system as a proof of principal, additional ligand-receptor systems can be developed for other therapies, and to target other tissues.

REFERENCES

Anderson WF (1992): Human gene therapy. *Science* 256:808-813

Arnon R, Sela M (1982): In vitro and in vivo efficacy of conjugates of daunomycin with anti-tumor antibodies. *Immunol Rev* 62:5-27

Ashwell G, Harford J (1982): Carbohydrate-specific receptors of the liver. *Ann Rev Biochem* 51:531-554

Ashwell G, Morell AG (1974): The role of surface carbohydrates in the hepatic recognition and transport of circulating glycoproteins. *Adv Enzymol Relat Areas Mol Biol* 44:99-129

Baümler E (1984): *Paul Ehrlich, Scientist for Life*. New York: Holmes & Meier p. 108

Braslawsky GR, Edson MA, Pearce W, Kaneko T, Greenfield RS (1990): Antitumor activity of adriamycin (hydrazone-linked) immunoconjugates compared with free adriamycin and specificity of tumor cell killing. *Cancer Res* 50:6608-6614

Chowdhury JR, Hays RM, Wu CH, Bommanani VR, Yerneni PC, Mukhopadhyay B, Wu GY, Chowdhury NR (1993): Disruption of microtubules results in prolonged persistence and expression of genes targeted to the liver in vivo by receptor-mediated endocytosis. *Gastroenterology* 104:A981

Cotten M, Längle-Rouault F, Kirlappos H, Wagner E, Mechtler K, Zenke M, Beug H, Birnstiel ML (1990): Transferrin-polycation-mediated introduction of DNA into human leukemic cells: Stimulation by agents that affect the survival of trasnfected DNA or modulate transferrin receptor levels. *Proc Natl Acad Sci USA* 87:4033-4037

Cotten M, Wagner E, Zatloukal K, Phillips S, Curiel DT, Birnstiel ML (1992): High-efficiency receptor-mediated delivery of small and large (48 kilobase) gene constructs using the endosome-disruption activity of defective or chemically inactivated adenovirus particles. *Proc Natl Acad Sci USA* 89:6094-6098

Cristiano RJ, Smith LC, Woo SLC (1993): Hepatic gene therapy: adenovirus enhancement of receptor-mediated gene delivery and expression in primary heaptocytes. *Proc Natl Acad Sci USA* 90:2122-2126

Curiel DT, Agarwal S, Wagner E, Cotten M (1991): Adenovirus enhancement of transferrin-polylysine-mediated gene delivery. *Proc Natl Acad Sci USA* 88: 8850-8854

Ewel CH, Urba WJ, Kopp WC, Smith JW, Steis RG, Rossio JL, Longo DL, Jones MJ, Alvord WG, Pinsky CM, Beveridge JM, McNitt KL, Creekmore SP (1992): Polyinosinic-polycytidylic acid complexed with poly-L-lysine and carboxymethylcellulose in combination with interleukin 2 in patients with cancer: clinical and immunological effects. *Cancer Res* 52:3005-3010

Felgner PL (1993): Genes in a bottle. *Lab Invest* 68:1-3

Findeis MA, Merwin JR, Spitalny GL, Chiou HC (1993): Targeted delivery of DNA for gene therapy via receptors. *Trends Biotechnol* 11:202-205

Freeman AI, Mayhew E (1986): Targeted drug delivery. *Cancer* 58:573-583

Guyton AC (1981): *Medical Physiology*, Philadelphia: W.B. Saunders Company, p. 875

Hartmann D, Schneider MA, Lenz BF, Talmadge JE (1987): Toxicity of polyinosinic-polycytidylic acid admixed with poly-L-lysine and solubilized with carboxymethylcellulose in mice. *Pathol Immunopathol Res* 6:37-50

Homewood CA, Warhurst DC, Peters W, Baggaley VC (1972): Lysosomes, pH and the anti-malarial action of chloroquine. *Nature* 235:50-52

Lampkin BC, Levine AS, Levy H, Krivit W, Hammond D (1985): Phase II trial of a complex polyriboinosinic-polyribocytidylic acid with poly-L-lysine and carboxymethyl cellulose in the treatment of children with acute leukemia and neuroblastoma: a report from the Children's Cancer Study Group. *Cancer Res* 45:5904-5909

Lee RT, Lee YC (1987): Preparation of cluster glycosides of N-acetylgalactosamine that have subnanomolar binding constants towards the mammalian hepatic Gal/GalNAc-specific receptor. *Glycoconjugate J* 4:317-328

Michael SI, Huang C-H, Rømer MU, Wagner E, Hu P-C, Curiel DT (1993): Binding-incompetent adenovirus facilitates molecular conjugate-mediated gene transfer by the receptor-mediated endocytosis pathway. *J Biol Chem* 268:6866-6869

Miller AD (1992): Human gene therapy comes of age. *Nature* 357:455-460

Mulligan RC (1991): Gene transfer and gene therapy: principles, prospects, and perspective. In: *Etiology of Human Disease at the DNA Level*, Lindsten J, Pettersson U, eds. New York:Raven Press, pp 143-189

Mulligan RC (1993): The basic science of gene therapy. *Science* 260:926-932

Neda H, Wu CH, Wu GY (1991): Chemical modification of an ecotropic murine leukemia virus results in redirection of its target cell specificity. *J Biol Chem* 266:14143-14146

Ochsner M, Creba J, Walker J, Bentley P, Muakkassah-Kelly SF (1990): Nafenopin, a hypolipidemic and non-genotoxic hepatocarcinogen increases intracellular calcium and transiently decreases intracellular pH in hepatocytes without generation of inositol phosphates. *Biochem Pharmacol* 40:2247-2257

Orton TC, and Parker GL (1982): The effect of hypolipidemic agents on the hepatic microsomal enzyme systems in the rat. *Drug Metab Dis* 10:110-115

Pastan I, Chaudhary V, FitzGerald DJP (1992): Recombinant toxins as novel therapeutic agents. *Annu Rev Biochem* 61:331-354

Plank C, Zatloukal K, Cotten M, Mechtler K, Wagner E (1992): Gene transfer into hepatocytes using asioaloglycoprotein receptor mediated endocytosis of dna complexed with an artificial tetra-antennary galactose ligand. *Bioconjugate Chem* 3:533-539

Rappaport AM (1987): In: *Diseases of the Liver*, Schiff L, Schiff ER, eds. Philadelphia: J.B. Lippincott Co., p. 22

Rosenfeld MA, Yoshimura K, Trapnell BC, Yoneyama K, Rosenthal ER, Dalemans W, Fukayama M, Bargon J, Stier LE, Stratford-Perricaudet L, Perricaudet M, Guggino WB, Pavirani A, Lecocq J-P, Crystal RG (1992): In vivo transfer of the human cystic fibrosis transmembrane conductance regulator gene to the airway epithelium. *Cell* 68:143-155

Schmid K (1975): In *The Plasma Proteins, Structure, Function, and Genetic Control. 2nd edition*. Putnam FW, ed. New York: Academic Press. Chapter 4

Schmid K, Polis A, Hunziker K, Fricke R, Yayoshi M (1967): Partial characterization of the sialic acid-free forms of a_1-acid glycoprotein from human plasma. *Biochem J* 104:361-368

Schwartz AL (1984): The hepatic asialoglycoprotein receptor. *CRC Crit Rev Biochem* 16:207-233

Schwartz AL (1991): Trafficking of asialoglycoproteins and the asialoglycoprotein receptor. In: *Liver Diseases: Targeted Diagnosis and Therapy Using Specific Receptors and Ligands*, Wu GY, Wu CH, eds. New York: Marcel Dekker, Inc. pp. 3-39

Soriano P, Dijkstra J, Legrand A, Spanjer H, Londos-Gagliardi D, Roerdink F, Scherphof G, Nicolau C (1983): Targeted and non-targeted liposomes for in vivo transfer to rat liver cells of a plasmid containing the preproinsulin I gene. *Proc Natl Acad Sci USA* 80:7128-7131

Spiess M (1990): The asialoglycoprotein receptor: a model for endocytic transport receptors. *Biochemistry* 29:10009-10018

Stribling R, Brunette E, Liggitt D, Gaensler K, Debs R (1992): Aerosol gene delivery in vivo. *Proc Natl Acad Sci USA* 89:11277-11281

Thompson L (1992): At age 2, gene therapy enters a growth phase. *Science* 258:744-746

Vitetta ES (1990): Immunotoxins: New therapeutic reagents for autoimmunity, cancer, and AIDS. *J Clin Immunol* 10:15S-18S

Wagner E, Cotten M, Foisner R, Birnstiel ML (1991): Transferrin-polycation-DNA complexes: the effect of polycations on the structure of the complex and DNA delivery to cells. *Proc Natl Acad Sci USA* 88:4255-4259

Wagner E, Plank C, Zatloukal K, Cotten M, Birnstiel ML (1992b): Influenza virus hemaglutinin HA-2 N-terminal fusogenic peptides augment gene transfer by transferrinpolylysine-DNA complexes: Toward a synthetic virus-like gene-transfer vehicle. *Proc Natl Acad Sci USA* 89:7934-7938

Wagner E, Zatloukal K, Cotten M, Kirlappos H, Mechtler C, Curiel DT, Birnstiel ML (1992a): Coupling of adenovirus to transferrin-polylysine/DNA complexes greatly enhances receptor-mediated gene delivery and expression of transfected genes. *Proc Natl Acad Sci USA* 89:6099-6103

Wagner E, Zenke M, Cotten M, Beug H, Birnstiel ML (1990): Transferrin-polycation conjugates as carriers for DNA uptake into cells. *Proc Natl Acad Sci USA* 87:3410-3414

Whitehead PH, Sammons HG (1966): A simple technique for the isolation of orosomucoid from normal and pathological sera. *Biochim Biophys Acta* 124:209-211

Wilson JM, Grossman M, Wu CH, Chowdhury NR, Wu GY, Chowdhury JR (1992): Hepatocyte-directed gene transfer in vivo leads to transient improvement of hypercholesterolemia in low density lipoprotein receptor-deficient rabbits. *J Biol Chem* 267:963-967

Wong, SS (1993): *Chemistry of Protein Conjugation and Cross-Linking.* Boca Raton: CRC Press

Wu GY, Wilson JM, Shalaby F, Grossman M, Shafritz DA, Wu CH (1991): Receptor-mediated gene delivery in vivo: Partial correction of genetic analbuminemia in Nagase rats. *J Biol Chem* 266:14338-14342

Wu CH, Wilson JM, Wu GY (1989): Targeting genes: delivery and persistent expression of a foreign gene driven by mammalian regulatory elements in vivo. *J Biol Chem* 264:16985-16987

Wu GY, Tangco MV, Wu CH (1990): Targeted gene delivery: persistence of foreign gene expression achieved by pharmacological means. *Hepatology* 12:871

Wu GY, Wu CH (1987): Receptor-mediated in vitro gene transformation by a soluble DNA carrier system. *J Biol Chem* 262:4429-4432

Wu GY, Wu CH (1988a): Receptor-mediated gene delivery and expression in vivo. *J Biol Chem* 263:14621-14624

Wu GY, Wu CH (1988b): Evidence for targeted gene delivery to Hep G2 hepatoma cells in vitro. *Biochemistry* 27:887-892

Wu GY, Wu CH (1992): Specific inhibition of hepatitis B viral gene expression in vitro by targeted antisense oligonucleotides. *J Biol Chem* 267:12436-12439

Wu GW, Zhan P, Rowell DL, Wu CH (1992): Modification of inactivated adenovirus with a targetable DNA carrier enhances foreign gene expression in vitro and in vivo. *Hepatology* 16:112A

Zenke M, Steinlein P, Wagner E, Cotten M, Beug H, Birnstiel ML (1990): Receptor-mediated endocytosis of transferrin-polycation conjugates: An efficient way to introduce DNA into hematopoietic cells. *Proc Natl Acad Sci USA* 87:3655-3659

CALCIUM PHOSPHATE-MEDIATED DNA TRANSFECTION

Patricia L. Chang

INTRODUCTION

The ability to express foreign genes introduced into cultured cells is a powerful tool for studying gene expression. It permits monitoring not only the transcriptional and translational activities of exogenous DNA but also the regulation of gene expression by other genetic elements. Furthermore, the approach to somatic gene therapy is entirely based on introducing genes either to correct a prior genetic defect or to augment the genetic repertoire of the recipient cell. The technology of gene transfer is truly one of the cornerstones in molecular genetics.

Methods for introducing foreign genes can be broadly grouped into four categories: a) direct introduction of cloned DNA (Capecchi, 1980; Zimmermann, 1982; Wu et al., 1989); b) use of viral vectors (Mulligan, 1982; Rosenfeld et al., 1991); c) encapsulation within a carrier system (Straubinger and Papahadjopoulos, 1983; Stewart et al., 1992); and d) use of facilitators such as calcium phosphate (CaPi) (Graham and Van der Eb, 1973) or DEAE-dextran (McCutchan and Pagano, 1968). The more recent developments in the first three categories are reviewed elsewhere in this book. The method for DNA transfection via facilitators, of which CaPi being the most widely used one, will be the subject of review in this chapter.

The earliest facilitator used was the polycationic diethylaminoethyl (DEAE) - dextran (McCutchan and Pagano, 1968). It improved the efficiency of assaying for viral infectivity by replacing the hypotonic salt solutions or dimethylsulfoxide used previously (Black and Rowe, 1965). Soon after this development, Graham and Van der Eb (1973) published their landmark paper on transfecting viral DNA co-precipitated with the facilitator CaPi. Since then, many other facilitators have been used to overcome some of the disadvantages associated with the CaPi technique (Morgan et al., 1986; Brash et al., 1987 ; Bond and Wold, 1987; Appel et al., 1988). However, of all these reagents, CaPi co-precipitation of DNA remains the most widely used because of its simplicity and general effectiveness for a wide variety of cell types (Graham et al., 1980; Chen and Okayama, 1987). This chapter will review the mechanism and the cellular pathways by which CaPi-precipitated DNA is transferred into the cell for eventual expression.

Gene Therapeutics: Methods and Applications of Direct Gene Transfer
Jon A. Wolff, Editor • ©1994 *Birkhäuser Boston*

DEVELOPMENT OF DNA-MEDIATED GENE TRANSFER WITH THE CAPI TECHNIQUE

The original goal of the CaPi technique was to develop an efficient method to assay for infectivity of adenoviral DNA in mammalian cells (Graham and Van der Eb, 1973). The low efficiency of this procedure permitted only one in $10^{3\text{-}5}$ cells to be transformed for stable expression of the transfected gene. Therefore, success in using this method depended on the transfected gene(s) either having some visible phenotype for scoring, e.g. lytic foci after transformation by viral DNA, or encoding a selectable marker such as thymidine kinase, which allowed the transformants to grow in an otherwise toxic medium (Littlefield, 1963). Thus, this method was used initially for studying the infectivity of viral DNA or expression of cloned viral DNA fragments (Bacchetti and Graham, 1977; Wigler et al., 1977; Graham et al., 1980), or total cellular DNA (Wigler et al., 1978) encoding sequences for thymidine kinase. Subsequently, it was shown that genes or total genomic DNA even without any biochemical selection function could be selected after transfection as long as a selectable marker gene was included in the transfecting DNA (Wigler et al., 1979b). The utility of this method of DNA transfection was expanded vastly by allowing for selection and expression of genes which did not encode a biochemically selectable property or visible phenotype.

Several advantages in the CaPi precipitation method account for its enduring popularity (Basolo et al., 1990). It is simple to perform, requires no special apparatus, tolerates a variety of DNA preparations and is effective for many different target cell types. Since its inception, this method has undergone a few minor refinements (Wigler et al., 1979a; Chen and Okayama, 1987) and the technique has been reviewed in great detail elsewhere (Graham et al., 1980; Graham and Bacchetti, 1983; Gorman, 1985; McKinnon and Graham, 1986). Hence, the technical details will not be covered further in this chapter. The readers are referred to these publications for the procedure and Appendix 1 (at the end of this chapter) developed from the above publications for the protocol currently used in our laboratory. This protocol has been applied successfully to the transfection of rat and human primary fibroblasts, mouse Ltk⁻ fibroblasts or their derivatives and mouse myoblasts.

There are also disadvantages inherent to the CaPi method of transfection, namely its cytotoxicity with prolonged exposure, its relative inefficiency, and its inability to transfect certain cell types such as cells that are differentiated (Muller et al., 1990) or grow in suspension (Pahl et al., 1991). The development of this technique has been largely through empirical optimizations of the various steps in the transfection protocol. It is a technique also well known for difficulties in reproducing comparable results from experiment to experiment. However, a few invariant themes have emerged from many studies and are briefly summarized as follows.

Efficiency of gene transfer is clearly dependent on the amount of DNA used, 10-20 µg/100-mm dish being the optimum (Graham and Bacchetti, 1983; DiNocera and Dawid, 1983). Higher or lower amounts of DNA will result in lower efficiency (Berger et al., 1985) but the exact optimal concentration varies with the cell line under study (Chen and Okayama, 1987). The physical condition of the CaPi-DNA precipitate also plays a critical role. Coarse or flocculant precipitate is more effective than cloudy suspensions (Graham and Bacchetti, 1983; Graham et al., 1980; Reeves et al., 1985) but exceptions do occur, depending on the exact transfection conditions (Chen and Okayama, 1987). The physical condition of the precipitate in turn is affected by many conditions (Graham and Van der Eb, 1973; Wigler et al., 1979a; Graham and Bacchetti, 1983; Chen and Okayama, 1987): the relative amount of high-molecular-weight carrier DNA in the transfection mixture (the more carrier, the coarser the precipitate); the pH of the buffer during the precipitation (pH 6.9-7.1 being optimal); and the rate at which the precipitate is formed (slowly, either by bubbling air through the forming precipitate or swirling the dish as the precipitate is being formed).

The conditions used to produce the CaPi-DNA precipitate varied widely among different laboratories (Kjer and Fallon, 1991; Chen and Okayama, 1987). Even within the same laboratory, the conditions could not always be sufficiently controlled to be absolutely reproducible from experiment to experiment (Corsaro and Pearson, 1981; P.L.C., unpublished observation). Furthermore, the cell density at the time of transfection (Graham and Bacchetti, 1983), the cell cycling conditions of the recipient cells (Rippe et al., 1990), the duration of exposure to the precipitated DNA (DiNocera and Dawid, 1983; McKinnon and Graham, 1986; Rippe et al., 1990), the species from which the cells are derived (Burke et al., 1984), the types of tissue from which the cells are derived (Basolo et al., 1990), and the cell lines used (Graham, 1977; Graham et al., 1980; Berger et al., 1985; Burke et al., 1984) all affect the ultimate transfection efficiency.

Because of the many variables, this method of gene transfection ideally should be optimised for the particular cell line under study, particularly when the goal is to quantify transient expression. Hence, the growth conditions of the cells during transfection, the amount of carrier DNA and transfecting DNA, the pH for the precipitate formation, the duration of exposure to the CaPi-DNA precipitate, the use of additional boostering agents such as DMSO (Lewis et al., 1980), glycerol (Basolo et al., 1990), or sodium butyrate (Gorman et al., 1983) all need to be customized. Furthermore, if transfection efficiency and expression levels are to be compared among different input DNA or different cell types, such experiments should be performed at the same time with all other variables being identical. This would minimize the day-to-day variations and render the results more reliable for comparison.

In practice, if the goal is simply to obtain stably transfected cell clones expressing the gene of choice, such optimization is usually not necessary. This is particularly true when adherent cell lines with good growth potential are the target cells for transfection. The technique according to generic protocols such as described by Graham and Bacchetti (1983) usually suffices. In some protocols for somatic gene therapy in which an abundant source of target cells such as fibroblasts is available for gene transfer (Selden et al., 1987; Chang et al., 1990), such customising is rarely necessary. Transfected cells and clonal isolates of stable transformants can be obtained even when the efficiency is as low as 10^{-6} (Chang et al., 1986).

In spite of the variability (Corsaro and Pearson, 1981) , the cytotoxic side-effects in some cell types (Ege et al., 1984; Brash et al., 1987) and low efficiency intrinsic to the CaPi transfection technique, this method has been widely used because it allows the transferred genes to be assayed in many different ways, i.e. transformation potential, transient expression as well as stable integration (McKinnon and Graham, 1986). Consequently, much of the effort in elucidating the mechanism of DNA-mediated transfection has been focused on the CaPi precipitate technique. Even though the details of many intervening steps are not clear still, some general understanding of the cellular and molecular processes leading to the final expression and integration of the CaPi-precipitated DNA has emerged.

MECHANISM OF DNA TRANSFER WITH CAPI

Role of Endocytosis

Most cultured cells engage in constitutive endocytic activities and the endocytic pathway has been well delineated (Besterman et al., 1983; Helenius et al., 1983; Goda and Pfeffer, 1989). DNA macromolecules, among other ligands, are known to be endocytosed in large amounts under some conditions (Szybalska and Szybalski, 1962; Bhargava and Shanmugam, 1971; Farber et al., 1975; Strain and Wyllie, 1984). Addition of calcium ions increased the rate of DNA endocytosis and the efficiency of gene transfer (Loyter et al., 1982a). This was thought to result from the ability of the nascent CaPi to promote fusion between biological membranes and cause local solubilization of phospholipid bilayers (Zakai et al., 1977). The plasma membrane is rendered more fluid to initiate formation of endocytic vesicles (Loyter et al., 1982b). Alternatively, the local partial solubilization of the plasma membrane may permit a facilitated passive diffusion of the DNA molecules directly into the cytosolic intracellular compartments (Loyter et al., 1982b). Hence, CaPi was thought to booster the uptake of exogenous DNA into the cell by either an active endocytic process or a passive diffusion event (Loyter et al., 1982a; Strain, 1987).

The relative importance of these two processes, active endocytosis and passive diffusion, to effect gene transfer and expression was resolved recently (Orrantia et al., 1990). They compared the transient and stable expression of exogenous CaPi-precipitated genes when the endocytic pathway was either functioning or inhibited. When endocytosis was inhibited by ATP-depletion, any DNA-uptake and subsequent gene expression would have been mediated by an energy-independent, and hence passive diffusion process. When this was achieved by feeding the cells with the metabolic inhibitor sodium azide and 2-deoxyglucose, only 2% of the normally-endocytosed DNA was internalized. However, because only 1 in 10^5 internalized DNA molecules was sufficient to account for the ultimate expression, this 2% of passively internalized DNA could have accounted for the effective expression of the CaPi-DNA complex. But this was shown not to be the case. Both transient expression of a *human growth hormone* gene or stable expression of a *G418-resistance* gene in mouse Ltk⁻ cells were reduced to almost background levels when the endocytic pathway was blocked. Therefore, the DNA responsible for transient expression or stable integration must have been transferred through an energy-dependent endocytic pathway.

Transfer of CaPi-DNA from endosome to nucleus

The transit of the internalized DNA between the plasma membrane and the nucleus seemed to occur together with the CaPi as a complex (Loyter et al., 1982a). Stains specific for the DNA (DAPI) and complex salts of calcium (chlorotetracycline) showed co-localization in the same punctate cytoplasmic pattern - consistent with a vesicular distribution of the two components of the CaPi-DNA complex together. For a population of Ltk⁻ Aprt⁻ cells, it appeared that all cells were able to demonstrate endocytic activities. However, because only 1 in 10^3 to 10^5 cells becomes effectively transformed, the ability to endocytose the CaPi-DNA complex is not a sufficient condition for gene expression. When an easily transformed mouse Ltk⁻ cell line with a transfection efficiency of 1 in 10^3 was compared with a transformation-resistant human primary fibroblast cell strain with a transfection efficiency of 1 in 10^6, the rate of endocytosis of exogenous DNA, although elevated about three-fold in the mouse cells (Orrantia, 1990), certainly was not sufficient to account for the 1000-fold increase in transfection efficiency. Hence, both qualitative cytological staining for endocytosed ligands (Loyter et al., 1982a) and quantitative uptake studies (Orrantia et al., 1990) showed that endocytosis is critically important but cannot account totally for successful transfection (Burke et al., 1984; Orrantia, 1990).

It is thus important to understand what happens to the CaPi-DNA complex after its initial entry to the cell. A general belief on the sequence of events was that after endocytosis, in which most cells participate (Loyter et al., 1982a), the endocytic vesicles containing the CaPi-DNA fused with lysosomes (Strain and Wyllie, 1984). This was indirectly supported by the increased efficiency of transfection in the presence of lysosomotropic agents (Fraley et al., 1981; Luthman and Magnusson, 1983; Ege et al., 1984). These reagents interfered with the acidification of the lysosomes by an ATP-driven proton pump and effectively raised the intralysosomal pH (de Duve, 1983). This presumably rendered the lysosomal nucleases less effective in degrading the internalized CaPi-DNA complexes (Strain and Wyllie, 1984). In the presence of the lysosomotropic drugs such as chloroquine, the frequency of gene transfer was significantly increased (Fraley et al., 1981; Luthman and Magnusson, 1983). However, the effect of lysosomotropic agents is open to question because its ability to increase transfection efficiency was not always observed (Ege et al., 1984). The role of lysosomotropic agents such as chloroquine is also subject to debate as it is both a lysosomotropic as well as a DNA-chelating agent (Cohen and Yielding, 1965; Pruitt and Reeder, 1984).

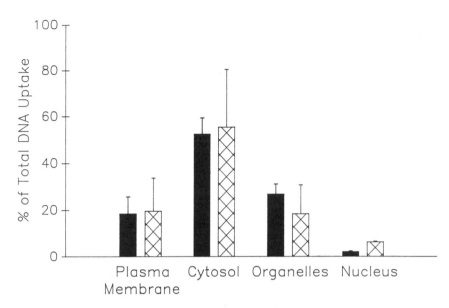

FIGURE 1. Distribution of internalized DNA in subcellular fractions from human and mouse cells. Human primary fibroblasts or mouse Ltk⁻ fibroblasts were transfected with ^{32}P-labelled high-molecular-weight DNA-CaPi precipitate for 4 h and washed stringently with EDTA, micrococcal nuclease and DNase I to remove absorbed DNA. After the cells were disrupted by nitrogen cavitation, the four subcellular fractions were prepared enriched in plasma membrane, cytosol, vesicular organelles (lysosomes, endosomes, mitochondria, microsomes) and nuclei. Acid-precipitable radioactivity in each fraction was monitored and expressed as percentage of the total recovered radioactivity. Adapted with permission of Academic Press from Orrantia and Chang, 1990. ■ : human primary fibroblast; ▨ : mouse Ltk⁻ fibroblast.

If the endocytosed DNA was indeed sequestered in the lysosomes, the entrapped DNA eventually must enter the nucleus. It was thought that the lysosomal DNA could escape somehow from the lysosomes into the cytoplasm and then enter the nuclei of a small proportion of the recipient cells (Loyter et al., 1982a). Alternatively, the CaPi precipitate may facilitate the dissolution of either the phagocytic vesicle membrane or the plasma membrane, allowing the CaPi-DNA precipitate to gain direct access into the cytoplasm and then the nucleus without passing through the endosome-lysosome pathway (Loyter et al., 1982b). Although the overall direction of DNA traffic is probably correct, the supporting evidence is circumstantial, and some of the assumptions have proven incorrect.

There is no doubt that the internalized CaPi-DNA is present in membrane-bound organelles. This was supported qualitatively by the cytoplasmic staining of the DNA complex in a punctate vesicular pattern (Loyter et al., 1982a). Quantitatively, about 40% of internalized DNA was sedimented in two membranous fractions (Fig. 1, Plasma Membrane and Organelles). These fractions were equally

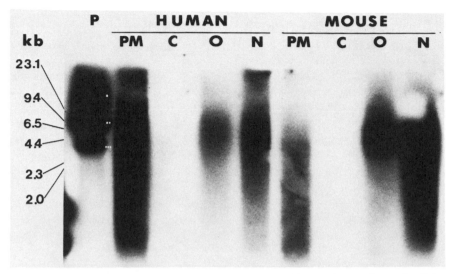

FIGURE 2. Southern blot analysis of internalized plasmid DNA into various subcellular fractions from human and mouse cells. Each 100-mm dish of human primary fibroblasts or mouse Ltk⁻ fibroblasts was transfected with 10 μg of DNA from a 9.6 kb plasmid, pNMG-2, and 10 μg of carrier salmon sperm DNA for 4 h. The cells were then processed for subcellular fractionation. DNA from each fraction was extracted and the integrity of the plasmid DNA was assessed with Southern blot analysis, using pNMG-2 as a probe. Adapted with permission of Academic Press from Orrantia and Chang, 1990. PM: plasma membrane; C: cytosol; O: organelles; N: nuclei; P: plasmid used for transfection, tentatively identified as monomers that were dimerized (•), relaxed (••) and supercoiled (•••). Markers on the left are from λ-HindIII digest.

enriched in marker enzymes for plasma membrane, microsomes and lysosomes (Orrantia and Chang, 1990). The lower density "Organelles" fraction isolated from either mouse or human fibroblasts showed only the intact plasmid DNA used for the CaPi transfection (Fig. 2, fraction O). It is possible that this fraction corresponded to the early endosomes containing the first endocytosed DNA molecules before the endosomes fused with the lysosomes. The biochemically similar but of a higher density "Plasma membrane" fraction contained not only the intact plasmid DNA but also plasmid fragments degraded to a continuous spectrum of sizes to less than 1 kb (Fig. 2, fraction PM). This fraction probably contained the degradative secondary lysosomal compartments whose nucleases were responsible for the DNA hydrolysis.

Apart from the localization of the CaPi-DNA complex in vesicular organelles, it is also widely believed that such a complex must traverse the cytoplasm before entering the nucleus. This was supported by the observation that CaPi-DNA signals from radioactively-labelled DNA were observed in situ in the cytoplasm with electron microscopic autoradiography (Loyter et al., 1982b). This mandatory passage through the cytoplasm was thrown into doubt when it was found that, al-

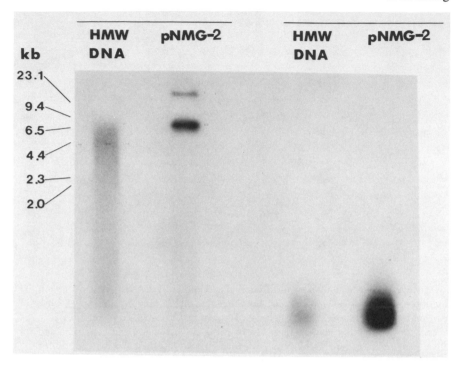

FIGURE 3. Integrity of DNA in the cytosolic fractions. ^{32}P-labelled high-molecular-weight DNA or plasmid DNA was used to transfect mouse Ltk⁻ cells. After a 4h transfection, cells were washed and processed to produce the cytosolic fraction. DNA was extracted, separated by electrophoresis in agarose, transferred to nylon membranes, and examined with autoradiography. Adapted with permission of Academic Press from Orrantia and Chang, 1990. Before: DNA used for transfection; After: DNA recovered from the cytosolic fraction after transfection; HMW DNA: high-molecular-weight DNA; pNMG-2: plasmid DNA tentatively identified as monomers that were (•) dimerized and (••) relaxed. Markers on the left are from λ-*Hind*III digest.

though the cytosolic fraction did contain over 50% of the endocytosed DNA (Fig. 1), all of it was degraded to tiny fragments of less than 100 bp (Fig. 3). It was thus obvious that in order for effective gene expression to occur, intact DNA fragments could not have been in the cytosolic compartment before reaching the nucleus.

On the basis of the above observation, Orrantia and Chang (1990) proposed that for the CaPi-DNA to enter the nucleus, it must have been transferred via some vesicular transport mechanism which allows direct fusion between the vesicle containing the DNA fragments with the nuclear compartment (Fig. 4). It is not known if the endosomal or lysosomal fractions were involved in this fusion. However, since the profile of the plasmid DNA in the nucleus fraction included both intact and partially degraded DNA (Fig. 2, fraction N), it is likely that vesicles derived from secondary lysosomes are responsible for the vesicular transfer of DNA frag-

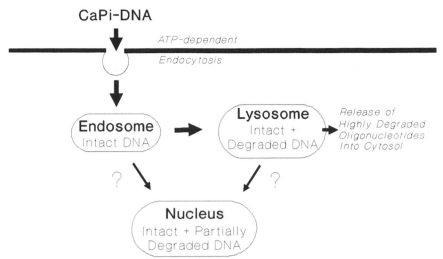

FIGURE 4. Proposed model for transport of CaPi-DNA to the nucleus. CaPi-DNA is internalized through endocytosis which requires ATP. After sequestering in endosomes, it may be delivered to lysosomes where degradation by nucleases occurs. DNA molecules degraded beyond a specific size limit, *eg.* <100 bp, will be excreted through the lysosomal membrane into the cytoplasm. DNA fragments above this size limit are retained in the lysosome. Transfer of DNA macromolecules to the nucleus may occur through intermediary transport vesicles originating from lysosomes and/or endosomes but the exact pathway is unknown. Adapted with permission of Academic Press from Orrantia and Chang, 1990.

ments into the nucleus. Vesicular transport among subcellular organelles in the endocytic pathway has been re-constituted in vitro to show that fusion between endocytic vesicles themselves (Braell, 1987) or between endosomes and lysosomes (Mullock et al., 1989) readily occurred. However, none of the vesicular organelles has been shown to fuse with the nuclear membrane except for the physical continuity between the endoplasmic reticulum and the nuclear membrane. Only two pathways have been identified for targeting into the nucleus. The first was through diffusion *via* the nuclear membrane pores, a process limited to molecules with sizes of 20-60 kDa (Peters et al., 1986; Langford et al., 1986). Another pathway was through nuclear targeting signal sequences (Wolff et al., 1988; Yoneda et al., 1988). They were thought to interact with receptors on the nuclear pore membrane so that larger molecules can pass through (Dworetzky and Feldherr, 1988). The existence of vesicular transport into the nucleus, in contrast, has never been demonstrated. However, the idea of transfer of contents from the endosomal compartment to the nucleus is not totally unfounded. After SV40 viral particles were endocytosed, they were localized in the endoplasmic reticulum, an organelle not previously thought to be acceptors for endosomal contents (Kartenbeck et al., 1989). Since the endoplasmic reticulum was in close proximity with the nucleus and the SV40 viral particles eventually were localized in the nucleus, this pathway may be part of a yet-to-be discovered vesicular transport system leading into the nuclear compartment *via* the endoplasmic reticulum network.

A property of CaPi that may be responsible for increasing the efficiency of gene transfer is its protective role for the DNA against nuclease degradation. When DNA was complexed with the CaPi, it was rendered resistant to serum nuclease digestion (Loyter et al., 1982a), presumably due to formation of a tight complex between the DNA and the calcium ions. If the calcium was removed by chelation with EDTA, some of the DNA then became susceptible to nuclease degradation again (Loyter et al., 1982b). Hence, the CaPi-DNA could be protected from the nucleases. However, this protection was not complete. SV40 DNA digested with DNase I in the presence of CaPi still was converted from the supercoiled and nicked circular relaxed forms into linearized forms (Strain and Wyllie, 1984), showing that slight degradative changes still could occur. Nevertheless, the protection provided by the CaPi precipitate was thought to contribute to the efficiency of gene transfer by increasing the structural integrity of the internalised DNA on its arrival to the nuclei. However, this role for CaPi in DNA transfection has not been verified with direct experimental evidence.

What happens in the nucleus

Although all cells were observed to engage in endocytosis, autoradiographic studies showed that only 20% of transfected cells expressed a transfected *gpt* gene (Burke et al., 1984), and only 1-5% of the cells incorporated the exogenous CaPi-DNA complexes into their nuclei (Loyter et al., 1982a). Therefore, only a small fraction of the recipient cells seemed to be competent for transcription and integration of exogenous DNA. This was supported by the observation that, on co-transfection with two unlinked genes, both genes tended to be either integrated into the same clones or not integrated at all (Wigler et al., 1979b). Thus, when a mouse thymidine kinase-negative cell line was co-transfected with the non-selectable øX DNA, of the 16 thymidine kinase-positive clones, 15 also had integrated the øX sequences. In contrast, when 15 clones were picked at random without selecting for thymidine kinase activity, none showed any sequences from the øX genome (Wigler et al., 1979b). This is consistent with the interpretation that if the cell internalizing the exogenous DNA is competent for transformation, genes present in the input DNA have a high probability of being integrated simultaneously even if they are not physically linked. In contrast, if the cell internalizing the exogenous DNA is not in a competent state, integration of the input genes, either independently or together, is unlikely to occur. In addition, this state of competence is not a heritable trait of a particular cell clone. Clones that have integrated exogenous DNA were not necessarily more competent in subsequent rounds of transfections (Wigler et al., 1979b).

Transient expression in the short term (within days of transfection) differs substantially from stable integration in the long term (weeks and months) in several important aspects. These include the conformation acquired by the input DNA,

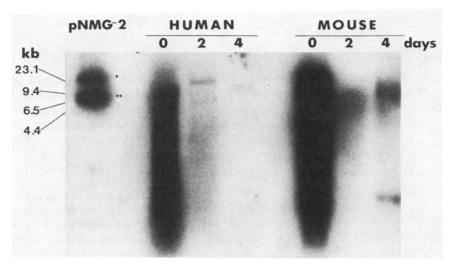

FIGURE 5. Loss of internalized plasmid DNA in the enriched nuclear fractions from human and mouse cells at various times post-transfection. After transfection for 4 h with DNA from a 9.6 kb plasmid pNMG-2, enriched nuclear fractions were prepared from 5 x 100mm-dishes of either a primary human fibroblast cell strain (Human) or a mouse Ltk⁻ transformed cell line (Mouse) on 0, 2, and 4 days post-transfection. DNA was extracted, separated by electrophoresis and transferred to nylon membranes for Southern blot analysis with a radioactive pNMG-2 probe at 10^7cpm/µg. The band at the mouse lane 4 in the very small molecular weight range was an artifact as it was not seen in replicate experiments. Adapted with permission from Orrantia, 1990. pNMG-2: plasmid DNA used for transfection. Markers on the left are from λ-*Hind*III digest.

the replication status of the exogenous DNA and the mechanisms leading to the two modes of expression.

Shortly after transfection within the first few days, transfected DNA remained in an extrachromosomal state (Sinclair et al., 1983) and was not replicated (Burke et al., 1984). The evidence for this came from several laboratories showing that the plasmid DNA remained in its original form and was not integrated into high-molecular weight chromosomal DNA (Sinclair et al., 1983; Orrantia and Chang, 1990). When a methylated version of the plasmid DNA was introduced into recipient cells which did not methylate DNA, the plasmid DNA remained uncut by methylation-sensitive restriction enzymes, thus showing that the exogenous DNA has not been replicated by the host DNA polymerase.

Not only that the extrachromosomal DNA was not replicated, it was also rapidly lost (Sinclair et al., 1983). This loss coincided with loss of DNA from the cell and specifically from the nuclear fractions (Fig. 5). It is noteworthy that in spite of the rapid loss, a significant amount of endocytosed plasmid DNA in its intact form is recoverable from the nuclear fraction of the easily transfected mouse Ltk⁻ cell line even 4 days after transfection. In the same compartment of the transfection-

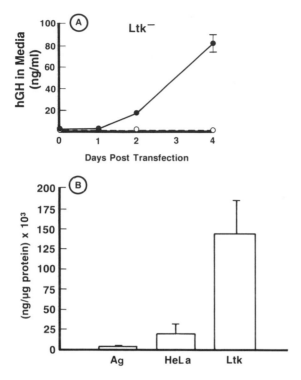

FIGURE 6. Transient expression of human growth hormone in transfected cells. Human primary fibroblasts, transformed human HeLa cells, or mouse Ltk⁻ fibroblasts were transfected with the plasmid pNMG-2 encoding the *human growth hormone* gene. Aliquots of the culture media were removed on various days post-transfection for radioimmunoassay of hGH. Controls were transfected with 20 μg of salmon sperm DNA. Adapted with permission from Orrantia, 1990). A. Ltk⁻: transformed mouse fibroblasts; ●——● = transfected; ○– –○ = control. B. On day 4 post-transfection, cells were harvested to assay for total cell proteins and the media was assayed for human growth hormone.

resistant human primary fibroblast, negligible amount of plasmid DNA was recovered (Fig. 5). In some cases, the early loss was correlated with quickly diminishing levels of transient expression from transfected genes such as those encoding chloramphenicol acetyl-transferase (Kjer and Fallon, 1991), xanthine guanine phosphoribosyl transferase (*gpt*) (Sinclair et al., 1983) and luciferase (Rippe et al., 1990). After peaking at about 96 hr, expression of the transfected *gpt* decreased to <50% by ~130 hr and to background levels by 4-6 days post-transfection (Burke et al., 1984; Kjer and Fallon, 1991). However, this early peaking was not invariable. The transcription and translation competence of a cell line also depended on the cell type, the vectors used (Burke et al., 1984; Chen and Okayama, 1987), and the exact transfection conditions (Rippe et al., 1990). In other cases, such as the mouse Ltk⁻ cells transfected with a *human growth hormone* gene driven by a mouse metallothionein promoter, the level of human growth hormone produced increased almost linearly up to day 4 (Fig. 6A) even as the DNA in the nuclear fraction was diminishing beginning from day 2 post-transfection (Fig. 5). Hence, even though the exogenous DNA at these early times was not integrated into the chromosome, the persistence of transient gene expression was not always correlated simply with the amount of DNA retained. It depended on the target cell line, the promoter and enhancers used (Burke et al., 1984; Weintraub et al., 1986), and the transfection conditions (Rippe et al., 1990).

The topology of the exogenous DNA may play an important role in regulating its expression. In spite of its extrachromosomal state, 60-70% of the incoming plasmid DNA in the nuclear compartment can assemble into chromatin (Weintraub et al., 1986; Reeves et al., 1985) and incorporate into minichromosomes with a typical nucleosomal repeat of about 190 bp (Reeves et al., 1985). While assembly into chromatin may not be sufficient to elicit gene expression, it may be a prerequisite for subsequent acquisition of an active chromatin conformation open for transcription. Evidence for this came from direct oocyte injection of plasmid DNA (Mertz, 1982). When circular SV40 DNA was microinjected, it was reconstituted into a regularly spaced nucleosomal form of negatively supercoiled chromatin. Transcription of this form of exogenous DNA was several orders of magnitude more efficient than microinjection of the linearized version that failed to assemble into minichromosome structures. It is possible that in order for the exogenous DNA to interact with appropriate transcription factors and RNA polymerase, it needs to assume an organized conformation provided within the chromatin such that it is open for transcription. This hypothesis is supported by the fact that the histones associated with the open and nuclease-sensitive form of the minichromosomes containing the exogenous DNA were typically those enriched in actively transcribed chromatin (Reeves et al., 1985).

The importance of the topology of the incoming DNA being in a supercoiled conformation and the efficiency with which supercoiled rather than linearized plasmid DNA can function as templates for gene expression are attributed to their interaction with limiting transcription factors. It was postulated that the supercoiling permitted a more efficient interaction between the host cell transcription factors with the promoters on the incoming DNA, thus leading to a higher level of expression (Weintraub et al., 1986).

The events during the early phase of transient expression can be summarised as follows. About 5% of the endocytosed CaPi-DNA complexes, together with partially degraded DNA fragments, became sequestered in the nucleus within the first day of transfection. A fraction of the intact DNA was assembled into chromatin nucleosomes, while most of the DNA and all the partially degraded fragments were completely lost by day 2 post-transfection. Assembly into the transcriptionally active form of chromatin might be pre-requisite for gene expression and supercoiled DNA was more effective than linearised plasmid DNA in enhancing the transcriptional activity of the template. However, the relative efficacy of supercoiled vs. linearized plasmid DNA may be subject to the experimental conditions used (S. Bacchetti, pers. comm.). During this early phase within the first week of transfection, the exogenous DNA remained extra-chromosomal and non-replicated. In addition, it was rapidly degraded and lost from the nuclear compartment. The level of transient expression was usually correspondingly diminished but exceptions also occurred (Fig. 6A) as this might be characteristic of the specific promoter and cell lines used.

An important difference between transient expression and stable integration of CaPi-DNA mediated gene transfer is the status of the DNA. When a gene is stably expressed, it no longer remains in an extra-chromosomal state. Instead, it is incorporated into the high-molecular weight chromosomal DNA with a chromatin structure typical of the host DNA (Camerini-Otero and Zasloff, 1980). In one reported study, large number of gene copies (1000-3000 per cell) was incorporated as head-to-tail tandem repeats (Bourouis and Jarry, 1983). However, this is not always the case. Low copy number (1-6) copies of integrated sequences were obtained when primary rat fibroblasts (Chang et al., 1990) or various established cell lines were transfected with the CaPi technique (P.L.C., unpublished observation; Chen and Okayama, 1987). In another report, gene rearrangement also occurred when the exogenous gene did not carry its own usable promoter (Sinclair et al., 1983).

Although it is reasonable to speculate that successful transient expression should facilitate eventual stable integration of the transgene, the correlation is not always present. It has been observed repeatedly that high transient expression level did not always lead to a similarly enhanced rate of stable integration. Hence, while the level of transient expression of a *human growth hormone* transgene was in the order of mouse Ltk⁻ > HeLa > human primary fibroblasts (Fig. 6B), the stable integration of a *neo^R* gene present in the same plasmid transfected at the same time resulted in a frequency of stable integration in the order of HeLa > Ltk⁻ > human primary fibroblasts (Table I). Obviously, the mechanisms leading to stable integration of a transgene introduced through CaPi precipitation are not totally identical to those required for transient expression. That the two processes are mediated through different mechanisms is indirectly supported by the empirical observation that transfection techniques leading to efficient transient expression do not always produce stable transformants. A good example is the DNA-mediated transfection using DEAE-dextran as facilitator. This method usually produces transient expression levels higher than that by CaPi precipitation. However, it is seldom effective in producing stable integration of the transgene (Sussman and Milman, 1984; Lopata et al., 1984; Reeves et al., 1985).

TABLE 1. Stable integration of NEO^R gene in different cell lines.

	Mouse Ltk⁻	HeLa	Human fibroblasts
	(No. x 10^{-3} resistant colonies/10^6 cells)		
Expt. 1	2.1 ± 1.0	n.d.	0.0004 ± 0.0004
Expt. 2	37.9 ± 16.5	92.8 ± 9.6	n.d.
Expt. 3	9.3 ± 2.4	189 ± 24	n.d.

n.d.: not determined. Culture cells (1.5 x 10^6/plate) were transfected with 10 µg of pNMG-2 and 10 µg of carrier high-molecular-weight salmon sperm DNA per plate with the CaPi precipitation method. Following a 4 h incubation at 37°C, cells were washed, glycerol shocked, refed with normal media and then seeded at lower density for selection with G418 for NEO^R expression. After 3 weeks, colonies were stained and counted. Adapted with permission from Orrantia, 1990.

Summary

Several factors are important for successful expression and integration of CaPi-precipitated DNA. Supercoiled DNA formed into a CaPi precipitate under empirically defined conditions should be used. A high rate of endocytic activity of the recipient cell is critical but not sufficient for transfection. The successful transfer of the internalized DNA from the endocytic compartment into the nucleus without degradation is also important. The transfer is not mediated by DNA traversing the cytosolic compartment *per se* but the DNA probably entered the nuclei via some intermediary vesicular transport. After entry into the nuclear compartment, prolonged retention and incorporation into chromatin are also associated with successful gene expression. The ultimate level of expression should reflect characteristics of the incoming DNA, the promoters and enhancers used, as well as the cell line used as recipients.

COMPARISON WITH OTHER DNA-MEDIATED GENE TRANSFER TECHNIQUES

In spite of the enduring popularity of the CaPi technique and considerable understanding of some of the cellular mechanisms responsible for the expression of CaPi-precipitated DNA, this method is not without its short-comings. For example, it is toxic to certain cell types, the efficiency of transformation is usually low, and some cell types such as myeloid cell lines (Pahl et al., 1991), pherochromocytoma cells (Muller et al., 1990) and mosquito cells (Fallon, 1986) are resistant to this method of gene transfer. Consequently, many different methods, some similar to, some drastically different from this procedure have been developed over the years. A variation of the CaPi precipitation was to substitute strontium for calcium (Basolo et al., 1990). This was reported to decrease the toxicity of the procedure and result in higher efficiency of gene transfer. Another variation was to use polybrene (Fallon, 1986), polyornithine (Farber et al., 1975; Bond and Wold, 1987), lipofectin (Felgner et al., 1987) or DEAE-dextran (McCutchan and Pagano, 1968; Lopata et al., 1984) instead of CaPi. These methods have been reported to give higher efficiency of transfection, and more reproducible results. Cell lines resistant to CaPi transfection were sometimes amenable to transfection through these alternate techniques. The exact mechanisms whereby these methods introduce DNA are not clear, other than that they must first be mediated through some endocytic event and that they have varying efficiencies for transient or stable integration of exogenous DNA.

Other more fundamentally different approaches include direct microinjection of DNA (Capecchi, 1980), electroporation (Zimmermann, 1982) and conjugation of DNA through polylysine linkage to ligands which enter the recipient cells *via* receptor-mediated endocytosis (Wu et al., 1989; Curiel et al., 1992). Direct injection of DNA is still commonly used for expression in oocytes, and has been applied in the development of somatic gene therapy (*see* chapter by Wolff). It has the advantage that all treated cells are assured of receiving the designated DNA fragments and is free from problems of toxicity of the carrier/ facilitator and virulence of the vectors. The disadvantage is that it is labour-intensive and becomes impractical when large number of cells are to be injected. The level of expression still needs to be improved for it to become a feasible therapeutic application. Electroporation by subjecting the cells to a high voltage discharge has been used successfully for gene transfection in cell lines that were anchorage-independent and recalcitrant to CaPi transfection (Potter et al., 1984). It has the advantages of being simple, reproducible, and suitable for many cell types that are either anchorage-dependent or growing in suspension. The disadvantage is that it can be a highly cytotoxic procedure for the cells. The protocol has to be truly optimised for each cell line to ensure an acceptable compromise between effective DNA transfer and cell survival.

CONCLUSIONS

Most of the currently approved clinical protocols for human gene therapy rely on viral vectors to transduce exogenous DNA into autologous cells derived from the recipient. The target cells are limited mainly to lymphocytes, hepatocytes and bone marrow cells. Because of the relatively restricted life-span or quantity of the target cells, a highly efficient method of gene transduction such as provided by the viral vectors is critical for success. Methods of DNA-mediated gene transfection such as that by CaPi are far less efficient. They are not anticipated to play any significant role in the first round of human gene therapy. However, as more efficient and cost-effective methods of gene therapy are developed, particularly the use of explantable tissue such as fibroblasts with a potentially unlimited supply, nonviral DNA-mediated gene transfer may be the method of choice. Methods of DNA-mediated gene transfer are relatively simple to perform. More important, their innocuous nature may be considered less of a risk factor for long-term safety. Chemical reagents such as CaPi are physiological constituents that are unlikely to elicit undesirable somatic changes such as those attributed to viral vectors (Pathak and Temin, 1991a,b; Donahue et al., 1992). An added advantage is that, unlike virally transduced cells, stable transfected cell strains can be thoroughly characterized before implantation. With our increasing understanding of the mechanisms by which gene transfer is effected through such chemical means and the developing repertoire of alternative cell types for somatic gene therapy, it may be time to consider the advantages they have to offer, and to exploit them more fully for therapeutic purposes in the near future.

ACKNOWLEDGMENT

Support from the Ontario Mental Health Foundation, Medical Research Council and the National Science and Engineering Research Council of Canada, and helpful comments on the manuscript by Drs. S. Bacchetti and J.R. Smiley are gratefully acknowledged.

REFERENCES

Appel JD, Fasy TM, Kohtz DS, Kohtz, JD, Johnson EM (1988): Asbestos fibers mediate transformation of monkey cells by exogenous plasmid DNA. *Proc Natl Acad Sci USA* 85:7670-7674

Bacchetti S, Graham FL (1977): Transfer of the gene for thymidine kinase to thymidine kinase-deficient human cells by purified herpes simplex viral DNA. *Proc Natl Acad Sci USA* 74:1590-1594

Basolo F, Elliott J, Russo J (1990): Transfection of human breast epithelial cells with foreign DNA using different transfecting techniques. *Tumori* 76:455-460

Berger EM, Marino G, Torrey D (1985): Expression of Drosophila hsp 70-Cat hybrid gene in *Aedes* cells induced by heat shock. *Som Cell Mol Genet* 11:371-377

Besterman JM, Low RB (1983): Endocytosis: a review of mechanisms and plasma membrane dynamics. *Biochem J* 210:1-13

Bhargava PM, Shanmugam G (1971): Uptake of nonviral nucleic acids by mammalian cells. *Nuc Acids Res Mol Biol* 11:103-192

Black PH, Rowe WP (1965): Increase of malignant potential of BHK-21 cells by SV40 DNA without persistant new antigen. *Proc Natl Acad Sci USA* 54:1126-1133

Bond CV, Wold B (1987): Poly-L-ornithine-mediated transformation of mammalian cells. *Mol Cell Biol* 7:2286-2293

Bourouis M, Jarry B (1983): Vectors containing a prokaryotic dihydrofolate reductase gene transform *Drosophila* cells to methotrexate-resistance. *EMBO J* 2:1099-1104

Braell WA (1987): Fusion between endocytic vesicles in a cell-free system. *Proc Natl Acad Sci USA* 77:3870-3874

Brash DE, Reddel RR, Quanrud M, Yang K, Farrell MP, Harris CC (1987): Strontium phosphate transfection of human cells in primary culture: stable expression of the simian virus 40 large-T-antigen gene in primary human bronchial epithelial cells. *Mol Cell Biol* 7:2031-2034

Burke JF, Sinclair JH, Sang JH, Ish-Horowicz D (1984): An assay for transient gene expression in transfected *Drosophila* cells, using [³H]guanine incorporation. *EMBO J* 3:2549-2554

Camerini-Otero RD, Zasloff MA (1980): Nucleosomal packaging of the thymidine kinase gene of herpes simplex virus transferred into mouse cells: an actively expressed single-copy gene. *Proc Natl Acad Sci USA* 77:5079-5083

Capecchi MR (1980): High efficiency transformation by direct microinjection of DNA into cultured mammalian cells. *Cell* 22:479-488

Chang PL, Gunby JL, Tomkins DJ, Mak I, Rosa NE, Mak S (1986): Transformation of human cultured fibroblasts with plasmids carrying dominant selection markers and immortalizing potential. *Exp Cell Res* 167:407-416

Chang PL, Capone JP, Brown GM (1990): Autologous fibroblast implantation-feasibility and potential problems in gene replacement therapy. *Mol Biol Med*

7:461-470

Chen C, Okayama H (1987): High-efficiency transformation of mammalian cells by plasmid DNA. *Mol Cell Biol* 7:2745-2752

Cohen SN, Yielding KL (1965): Spectrophotometric studies of the interaction of chloroquine with deoxyribonucleic acid. *J Biol Chem* 240:3123-3131

Corsaro CM, Pearson ML (1981): Enhancing the efficiency of DNA-mediated gene transfer in mammalian cells. *Som Cell Genet* 7:603-616

Curiel DT, Wagner E, Cotten M, Birnstiel ML, Agarwal S, Li C-M, Loechel S, Hu P-C (1992): High-efficiency gene transfer mediated by adenovirus coupled to DNA-polylysine complexes. *Hum Gene Ther* 3:147-154

de Duve C (1983): Lysosomes revisited. *Eur J Biochem* 137:391-397

DiNocera PP, Dawid IB (1983): Transient expression of genes introduced into cultured cells of Drosophila. *Proc Natl Acad Sci USA* 80:7095-7098

Donahue RE, Kessler SW, Bodine D, McDonagh K, Dunbar C, Goodman S, Agricola B, Byrne E, Raffeld M, Moen R, Bacher J, Zsebo KM, Nienhuis AW (1992): Helper virus induced T cell lymphoma in nonhuman primates after retroviral mediated gene transfer. *J Exp Med* 176:1125-1135

Dworetzky SI, Feldherr CM (1988): Translocation of RNA-coated gold particles through the nuclear pores of oocytes. *J Cell Biol* 106:575-584

Ege T, Reisbig RR, Rogne S (1984): Enhancement of DNA-mediated gene transfer by inhibitors of autophagic-lysosomal function. *Exp Cell Res* 155:9-16

Fallon AM (1986): Factors affecting polybrene-mediated transfection of cultured *Aedes albopictus* (Mosquito) cells. *Exp Cell Res* 166:535-542

Farber FE, Melnick JL, Butel JSA (1975): Optimal conditions for uptake of exogenous DNA by Chinese-Hamster lung cells deficient in hypoxanthine-guanine phosphoribosyltransferase. *Biochim Biophys Acta* 390:298-311

Felgner PL, Gadek TR, Holm M, Roman R, Chan HW, Wenz M, Northrop JP, Ringold GM, Danielsen M (1987): Lipofection: a highly efficient, lipid-mediated DNA-transfection procedure. *Proc Natl Acad Sci USA* 84:7413-7417

Fraley R, Straubinger RM, Rule G, Springer EL, Papahadjopoulos D (1981): Liposome-mediated delivery of deoxyribonucleic acid to cells: enhanced efficiency of delivery related to lipid composition and incubation conditions. *Biochemistry* 20:6978-6987

Goda Y, Pfeffer SR (1989): Cell-free systems to study vesicular transport along the secretory and endocytic pathways. *FASEB* 3:2488-2495

Goldstein S, Fordis CM, Howard BH (1989): Enhanced transfection efficiency and improved cell survival after electroporation of G2/M-synchronized cells and treatment with sodium butyrate. *Nuc Acids Res* 17:3959-3971

Gorman C, Padmanabhan R, Howard B (1983): High efficiency DNA-mediated transformation of primate cells. *Science* 221:551-553

Gorman C (1985): High efficiency gene transfer into mammalian cells. In: *DNA cloning - a practical approach*. Glover DM, ed. IRL Press, Oxford. Vol II, Chapter 6, pp. 143-190

Graham FL, Van der Eb AJ (1973): A new technique for the assay of infectivity of human adenovirus 5 DNA. *Virology* 52:456-467

Graham FL (1977): Biological activity of tumor virus DNA. In: *Advances in Cancer Research*. Klein G, Weinhouse S, eds., Academic Press, New York, pp. 1-51

Graham FL, Bacchetti S, McKinnon R, Stanners C, Cordell B, Goodman HM (1980): Transformation of mammalian cells with DNA using the calcium technique. In: *Introduction of Macromolecules into Viable Mammalian Cells*. Baserga R, Croce C, Rovera G, eds., Alan R. Liss Inc., New York, pp. 3-25

Graham FL, Bacchetti S (1983): DNA mediated gene transfer using the calcium technique. *Nucl Acid Biochem* B506:1-14

Helenius A, Mellman I, Wall D, Hubbard A (1983): Endosomes. *TIBS* 7:245-250

Kartenbeck J, Stukenbrok H, Helenius A (1989): Endocytosis of Simian virus 40 into the endoplasmic reticulum. *J Cell Biol* 109:2721-2729

Kjer KM, Fallon AM (1991): Efficient transfection of mosquito cells is influenced by the temperature at which DNA-calcium phosphate coprecipitates are prepared. *Arch Insect Biochem Physiol* 16:189-200

Langford RE, Kanda P, Kennedy RC (1986): Induction of nuclear transport with a synthetic peptide homologous to the SV40 T antigen transport signal. *Cell* 46:575-582

Lewis WH, Srinivasan PR, Stokoe N, Siminovitch L (1980): Parameters governing the transfer of the genes for thymidine kinase and dihydrofolate reductase into mouse cells using metaphase chromosomes or DNA. *Som Cell Genet* 6:333-347

Littlefield, J (1963): The inosinic acid pyrophosphorylase activity of mouse fibroblasts partially resistant to 8-azaguanine. *Proc Nat Acad Sci USA* 50:568-573

Lopata MA, Cleveland DW , Sollner-Webb B (1984): High level transient expression of a chloramphenicol acetyl transferase gene by DEAE-dextran mediated DNA transfection coupled with a dimethyl sulfoxide or glycerol shock treatment. *Nuc Acids Res* 12:5707-5717

Loyter A, Scangos GA, Ruddle FH (1982a): Mechanisms of DNA uptake by mammalian cells-fate of exogenously added DNA monitored by the use of fluorescent dyes. *Proc Natl Acad Sci USA* 79:422-426

Loyter A, Scangos G, Juricek D, Keene D, Ruddle FH (1982b): Mechanisms of DNA Entry into Mammalian Cells II. Phagocytosis of Calcium Phosphate DNA Co-precipitate Visualized by Electron Microscopy. *Exp Cell Res* 139:223-234

Luthman H, Magnusson G (1983): High efficiency polyoma DNA transfection of chloroquine treated cells. *Nuc Acids Res* 11:1295-1308

McCutchan JH, Pagano JS (1968): Enhancement of the infectivity of Simian Virus 40 deoxyribonucleic acid with diethyl-aminoethyl-dextran. *J Natl Cancer Inst* 41:351-356

McKinnon RD, Graham FL (1986): Transformation of mammalian cells with DNA using the calcium technique. In: *Microinjection and Organelle Transplantation Technique*. Celis JE, Graessmann A, Loyter A, eds. Academic Press, San

Diego, CA, pp. 199-236

Mertz J (1982): Linear DNA does not form chromatin containing regularly spaced nucleosomes. *Molec Cell Biol* 2:1608-1618

Morgan TL, Maher VM, McCormick JJ (1986): Optimal parameters for the polybrene-induced DNA transfection of diploid human fibroblasts. *In Vitro Cell Dev Biol* 22:317-319

Muller SR, Sullivan PD, Clegg DO, Feinstein SC (1990): Efficient transfection and expression of heterologous genes in PC12 cells. *DNA Cell Biol* 9:221-229

Mulligan RC (1982): Development of new mammalian transducing vectors In: *Eukaryotic Viral Vectors.* Gluzman Y, ed. Cold Spring Harbor Laboratory, Cold Spring Harbor, NY, pp. 133-137

Mullock BM, Branch WJ, van Schaik M, Gilbert LK, Luzio JP (1989): Reconstitution of an endosome-lysosome interaction in a cell-free system. *J Cell Biol* 108:2093-2099

Orrantia E (1990): Internalization of exogenous DNA through calcium phosphate precipitation. MSc Thesis, McMaster University, Hamilton, Ontario

Orrantia E, Chang PL (1990): Intracellular distribution of DNA internalized through calcium phosphate precipitation. *Exp Cell Res* 190:170-174

Orrantia E, Li Z, Chang PL (1990): Energy dependence of DNA-mediated gene transfer and expression. *Som Cell Mol Genet* 16:305-310

Pahl HL, Burn TC, Tenen DG (1991): Optimization of transient transfection into human myeloid cell lines using a luciferase reporter gene. *Exp Hematol* 19:1038-1041

Pathak VK, Temin HM (1991a): Broad spectrum of in vivo forward mutations, hypermutations, and mutational hotspots in a retroviral shuttle vector after a single replication cycle-Substitutions, frameshifts and hypermutations. *Proc Natl Acad Sci USA* 87:6019-6023

Pathak VK, Temin HM (1991b): Broad spectrum of in vivo forward mutations-hypermutations, and mutational hotspots in a retroviral shuttle vector after a single replication cycle-Deletions and deletions with insertions. *Proc Natl Acad Sci USA* 87:6024-6028

Peters R, Lang I, Scholz M, Schulz B, Kayne F (1986): Fluorescence microphotolysis to measure nucleocytoplasmic transport in vivo et vitro. *Biochem Soc Trans* 14:821-822

Potter H, Weir L, Leder P (1984): Enhancer-dependent expression of human K immunoglobulin genes introduced into mouse pre-B lymphocytes by electroporation. *Proc Natl Acad Sci USA* 81:7161-7165

Pruitt SC, Reeder RH (1984): Effect of intercalating agents on RNA polymerase I promoter selection in *Xenopus laevis. Mol Cell Biol* 4:2851-2857

Reeves R, Gorman CM, Howard B (1985): Minichromosome assembly of non-integrated plasmid DNA transfected into mammalian cells. *Nucl Acids Res* 13:3599-3615

Rippe RA, Brenner DA, Leffert HL (1990): DNA-Mediated gene transfer into adult rat hepatocytes in primary culture. *Mol Cell Biol* 10:689-695

Rosenfeld MA, Siegfried W, Yoshimura K, Yoneyama K, Fukayama M, Stier LE, Pääkkö PK, Gilardi P, Stratford-Perricaudet LD, Perricaudet M, Jallat S, Pavirani A, Lecocq J-P, Crystal RG (1991): Adenovirus-mediated transfer of a recombinant α1-antitrypsin gene to the lung epithelium in vivo. *Science* 252:431-434

Selden RF, Skoskiewicz MJ, Howie KB, Russell PS, Goodman HM (1987): Implantation of genetically engineered fibroblasts into mice-implications for gene therapy. *Science* 236:714-718

Sinclair JH, Sang JH, Burke JF Ish-Horowicz D (1983): Extrachromosomal replication of *copia*-based vectors in cultured *Drosophila* cells. *Nature* 306:198-200

Stewart MJ, Plautz GE, Del Buono L, Yang ZY, Xu L, Gao X, Huang L, Nabel EG, Nabel GJ (1992): Gene transfer in vivo with DNA-liposome complexes: Safety and acute toxicity in mice. *Hum Gene Ther* 3:267-275

Strain AJ, Wyllie AH (1984): The uptake and stability of simian-virus-40 DNA after calcium phosphate transfection of CV-1 cells. *Biochem J* 218:475-482

Strain AJ (1987): The uptake and fate of DNA transfected into mammalian cells in vitro. *Develop Biol Std* 68:27-32

Straubinger RM, Papahadjopoulos D (1983): Liposomes as carriers for intracellular delivery of nucleic acids. *Meth Enzym* 101:512-527

Sussman DJ, Milman G (1984): Short-term, high efficiency expression of transfected DNA. *Molec Cell Biol* 4:1641-1643

Szybalska EH, Szybalski W (1962): Genetics of human cell lines IV. DNA-mediated heritable transformation of a biochemical trait. *Proc Natl Acad Sci USA* 48:2026-2034

Weintraub H, Cheng PF, Conrad K (1986): Expression of transfected DNA depends on DNA topology. *Cell* 46:115-122

Wigler M, Silverstein S, Lee L-S, Pellicer A, Cheng Y-C, Axel R (1977): Transfer of purified herpes virus thymidine kinase gene to cultured mouse cells. *Cell* 11:223-232

Wigler M, Pellicer A, Silverstein S, Axel R (1978): Transfer of single copy eucaryotic genes using total cellular DNA as donor. *Cell* 14:725-731

Wigler M, Pellicer A, Silverstein S, Axel R, Urlaub G, Chasin L (1979a): DNA-mediated transfer of the APRT locus into mammalian cells. *Proc Natl Acad Sci USA* 76:1373-1376

Wigler M, Sweet R, Kee Sim G, Wold B, Pellicer A, Lacy E, Maniatis T, Silverstein S, Axel R (1979b): Transformation of Mammalian Cells with Genes from Procaryotes and Eucaryotes. *Cell* 16:777-785

Wolff B, Willingham MC, Hanover JA (1988): Nuclear protein import: specificity for transport across the nuclear pore. *Exp Cell Res* 178:318-334

Wu CH, Wilson JM, Wu GY (1989): Targeting genes-delivery and persistent expression of a foreign gene driven by mammalian regulatory elements in vivo. *J Biol Chem* 264:16985-16987

Yoneda Y, Imamoto-Sonobe N, Matsuoka Y, Iwamoto R, Kiho Y, Uchida T (1988): Antibodies to Asp-Asp-Glu-Asp can inhibit transport of nuclear proteins into the nucleus. *Science* 242:275-278

Zakai N, Kulka RG, Loyter A (1977): Membrane ultrastructural changes during calcium phosphate-induced fusion of human erythrocyte ghosts. *Proc Natl Acad Sci USA* 74:2417-2421

Zimmermann U (1982): Electric field mediated fusion and related electrical phenomena. *Biochem Biophys Acta* 694:227-277

APPENDIX 1: CALCIUM PHOSPHATE TRANSFECTION PROTOCOL

General Protocol

Day 1:   0.5 - 1 million cells seeded/100 mm dish.

Day 3:   First thing in the morning, change media.
4 hours later, transfection.
4 hours post-transfection, glycerol shock.
Refeed with media.

Day 4:   Cells may be harvested at any time after this for transient expression assays.

For stable integration, follow the remaining steps.

Day 5:   48-60 hours post-transfection, split into 150 mm dish with regular media.

Day 6:   Add ingredients for marker selection to the media.

Each week: half change with selection media.

When colonies are visible (usually within 2-3 weeks), transfer with cloning cylinder into 24-well plate, each well with 1 ml of nonselection media.

When wells are confluent, each is split into 25 cm^2-flask with 5 ml of selection media.

Detailed Protocol

Transfection: The amounts are calculated according to the requirement of each 100-mm dish but are normally scaled up 10 X to transfect at least 10 dishes.

1.   In a conical centrifuge tube, mix plasmid DNA and high-molecular-weight human placental DNA or salmon sperm DNA as carrier to a total of 20 μg. However, amount of plasmid DNA should not be less than 10 μg.

2.   Make up to 450 μl with DDW.

3.   Add 50 μl of 2.5M $CaCl_2$.

4. Bubble air into 0.5 ml of HeBS (2x) through a 1 ml sterilized plastic pipette with a pipettor controlled with a masking tape so that the rate is about 1 bubble/ second.

5. 1 drop/second of the Calcium-DNA mix is added with a 1 ml sterilized plastic pipette.

6. Let sit at room temp. for 30-45 minutes. Solution could vary from being cloudy to particulate.

7. 1 ml of the total mix is added per dish. Swirl to disperse over the cells.

Glycerol Shock:

1. Media discarded.

2. Rinse 2 X with serum free media, 5 ml each time.

3. 1 ml of 15% glycerol in serum free media added per dish. Swirl to mix. Remove after 30 seconds.

4. Wash with 5 ml serum free media twice.

5. Refeed with 10 ml of non-selection medium.

Solutions and media:
Human placental DNA: 1 mg/ml DDW (Type XIII, Sigma D-7011)

HeBS (2 X):	NaCl	8 gm
	KCl	0.37 gm
⎧	$Na_2HPO_4 \cdot 7H_2O$	0.376 gm
⎨	or	
⎩	$Na_2HPO_4 \cdot 2H_2O$	0.25 gm
	Dextrose	1 gm
	Hepes	5 gm
Dissolve in 500 ml		

pH adjusted from 6.2 to 7.1: 1 N NaOH about 70 drops.
Sterilize by filtration.

Glycerol (15%):	glycerol	3 ml
	serum free media	17 ml
	Sterilize by filtration.	

$CaCl_2$ (2.5M):	36.7 gm
	100 ml DDW
	Sterilize by filtration.

CELLULAR INTERNALIZATION OF OLIGODEOXYNUCLEOTIDES

Leonard M. Neckers

INTRODUCTION

Although the addition of oligodeoxynucleotides to cell cultures has been demonstrated to effectively inhibit intracellular gene expression, such findings have been in contrast to the prevailing view that cells are impermeable to negatively charged large molecules. With this in mind, several groups have attempted to modify oligos in order to circumvent the problem of negative charge. Thus, methylphosphonates are ionically neutral, and poly-L-lysine has been linked to oligos to supply a strong positive charge. Others have made various oligonucleotide-protein conjugates to aid internalization, while the benefits of oligo encapsulation into liposomes have also been explored. During the last several years, it has become clear that even highly negatively charged oligonucleotides (i.e., phosphodiesters and phosphorothioates) are actively internalized by cells in culture. Furthermore, it has become equally apparent that backbone or pendant oligonucleotide modifications can alter olionucleotide uptake characteristics, although not always in the way intended. In this chapter, we will review the current state of knowledge concerning internalization pathways for modified and unmodified oligonucleotides and how these pathways may affect the intracellular trafficking of oligonucleotides.

CELLULAR INTERNALIZATION OF UNMODIFIED OLIGONUCLEOTIDES

As early as 1986, Zamecnik and colleagues (Zamecnik and Stephenson, 1978) reported that cells exposed to 20 μM concentration of a 20-mer for 15 minutes contained 1.5 μM intracellular oligo. However, these experiments were performed with radioactively end-labelled oligos, and it is unclear how much of the cell-associated radioactivity was due to degraded radiolabelled nucleotides. In addition, the properties and specificity of the uptake mechanism were not investigated.

We have utilized fluorescently labelled oligos (initially labelled with acridine and more recently with fluorescein) to study uptake with the aid of flow cytometry. Glycine stripping, which removes externally bound, but not internalized oligo, revealed that greater than 95% of cell-associated oligo was bound to the extracel-

Gene Therapeutics: Methods and Applications of Direct Gene Transfer
Jon A. Wolff, Editor • ©1994 *Birkhäuser Boston*

lular cell membrane following a 90 minute incubation at 4° C (Neckers, 1989). Conversely, at 37° C, intracellular oligo accumulated until a plateau was reached within 1-2 hours. These experiments were performed in serum-free medium to prevent enzymatic degradation of the oligo by serum nucleases.

This approach allows for precise mathematical analysis of intracellular fluorescence due to the oligo and has been used to analyze the characterisitics of oligonucleotide uptake (Loke et al., 1989). We found that oligos up to 30 bases in length were taken up by cells in a saturable, temperature- and energy-dependent, sequence-independent manner compatible with receptor-mediated endocytosis. Any sequence or size of unlabelled oligo could compete with a fluorescently tagged oligo for uptake. All ribo- and deoxyribonucleotides competitively inhibited uptake in a concentration-dependent manner, with the number of terminal phosphates being unimportant. Both high molecular weight DNA (plasmid DNA) and yeast tRNA competed for uptake with a fluorescently tagged oligomer. However, neither free nucleosides nor deoxyribose-5'-phosphate were effective competitors. In addition, mononucleotides possessing a 5'phosphate linkage were more efficient competitors of uptake than were those with either a 2'- or 3'-phosphate linkage (Neckers, 1989). Taken together, these data demonstrate that the phosphate backbone is necessary for oligo uptake.

A striking feature of the dynamics of many cell surface receptors is their involvement in a pathway of either constitutive or ligand-induced endocytosis, in which receptors enter the cell via clathrin-coated vesicles and pass through an acidified endosomal compartment before either fusing with lysosomes and being degraded, or recycling to the cell surface (Krangel, 1987; Pastan and Willingham, 1981; Willingham and Pastan, 1980). In attempting to determine whether oligo uptake is endocytic, we made use of several characteristics of endosomal transport, including the ability of chloroquine, a lysosomatropic agent, to prevent acidification of endosomal vessicles; the ability of sodium azide to inhibit internalization of endocytic vessicles; and finally, the fact that fluorescently labelled ligands internalized by endocytosis typically display a punctate pattern of intracellular fluorescence. Using fluorescence microscopy, we in fact observed an intracellular punctate fluorescence upon addition of tagged oligos to cells. In addition, we were able to demonstrate that chloroquine treatment resulted in markedly elevated intracellular fluorescence, without altering the initial rate of oligo uptake or association with cells. Since fluorescein fluorescence is quenched at acid pH, these results suggest that fluorescent oligos are contained within endosomes which have entered an intracellular acidic compartment. Finally, we found that sodium azide significantly inhibited the amount of oligo accumulated intracellularly after 1 hour of incubation at 37° C, but that binding at 4° C was not affected. Taken together, these results support the hypothesis that uptake of unmodified oligos is an endocytic process. Similar results have been reported by Yabukov (Yakubov et al., 1989).

Interestingly, we have observed evidence of oligo recycling as well as oligo uptake (Loke et al., 1989). When fluorescently tagged extracellular oligo was removed from culture medium, or substituted with unlabelled oligo, the amount of detectable intracellular tagged oligo declined. A similar phenomenon has been reported for the endocytic uptake and recycling of a_2-macroglobulin by NRK cells and transferrin in several cell types (Dautry-Varsat, Ciechanover, and Lodish, 1983; Pastan et al., 1977; van Renswoude et al., 1982; Willingham et al., 1984). These data point out that at least some of the intracellular oligonucleotide pool is exchangeable with extracellular oligonucleotides (or their breakdown products), even several hours after addition of the oligos to the culture medium.

Using radioactively end-labelled oligos, we determined binding characteristics at 4° C. Receptor saturation was obtained within 90 minutes. Scatchard analysis revealed single dissociation constants in the low nanomolar range with most cells expressing 20,000 - 100,000 binding sites per cell. Oligo length did not affect binding affinity (Neckers, 1989; Zhang, Loke, and Neckers, 1990). Harel-Bellan (Harel-Bellan et al., 1988) reported similar results when studying labelled oligo association with T cells. They found a plateau in cell-associated radioactivity occurring within 1-2 hours after oligo addition.

CELLULAR INTERNALIZATION OF BACKBONE-MODIFIED OLIGONUCLEOTIDES

Methylphosphonates

The structural selectivity of oligonucleotide uptake led us to investigate the consequences of alterations to the phosphate backbone (Loke et al., 1989; Neckers, 1989). The two modified oligos we examined were phosphorothioates and methylphosphonates. We found that methylphosphonates could not compete with unmodified oligos for uptake, while phosphorothioates were found to be excellent competitors. Since methylphosphonates have increased hydrophobicity when compared to normal oligos and lack ionizable groups, while phosphorothioates retain the same negative charge as unmodified oligos, the ionic character of the oligonucleotide backbone may be critical for uptake through the mechanism described here.

Although on the surface these findings support the contention of Miller (Miller et al., 1981) that the hydrophobic nature of methylphosphonates allows them to be passively transported across cell membranes, this does not appear to be the case. In two recent reports from Juliano's laboratory, the transport of methylphosphonate oligonucleotides across lipid membranes was examined in detail (Akhtar et al., 1991; Shoji et al., 1991) Using either radioactively or fluorescently tagged oligos encapsulated in liposomes, Akhtar et al. (1991) demonstrated that passive diffusion of oligos out of the liposome was very slow (efflux $t_{1/2} > 4$ days). In fact, the rate of diffusion of methylphosphonate oligos was not significantly different from the rates of diffusion of unmodified phosphodiester or phosphorothioate oligos.

In another study, Shoji et al. (1991) demonstrated that cellular uptake of fluorescently tagged methylphosphonate oligos was temperature dependent and resulted in an intracellular pattern of punctate fluorescence, very similar to that previously demonstrated for unmodified oligos (Loke et al., 1989). Although this suggests energy dependent endocytic uptake, excess unlabeled methylphosphonate (or unmodified) oligo could not compete for uptake with a tracer amount of fluorescently tagged oligo. Taken together, these data point to non-specific endocytosis (i.e., fluid phase or adsorptive endocytosis) as the predominant means of cellular internalization of methylphosphonate oligos.

Phosphorothioates

Phosphorothioate oligos appear to be internalized similarly to unmodified oligos, although they take longer to reach intracellular equilibrium than do normal oligos (albeit at a higher final intracellular concentration). We have demonstrated that phosphorothioate oligos readily compete with unmodified oligos for uptake (Loke, et al., 1989; Stein, et al., 1988). Uptake characteristics of phosphorothioate and unmodified oligos are similar and internalized fluorescently tagged phosphorothioate oligos demonstrate a punctate pattern of fluorescence, as would be expected if uptake occured by endocytosis (Harewood et al., 1991).

CELLULAR INTERNALIZATION OF OLIGONUCLEOTIDES MODIFIED WITH PENDANT GROUPS

Poly L-lysine

There are now many examples of pendant modifications in the literature. Several pendant modifications have been reported to potentiate the cellular uptake of oligonucleotides. The effects on uptake of several of these modification will be described here. Poly L-lysine (PLL), a well-known polycationic drug carrier(Ryser and Shen, 1978) has been used to potentiate the antiviral effects of antisense oligos directed against VSV and HIV (Lemaitre, Bayard, and Lebleu, 1987; Stevenson and Iversen, 1989). The effects of PLL conjugation to oligos on their cellular uptake were recently described by Leonetti (Leonetti, Degols, and Lebleu, 1990). Using flow cytometric analysis of fluorescently tagged oligos as described above (Loke et al., 1989) these investigators demonstrated that PLL conjugation both accelerated the rate of oligo uptake and increased the total amount of oligo taken up. Interestingly, the uptake process nevertheless displayed characteristics of endocytosis in that intracellular fluorescence was punctate, uptake was temperature- and energy-dependent, and lysosomotropic amines prevented the sequence-specific cytotoxicity of the oligo (presumably by stabilizing the endosomal vessicle). PLL has been shown to be efficiently transported into mammalian cells by nonspecific adsorptive endocytosis (Ryser et al., 1978). That is, the positively charged PLL interacts nonspecifically with negatively charged molecules on the cell surface and is internalized along with those molecules. Such a higher capacity for cell membrane association could explain the efficacy of PLL-coupled oligos.

Avidin

Another cationic protein which has recently been coupled to oligonucleotides is avidin. Cells internalize avidin by adsorptive endocytosis. Association of a biotin-conjugated oligonucleotide with avidin is rapid and of high affinity (Pardridge and Boado, 1991). Cellular internalization of an avidin-biotin-oligo conjugate was shown to be approximately fourfold more efficient than of the biotin-oligo conjugate alone (Pardridge et al., 1991). The antisense efficacy of such an internalized complex has yet to be reported.

Cholesterol Or Phospholipid Moieties

Another pendant modification reported in the literature is the conjugation of cholesterol to oligonucleotides (Boutorin et al., 1989; Letsinger et al., 1989). Although experimental details concerning uptake of these compounds is sketchy, attachment of a single cholesterol moiety to an oligo appears to increase its intracellular concentration by up to 15-fold (Boutorin et al., 1989). Anti-HIV cholesteryl-conjugated oligos are more active than their unmodified counterparts (Letsinger et al., 1989). It is not known if endocytosis is involved in uptake of these modified oligos.

Other hydrophobic pendant modifications reported to increase oligo uptake and efficacy include the attachment of a phospholipid moiety to an oligo (Shea, Marsters, and Bischofberger, 1990). Similar modification of other chemotherapeutic agents appears to enhance their anti-tumor activity (Shea et al., 1990). When phospholipid was coupled to the 5'-terminus of an oligonucleotide, 8-10 times more oligo-lipid became cell associated than unmodified oligo (Shea et al., 1990). Maximal cell association occured within 4 hours of oligo addition to culture medium and reached levels approximately 8-fold greater than those seen with unmodified oligos. Whether an endocytic uptake mechanism is involved is not known. The antiviral activity of such oligos was found to be markedly potentiated. Perhaps significantly, anti-viral effects observed with lipid-oligos were not always sequence specific. Similar findings have been reported for cholesteryl-oligos as well (Letsinger et al., 1989). These studies raise the possiblity that, although efficacious for oligo uptake, hydrophobic pendant modifications to oligos might introduce non-sequence specific effects, particularly when viral systems are being examined.

CELLULAR INTERNALIZATION OF LIPOSOME-ENCAPSULATED OLIGONUCLEOTIDES

Macromolecules may be stably encapsulated within liposomes, resulting in restricted access of these molecules to the extracellular environment, and protecting such encapsulated molecules against enzymatic degradation. Thus, encapsulation of both DNA and RNA into liposomes has been shown to protect these species against nuclease attack (Leonetti et al., 1990; Milhaud et al., 1989). Liposomes have the added advantage of being able to target their contents to particular cells in a mixed population. This is accomplished by incorporating either an antibody or some other targeting ligand into the liposomal membrane. Use of such technology has been demonstrated to greatly increase the efficacy of both antisense oligos and antisense RNA (Leonetti et al., 1990; Renneisen et al., 1990) .

Liposomes are internalized via receptor-mediated endocytosis and their rate of uptake, degree of intracellular accumulation and intracellular fate are all determined by the fate of the cell surface molecules to which they bind. This may depend on both the cell type and target molecule. For example, liposomes targeted to MHC-encoded class I molecules on L cells are internalized via non-coated pits, whereas the same liposomes targeted to T cells are internalized via clathrin-coated pits (Leonetti et al., 1990; Machy et al., 1987).

Most non-targeted liposomes are internalized by non-specific endocytosis and eventually fuse with lysosomes. pH-sensitive liposomes have been developed as a way to circumvent this process (Chu et al., 1990). Before fusing with lysosomes, the pH of endocytic vesicles is reduced. pH-sensitive liposomes destabilize membranes or become fusogenic when exposed to acidic pH. Ideally, such liposomes can convey their contents to the cytoplasm before fusing with lysosomes. Although cytoplasmic delivery from pH-sensitive liposomes is much more efficient than that from non-pH-sensitive liposomes, cytoplasmic delivery still accounts for only 0.01% - 10% of the liposome contents that becomes cell associated (Chu et al., 1990).

OLIGONUCLEOTIDE BINDING PROTEINS

The characteristics of normal oligo transport into cells suggest that a cell surface receptor(s) may mediate this process. The fact that binding to cells is a saturable and specific process supports this contention. If oligo uptake is receptor-mediated, the intracellular fate of the oligo would depend in part on the route of internalization of the receptor complex. Once in the cytoplasm and/or nucleus, oligos might associate with other proteins, making their availability as antisense or triplex reagents problematic. For these reasons, it is important to characterize such oligo binding proteins.

Cell Surface

Recently, Bennett and his colleagues have described a 30-kD cell surface protein present on a wide variety of cells capable of binding and internalizing high molecular weight DNA (Bennett et al., 1983; Bennett, Gabor, and Merritt, 1985; Bennett, Kotzin, and Merritt, 1987; Bennett, Peller, and Merritt, 1986; Gabor and Bennett, 1984; Hefeneider et al., 1990). This protein initially attracted interest as perhaps being the "oligonucleotide receptor." However, oligos do not competitively inhibit the binding of DNA to this protein (Bennett et al., 1985), suggesting that it is not utilized for internalization of oligos. In addition, several of its characteristics are not compatible with the properties of oligonucleotide uptake as described above. For example, the 30-kD DNA binding protein is not inhibited by tRNA, but DNA binding is blocked by the polyanion heparin. On the other hand, oligo uptake is blocked by excess tRNA and is not affected by either the polyanions heparin or chondroitin sulfate (Loke et al., 1989; Yakubov et al., 1989).

We utilized oligo dT-cellulose beads as a tool for affinity purification of a putative plasma membrane oligo binding protein from surface-iodinated cells. Polyacrylamide gel electrophoresis of the material bound to such beads revealed a single 80-kD protein.(Loke et al., 1989). Binding of labelled membrane lysate to oligo dT beads could be prevented by prior incubation of the lysate with a large excess of random sequence oligomer. Similar results were obtained when oligo dG and dC beads were used as the affinity matrix (Loke et al., 1989). The 80-kD protein was identified in a number of different cell types, including neuroblastoma cells, myelomonocytic cells, fibroblasts and epithelial cells. Using a somewhat different approach, Yakubov et al. have identified a similar binding protein (Yakubov et al., 1989).

We recently developed a novel technique to confirm and extend these findings (Geselowitz and Neckers, 1992) This makes use of an iodinated, photoactivatible, heterobifunctional crosslinking reagent, termed the Denny-Jaffe reagent. The oligo can be crosslinked to the reagent via the NHS ester on the crosslinker and an aminolinker group on the oligo. The resultant conjugate can then be incubated with cells or subcellular fractions (in the dark) and then subjected to a brief exposure of UV light, photoactivating the aryl azide on the other end of the crosslinker and covalently coupling the oligo to associating proteins (or nucleic acids). Using this technique, we have confirmed the association of unmodified and phosphorothioate oligos with an 80 kD membrane protein (Geselowitz and Neckers, 1992). Isolation of an endosomal/lysosomal subcellular fraction from incubated intact cells again reveals the presence of oligo bound to an 80 kD protein, supplying direct evidence that the 80 kD surface protein is involved in endocytosis of the oligo.

Cytoplasm And Nucleus

Oligos in the cytoplasmic compartment but not in vesicles do not appear to be bound to protein, but also make up a small fraction of the total intracellular oligo concentration (see below) (Geselowitz and Neckers, 1992). Oligos isolated from the nucleus do appear to be in close proximity to several proteins. Whether nuclei are isolated from intact cells which have been incubated with a Denny-Jaffe crosslinked oligo, or whether such a derivatized oligo is incubated with purified intact nuclei, a series of similar low molecular weight proteins can be observed, none of which correspond to the 80-kD surface protein. In fact, if total nuclear oligo concentration is considered, the majority of the oligo (up to 80%) can be found associated with these proteins (Geselowitz and Neckers, 1992). Whether oligos are normally free to dissociate from nuclear proteins and associate with nucleic acids cannot be determined from these experiments. Nonetheless, these data suggest that it should not be assumed *a priori* that, once in the nucleus, oligos are free to hybridize with their targeted DNA or RNA.

INTRACELLULAR LOCALIZATION OF OLIGONUCLEOTIDES

The previous discussion on cell uptake of oligos and their binding proteins raises several questions. For example, what is the intracellular localization of oligos and is it altered by either oligo modification or method of delivery? Do oligos in fact prefer to be in the nucleus as opposed to the cytoplasm? These questions are only now being addressed and some of the answers available to date are contradictory.

Routes Of Internalization

It is now clear that unmodified phosphodiester oligos are taken up by endocytosis via specific receptors on the cell surface. Phosphorothioates are also taken up endocytically, but may bind to the cell surface more promiscuously than unmodified oligos. Methylphosphonate oligos do not compete with unmodified and phosphorothioate oligos for uptake but are probably endocytosed in a nonspecific fashion (similar to poly L-lysine or avidin). It is yet to be determined how chimeric oligos (i.e., part methylphosphonate and part phosphodiester) enter the cell, and the mode of uptake of other back-bone-modified oligos remains to be explored. It is also not yet known if pendant modification of an oligo with hydrophobic groups, such as cholesterol or phospholipid, alter the mode of uptake. Such oligos may be able to utilize both the receptor-mediated, endosomal uptake process as well as a passive diffusion or adsorptive endocytic process. The ability to fluorescently label, and otherwise modify, almost any type of oligo by automated synthesis will make such studies much simpler to carry out and more reproducible as well. Liposomal and poly L-lysine delivery of oligos is clearly mediated by endocytosis, although not via oligo binding proteins. Poly L-lysine randomly targets many negatively charged cell surface proteins, while liposomes can be targeted to specific receptors on the cell.

The intracellular fate of endocytic vessicles containing oligos will be dependent on the fate of the particular surface protein to which the oligo has been targeted. As described above, some receptors recycle through acidic compartments in the cytoplasm, releasing their contents and returning to the cell surface undegraded, while other receptors fuse with lysosomes following internalization and are degraded. The pathway which oligo binding proteins follow is not yet completely understood, yet fluorescence microscopy reveals a distinct punctate pattern of intracytoplasmic fluorescence. Because fluorescein fluorescence is quenched at acid pH, and because intracellular oligo fluorescence is markedly enhanced following chloroquine treatment (chloroquine raises intracellular pH), we can assume that the oligo receptor endocytic complex must enter an intracytoplasmic acidic compartment at some point in its cycle. Which of the pathways favors an oligo is not known, although one might suppose that association with a lysosome would not be ideal. Nonetheless, in the case of poly L-lysine-conjugated oligos, the poly-L-lysine must be cleaved from the oligo in order for the oligo to be effective, and such cleavage probably occurs intralysosomally. In fact, lysosomotropic amines block the effectiveness of poly L-lysineconjugated oligos (Leonetti et al., 1990).

Intracellular Fate

It is clear that if an oligo is in an endosome it cannot hybridize to its target, whether cytoplasmic or nuclear. The ease with which oligos can exit the endosome will play a major role in their usefulness. Once free in the cytoplasm, where does an oligo go? Recent, but still incomplete, data suggest that oligos in the cytoplasm migrate rapidly to the nucleus. Oligos microinjected intracytoplasmically have been reported to appear within the nucleus within seconds to minutes (Chin et al., 1990; Leonetti et al., 1991). Similarly, when cells are incubated with iodinated Denny-Jaffe-conjugated oligo for 1-3 hours, about 50% of the radioactively crosslinked oligo can be found in isolated nuclei, with very little free oligo detectable in cytosol. The remaining 50% of the material can be found associated with plasma membranes and intracytoplasmic membranes (Geselowitz and Neckers, 1992).

These results support the possiblity that very little hybridizable oligo exists in the cytoplasm and suggest that any cytoplasmically occuring, non-membrane associated oligo may rapidly translocate to the nucleus. The discrepancy between results such as these and those obtained with fluorescence microscopy is as yet difficult to explain. While fluorescence micrographs reveal little intracytoplasmic, nonpunctate fluorescence, as would be expected, little nuclear fluorescence is detectable as well. This is the case even when oligos are coupled to several different fluorochromes, including acridine, fluorescein or rhodamine. While acridine fluorescence may be quenched upon DNA intercalation, and fluorescein fluorescence is pH sensitive, no one explanation can yet explain this perplexing observation.

Rapid translocation of oligos to the nucleus is supported by some experimental observations. Antisense oligonucleoside methylphosphonates targeting the acceptor splice junction of herpes simplex virus type I immediate early mRNA 4 are effective inhibitors of virus growth if administered to cells within the first few hours of infection (Kulka et al., 1989). However, these authors did not study the intracellular distribution of the oligo. Boutorin (Boutorin et al., 1989) reported that up to 30% of an intracellularly localized cholesterolconjugated oligo could be found in the nucleus within 2 hours of oligo addition to the cell culture. In a recent study, Sburlati (Sburlati, Manrow, and Berger, 1991) determined the intracellular distribution of an unmodified 16-mer at 1, 6, 24 and 48 hours after addition to cells and found the majority of intact oligo in the nuclear fraction within 6 hours of administration. This study suffered from the fact that all oligos were 3'-end labelled. Since 3'-exonuclease seems to be the major degradative nuclease in fetal bovine serum, only the full-length oligo would be detectable by these investigators. This explains perhaps why only the antisense, and not a sense, oligo could be detected at all intracellularly, even within 1 hour of administration. Nonetheless, a strong nuclear signal from the antisense oligo was still visible at 6 hours.

CONCLUSIONS

Although the evidence is beginning to point to nuclear localization of free cytoplasmic oligos, final proof must still be obtained. The analysis of the intracellular whereabouts of photoactivatable, crosslinkable oligos - such as psoralen derivatives, Denny-Jaffe derivatives, or others - at various times after addition to intact cells should provide time exposure snapshots of oligo trafficking within the cell. With such information in hand, a complete understanding of oligonucleotide subcellular distribution will be possible.

REFERENCES

Akhtar S, Basu S, Wickstrom E, Juliano RL (1991): Interactions of antisense DNA oligonucleotide analogs with phospholipid membranes (liposomes). *Nucleic Acids Research* 19:5551-5559

Bennett RM, Davis J, Campbell S, Portnoff S (1983): Lactoferrin binds to cell membrane DNA. *J Clin Invest* 71:611-618

Bennett RM, Gabor GT, Merritt MM (1985): DNA binding to human leukocytes. *J Clin Invest* 76:2182-2190

Bennett RM, Kotzin BL, Merritt MJ (1987): DNA receptor dysfunction in systemic lupus erythematosus and kindred disorders. *J Exp Med* 166:850-863

Bennett RM, Peller JS, Merritt MM (1986): Defective DNA-receptor function in systemic lupus erythematosus and related diseases: evidence for an autoantibody influencing cell physiology. *The Lancet* Jan 25:186-188

Boutorin AS, Gus'kova, LV, Ivanova EM, Kobetz ND, Zarytova VF, Ryte AS, Yurchenko LV, Vlassov VV (1989): Synthesis of alkylating oligonucleotide derivatives containing cholesterol of phenazinium residues at their 3'-terminus and their interaction with DNA within mammalian cells. *FEBS Lett* 254:129-132

Chin DJ, Green GA, Zon G, Szoka FCJ, Straubinger RM (1990): Rapid nuclear accumulation of injected oligodeoxyribonucleotides. *New Biologist* 2:1091-1100

Chu C-J, Dijkstra J, Lai M-Z, Hong K, Szoka FC (1990): Efficiency of cytoplasmic delivery by pH-sensitive liposomes to cells in culture. *Pharmaceutical Research* 7:824-834

Dautry-Varsat A, Ciechanover A, Lodish HF (1983): pH and the recycling of transferrin during receptor-mediated endocytosis. *Proc Natl Acad Sci USA* 80:2258-2262

Gabor G, Bennett RM (1984): Biotin-labelled DNA: A novel approach for the recognition of a DNA binding site on cell membrane. *Biochem Biophys Res Commun* 122:1034-1039

Geselowitz DA, Neckers L (1992): Analysis of oligonucleotide binding, internalization and intracellular trafficking utilizing a novel radiolabeled crosslinker. *Antisense Res Dev* (In Press)

Harel-Bellan A, Ferris DK, Vinocour M, Holt JT, Farrar WL (1988): Specific inhibition of c-myc protein biosynthesis using an antisense synthetic deoxy-oligonucleotide in human lymphocytes. *J Immunology* 140:2431-2435

Harewood K, Pape K, Gabel C, Suleske R, Cunningham A (1991): Cellular uptake and localization of fluorescein-labelled, 15 mer phosphorothioate and phosphodiester oligonucleotides. *J Cell Biochem* 15D:35

Hefeneider SH, Bennett RM, Pham TQ, Cornell K, McCoy SL, Heinrich MC (1990): Identification of a cell-surface DNA receptor and its association with systemic lupus erythematosus. *J Invest Dermatol* 94:79S-84S

Krangel MS (1987): Endocytosis and recycling of the T3-T cell receptor complex. The role of T3 phosphorylation. *J Exp Med* 165:1141-1159

Kulka M, Smith CC, Aurelian L, Fishelevich R, Meade K, Miller P, Ts'o POP (1989): Site specificity of the inhibitory effects of oligo(nucleoside methylphosphonate)s complementary to the acceptor splice junction of herpes simplex virus type 1 immediate early mRNA 4. *Proc Natl Acad Sci USA* 86:6868-6872

Lemaitre M, Bayard B, Lebleu B (1987): Specific antiviral activity of a poly(L-lysine)-conjugated oligodeoxyribonucleotide sequence complementary to vesicular stomatitis virus N protein mRNA initiation site. *Proc Natl Acad Sci USA* 84:648-652

Leonetti J-P, Degols G, Lebleu B (1990): Biological Activity of Oligonucleotide-Poly (L-lysine) Conjugates: Mechanism of Cell Uptake. *Bioconj Chem* 1:149-153

Leonetti JP, Machy P, Degols G, Lebleu B, Leserman L (1990): Antibodytargeted liposomes containing oligodeoxynucleotides complementary to viral RNA selectively inhibit viral replication. *Proc Natl Acad Sci USA* 87:2448-2451

Leonetti JP, Mechti N, Degols G, Gagnor C, Lebleu B (1991): Intracellular distribution of microinjected antisense oligonucleotides. *Proc Natl Acad Sci USA* 88:2702-2706

Letsinger RL, Zhang GR, Sun DK, Ikeuchi T, Sarin PS (1989): Cholesteryl-conjugated oligonucleotides: synthesis, properties and activity as inhibitors of replication of human immunodeficiency virus in cell culture. *Proc Natl Acad Sci USA* 86:6553-6556

Loke SL, Stein CA, Zhang XH, Mori K, Nakanishi M, Subasinghe C, Cohen J S, Neckers LM (1989): Chacterization of oligonucleotide transport into living cells. *Proc Natl Acad Sci USA* 86:3474-3478

Machy P, Truneh A, Gennaro D, Hoffstein S (1987): Major histocompatibility complex class I molecules internalized via coated pits in T lymphocytes. *Nature* (London) 328:724-726

Milhaud PG, Machy P, Lebleu B, Leserman L (1989): Antibody targeted liposomes containing poly (rI). poly(rC) exert a specific antiviral and toxic effect on cells primed with interferons alpha, beta or gamma. *Biochim Biophys Acta* 987:15-20

Miller PS, McParland KB, Jayaraman K, Ts'o POP (1981): Biochemical and biological effects of nonionic nucleic acid methylphosphonates. *Biochemistry* 20:1874-1880

Neckers LM (1989): Antisense oligonucleotides as a tool for studying cell regulation: mechanism of uptake and application to the study of oncogene function. In: *Oligodeoxynucleotides: Antisense inhibitors of gene expression,* Cohen J, ed. London: Macmillan Press

Pardridge WM, Boado RJ (1991): Enhanced cellular uptake of biotinylated antisense oligonucleotide or peptide mediated by avidin, a cationic protein. *FEBS Letters* 288:30-32

Pastan I, Willingham M, Anderson W, Gallo M (1977): Localization of serum-derived a2 macroglobulin in cultured cells and decrease after Moloney sarcoma virus transformation. *Cell* 609-617

Pastan IH, Willingham MC (1981): Journey to the center of the cell: Role of the receptosome. *Science* 214:504-509

Renneisen K, Leserman L, Matthes E, Schroder HC, Muller WEG (1990): Inhibition of expression of human immunodefiency virus-1 in vitro by antibody-targeted liposomes containing antisense RNA to the env region. *J Biol Chem* 265:16337-16342

Ryser HJ-P, Shen W-C (1978): Conjugation of methotrexate to poly(Llysine) increases drug transport and overcomes drug resistance in cultured cells. *Proc Natl Acad Sci USA* 75:3867-3870

Sburlati AR, Manrow RE, Berger SL (1991): Prothymosin a antisense oligomers inhibit myeloma cell division. *Proc Natl Acad Sci USA* 88:253-257

Shea RG, Marsters JC, Bischofberger N (1990): Synthesis, hybridization properties and antiviral activity of lipid-oligodeoxynucleotide conjugates. *Nucl Acid Res* 18:3777-3783

Shoji Y, Akhtar S, Periasamy A, Herman B, Juliano RL (1991): Mechanism of cellular uptake of modified oligodeoynucleotides containing methylphosphonate linkages. *Nucl Acid Res* 19:5543-5550

Stein CA, Mori K, Loke SL, Subasinghe K, Cohen JS, Neckers LM (1988): Phosphorothioate and normal oligodeoxyribonucleotides with 5'-linked acridine: characterization and preliminary kinetics of cellular uptake. *Gene* 72:333-341

Stevenson M, Iversen PL (1989): Inhibition of human immunodeficiency virus type 1-mediated cytopathic effects by poly(L-lysine)-conjugated synthetic antisense oligodeoxyribonucleotides. *J Gen Virol* 70:2673

van Renswoude J, Bridges KR, Harford JB, Klausner RD (1982): Receptormediated endocytosis of transferrin and the uptake of Fe in K562 cells: identification of a nonlysosomal acidic compartment. *Proc Natl Acad Sci USA* 79:6186-6190

Willingham MC, Hanover JA, Dickson RB, Pastan I (1984): Morphologic characterization of the human pathway of transferrin endocytosis and recycling in human KB cells. *Proc Natl Acad Sci USA* 81:175-179

Willingham MC, Pastan I (1980): The receptosome: an intermediate organelle of receptor-mediated endocytosis in cultured fibroblasts. *Cell* 21:67-77

Yakubov LA, Deeva EA, Zarytova VF, Ivanova EM, Ryte AS, Yurchenko VL, Vlassov VV (1989): Mechanism of oligonucleotide uptake by cells: Involvement of specific receptors? *Proc Natl Acad Sci USA* 86:6454-6458

Zamecnik PC, Stephenson ML (1978): Inhibition of Rous sarcoma virus replication and cell transformation by a specific oligodeoxynucleotide. *Proc Natl Acad Sci USA* 75:280-284

Zhang XH, Loke SL, Neckers L (1990): unpublished observations

GENE TRANSFER VIA PARTICLE BOMBARDMENT: APPLICATIONS OF THE ACCELL GENE GUN

Ning-Sun Yang, Carolyn De Luna, and Liang Cheng

INTRODUCTION

Gene therapy has great potential for the treatment of a wide spectrum of genetic, neoplastic, and infectious diseases (Anderson, 1992; Miller, 1992). Advances in recombinant DNA and PCR technologies have significantly facilitated the identification of functional genes which cause, promote, control, or correct a variety of diseases. Gene transfer techniques must now be developed which can efficiently deliver candidate therapeutic genes into target somatic tissues where their therapeutic effects can be evaluated.

Two main experimental strategies for gene therapy are currently being actively explored. One approach is in vivo gene transfer into targeted somatic tissues; the other approach utilizes ex vivo gene transfer into tissue or cell explants or their derived primary cultures, which are then transplanted into host animals. Several gene transfer methods, initially developed for cell culture systems, were often ineffective or inefficient for certain of the targeted cell types, varying with animal species (Yang, 1992). A number of reasons, such as differences in membrane receptor properties between different cell types, tissue-specific anatomical features, or other biochemical mechanisms necessary for specific gene uptake, may account for these limitations. As a result, the utility of many cultured and explanted somatic tissues in gene therapy has not been realized. Alternative or improved gene transfer techniques are needed to advance the development of gene therapy research.

One alternative approach for mammalian gene therapy is a physical means for gene transfer called particle bombardment. Also known as the ballistic, microprojectile, or gene gun method of gene delivery, this technology was initially developed for the transformation of plants. Microscopic particles coated with the gene of interest are accelerated by a motive force to penetrate the cells and deliver the DNA (Klein et al., 1987; McCabe et al., 1988; Sanford, 1988). The motive force can be generated by a number of ways: high-voltage electric discharge (Accell®, McCabe et al., 1988; Christou et al., 1990), helium pressure discharge (Biolistics®, Williams et al., 1991; Fitzpatrick-McElligott, 1992), or other means (Klein et al., 1987; Sautter et al., 1991). Accell electric-discharge particle-medi-

Gene Therapeutics: Methods and Applications of Direct Gene Transfer
Jon A. Wolff, Editor • ©1994 *Birkhäuser Boston*

ated gene delivery has repeatedly resulted in high efficiency gene transfer in various plant systems, generating a wide variety of genetically engineered crops (Christou et al., 1990; Christou et al., 1993; Yang, 1993).

Using the Accell particle bombardment method, we demonstrated effective in vivo and ex vivo gene transfer in a variety of mammalian somatic tissues with minimal or no restrictions in cell-type or species specificity. Bombardment of skin, liver, pancreas, kidney, muscle, and other tissues of live rats resulted in readily detectable transgene activities. Likewise, in vivo gene transfer was successful in all of the mammalian species tested — mouse, rat, hamster, rabbit and rhesus monkey (Yang, 1992; Cheng et al., 1993). The Accell method is also effective for transfection of tissue explant systems and their derivative primary cell cultures. In addition, it can be conveniently used for transfection of monolayer or suspension cell lines in culture. In this chapter, we discuss its application to gene transfer studies in mammalian systems and its potential utility in human gene therapy.

MECHANICS AND FUNCTIONAL PARAMETERS OF THE ACCELL DEVICE

Two particle bombardment devices, marketed under the trade names Accell and Biolistics, have been successfully applied to systematic mammalian gene transfer experiments. Although these two devices utilize very different mechanisms for particle acceleration, experimental results obtained from each are quite comparable (Yang et al., 1990; Williams et al., 1991; Thompson et al., 1993; Jiao et al., 1993). Since our results are typical, we will focus our discussion mainly on the Accell particle bombardment device, for which we have established stringent protocols for its routine use.

The original Accell particle acceleration mechanism, designed by D. McCabe and co-workers (1988, 1992), is diagrammed in Fig. 1. A strong burst of shock waves, generated by a high voltage electric discharge, accelerates DNA-coated microscopic gold particles to a high velocity, resulting in efficient penetration of a target cell or tissue sample. The particles pass through the cell wall or membrane, delivering their DNA to targeted organs, tissues, or single cells. This method circumvents the cell wall or cell membrane receptors that often present physical or biochemical barriers for vector- and chemical-mediated gene transfer protocols.

Ballistic parameters can be modified to enhance gene expression in specific tissue or cell types. One important parameter, particle acceleration rate, is varied by the discharge voltage to give optimal penetration of monolayer cells or multiple-layered tissues and organs. Low particle acceleration resulting from a 5-8 kV discharge is generally sufficient to transfect cell samples in culture (Yang et al., 1990; Thompson et al., 1993; Jiao et al., 1993); a discharge voltage of 15-22 kV is optimal for bombardment of somatic tissues in vivo (Cheng et al., 1993).

The material used for the microprojectile is another important parameter. Gold particles are the most effective and the most commonly used for mammalian gene transfer. Gold is chemically inert, has no cytotoxic effects in cells, and its high

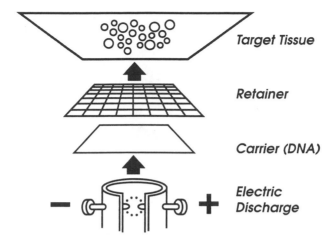

FIGURE 1. Diagram of the particle accleration mechanism of the Accell gene gun. The motive force is generated in a spark discharge chamber containing two electrodes. A 10 μl water droplet is placed in between the electodes, and a high-voltage capacitor is discharged through the water droplet that vaporizes instantly, creating a shock wave. We have found that a polyvinyl chloride pipe with an internal diameter of 13 mm is adequate for use at the spark discharge chamber. The electrodes are located opposite each other, project into the interior of the chamber approximately 5 mm below the top and are protected at the tips with an arc-resistant alloy. The gap between the two electrodes can be adjusted by appropriately threading them into or out of the spark chamber. A spacer ring is placed above the spark chamber that, in a fixed apparatus for transformations of a single crop species, can be a vertical extension of the spark discharge chamber. However, a removable spacer ring allows the distance from the spark discharge to the carrier sheet to be varied so that the force of the shock wave can be adjusted. The motive force can also be adjusted by varying the voltage of the discharge. The carrier sheet on which the DNA-coated gold particles are precipitated is placed on top of the spacer; the function of this sheet is to transfer the force of the shock wave from the spark discharge into acceleration of the carrier particles. Located above the carrier sheet is a 100-mesh stainless steel screen that retains the sheet so that it does not proceed to the target tissue. The target tissue can be placed on a water-agar plate in such a way that when the plate is inverted over the retaining screen, the tissue is in the direct path of the gold particles. The whole assembly is under a partial vaccum in order to minimize aerodynamic drag. (Reprinted by permission of the publisher from Christou et al., *Trends Biotechnol*, Elsevier, Cambridge, 1990.)

density permits greater momentum and, hence, deeper penetration. A range of gold particle sizes are commercially available for particle bombardment, including 0.95 μm, 1-3 μm, 2-5 μm, 5-7 μm and ~15 μm diameter beads. The 0.95 μm beads are suitable for bombarding most cell cultures and 1-3 μm beads are commonly used for bombardment of somatic tissues in vivo. The 5-7 μm beads can penetrate much deeper into somatic tissues, but are often too destructive for intracellular delivery. However, they can be used for intra-tissue DNA delivery and for passive DNA uptake into some tissue types.

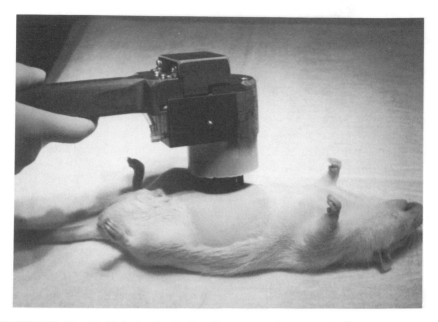

FIGURE 2. Hand-held device for the Accell gene gun. Courtesy of Dr. D. McCabe.

Gold particle loading rate has to be adjusted to optimize cell transfection efficiency. For confluent monolayer cell cultures with cells 15-20 μm in size, a density of 0.1 mg beads/cm^2 of the 0.95 μm beads delivers about two beads per cell. Using these variables, cell viability assays of bombarded cells show that the damaged cell membranes seal within 10 minutes. In general, more than 90% of monolayer cells and 75% of suspension cells in bombarded cultures are viable and healthy after this period (Yang et al., 1990; Jiao et al., 1993; Burkholder et al., 1993). For most tissue samples, a higher bead density level causes extensive cell and tissue damage.

In situ particle-mediated gene transfer into targeted tissues of live animals was first demonstrated by Yang et al. (1990) and Johnston et al. (1991). To perform in vivo gene transfer experiments on larger animals, D. McCabe and B. Martinell (1992) developed a hand-held version of the original Accell device, shown in Fig. 2. This new apparatus permitted effective in vivo gene transfer in mammalian systems.

IN VIVO AND IN SITU GENE TRANSFER

Particle bombardment of somatic tissues has been successfully applied to in situ and in vivo gene transfer in a variety of mammalian species (Yang et al., 1990; Williams et al., 1991; Cheng et al., 1993). The specific somatic tissue targeted for gene delivery is chemically or surgically exposed, positioned under the retaining screen of the hand-held particle acceleration device and bombarded. The gene transfer procedure typically takes less than one minute.

The most accessible somatic tissue is the skin. Bombardment of the epidermis is simple and can be easily adapted for multiple, routine operations. An area of skin is shaved and treated with Nair (a commercial depilatory) which removes the hair as well as the stratum corneum (the top layer of dead cells), exposing the living epidermal cells. Gene transfer efficiency and expression after bombardment of the epidermis are similar for different body locations, including the abdomen, ear, back, and leg. Using Biolistic technology, Williams et al. (1991) reported that minimal cell damage and inflammation were observed in bombarded mouse epidermal tissues exhibiting high-levels of transgene expression. Histological examination showed that marker DNA was retained on the gold microprojectiles which had penetrated deeply into the mouse skin tissue.

Bombardment of internal organs or tissues requires surgical procedures to expose the target site. For skin dermis, an incision is made to expose the underside of the dermal tissue, and the thick fascia layer is removed by scraping with a scalpel. Muscle tissues are exposed and scraped in a similar manner before bombardment. Other internal organs, including kidney, spleen, heart, pancreas, and liver, are exposed via incisions through skin and muscle layers using standard surgical procedures.

The efficiency and pattern of in vivo transgene expression in several bombarded rat somatic tissues were evaluated by Cheng et al. (1993). A plasmid containing the firefly luciferase (luc) gene driven by the cytomegalovirus (CMV) immediate early gene enhancer/promoter was employed for quantitative analysis of in vivo transgene expression. Significant CMV-luc activity was observed in various rat tissues. Pancreas, epidermis, and liver tissues expressed about 10^7 relative light units (RLU) per uniform size tissue (3.24 cm^2); dermis and kidney expressed slightly lower levels of activity ($\sim 10^6$ RLU), and spleen, heart, and abdominal muscles expressed the lowest levels (10^5 RLU) of all tested tissues. The reporter gene CAT was also used for bombardment of some of these tissues and similar trends in transgene expression levels were observed (Yang et al., 1990). When an *Escherichia coli* β-galactosidase (β-gal) gene was used to evaluate transgene expression at the cellular or tissue level, readily detectable levels were observed in bombarded skin, liver, and muscle tissues (Fig. 3 A-D, Page 199). As many as 20% of the bombarded epidermal cells demonstrated high levels of CMVβ-gal activity.

Time course studies of transient gene expression from four different somatic tissues bombarded in vivo had strikingly different results (Yang et al., 1990; Cheng et al., 1993). In epidermis and liver, transgene luc activity peaked between 1 and 3 days post-bombardment, declined quickly during the next few days, and was minimal (i.e., 1 to 10% of maximal activity) after 1-2 weeks. In contrast, rat dermis tissues' transgene CMV-luc activity was sustained for over one and a half years, with greater than 40% of original (day 1) activity maintained throughout this time. At six months post-bombardment, luc transgene sequences in bombarded rat dermis were detectible by PCR analysis. A muscle cell type present in the panniculus carnosus layer expresses high level CMVβ-gal activity in bombarded dermal tissues (Fig. 3D, Page 199) and may play a role in long-term expression of transgenes. Wolff et al. (1990) had previously achieved long-term transgene expression in striated mouse muscles by direct needle injection of plasmid DNA into target tissues. They demonstrated that the injected DNA was sustained as free, circular DNA without replication in the muscle cells for over a year (Wolff et al., 1990; Jiao et al., 1992). It is possible that a similar mechanism may be responsible for the long-term transgene expression observed in rat dermal tissue. Although bombarded rat abdominal muscle was able to sustain CMV-luc activity over a two week test period (Cheng et al., 1993), the expression levels were at least 20-fold less than those observed from dermal tissues. These observations suggest that dermal skin tissue may be a preferred vehicle for in vivo long-term transgene expression.

Recent experiments also revealed that secretory proteins synthesized from bombarded tissues in vivo can be effectively secreted into the circulatory system in transient expression experiments. A human growth hormone (hGH) gene was used to evaluate secretion of transgene products from bombarded skin and liver tissues. In mice, rats, and rhesus monkeys, 0.2 to 0.5 ng hGH protein/ml of serum was detected for 1 to 2 days after bombarding 6-10% of the epidermal skin surface area with CMV-hGH DNA (Cheng et al., unpublished results). Significant levels of hGH were also found in tissue extracts excised from the bombarded skin samples.

FIGURE 3. In vivo expression of transgenic CMVβ-gal activity in various rat somatic tissues bombarded in situ in live animals. (A) Epidermis; (B) Muscle; (C) Liver; and (D) Dermis; the arrows indicate β-gal expressing cells. X-gal staining of excised tissues or tissue sections revealed β-gal activity at the cellular or tissue level (adapted from Yang et al., 1990 *Proc Natl Acad Sci USA*, National Academy of Sciences, Washington DC, and from Cheng et al., 1993 *Proc Natl Acad Sci USA* Vol. 90).

FIGURE 4. Expression of transgenic β-gal or tyrosine hydroxylase (TH) activity in various [rat] somatic tissues bombarded ex vivo. (A) Fetal brain tissue clumps bombarded with pCMVβ-gal and plated in primary culture. (B) Fetal brain tissue was bombarded ex vivo with pCMV-TH gene then immediately transplanted into adult host brain. In vivo expression of transgenic TH protein in the graft 9 days after bombardment (arrows). Cells were labeled by immunoperoxidase staining, with anti-TH antibody. (C) Rat mammary gland organoids bombarded ex vivo with pCMVβ-gal. (D) Primary culture of peripheral blood lymphocytes bombarded with pCMVβ-gal (adapted with permission of Bio/Technology from Jiao et al.,1993, *Bio/Technology*; Nature Publishing, New York, and Yang et al., 1990 *Proc Natl Acad Sci USA*, National Academy of Sciences, Washington, DC).

FIGURE 5. Expression of transgenic CMVβ-gal activity in Accell-bombarded human mammary carcinoma cell line, MCF-7 cells. (A) low magnification; more than 15% of cells in culture express β-gal activity. (B) high magnification; arrows indicate single gold bead apparently localized in nucleus or cytosol of bombarded cells (adapted from Yang et al., 1990 *Proc Natl Acad Sci USA*, National Academy of Sciences, Washington, DC).

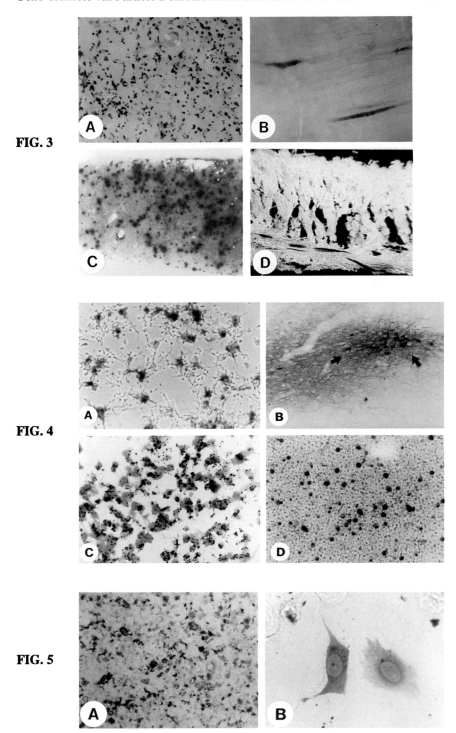

FIG. 3

FIG. 4

FIG. 5

Similarly, bombarded mouse or rat liver tissue also released transgenic hGH into serum.

Williams et al. (1991) also demonstrated effective in vivo gene transfer into mouse epidermis and liver tissues using the Biolistic method. The level and pattern of expression for marker genes (luc, hGH) were similar to those using the Accell method. Particle-bombardment mediated gene delivery appears to be generally applicable to in vivo gene transfer in a broad range of somatic tissues in rat, mouse, hamster, rabbit and rhesus monkey (Cheng et al., 1993), so it is an attractive option for studying transgene expression in vivo.

EX VIVO AND IN VITRO GENE TRANSFER

The most commonly used approach for gene therapy research today is ex vivo gene transfer into primary cell cultures derived from freshly isolated tissue or cell explants followed by transplantation or infusion into target organs of host animals. Various primary cultures, including those derived from liver hepatocytes, peripheral blood lymphocytes, tumor infiltrating lymphocytes, muscle cells, and others (Anderson, 1992; Yang, 1992), have been successfully transfected by different methods. As a clinical procedure, however, it is highly desirable that the tissue or cell explants be processed with minimal biochemical or tissue culture manipulation to facilitate rapid transfection and implantation. Particle bombardment is ideal for ex vivo procedures because it can transfect multiple cell layers of solid tissue or cell clumps (Williams et al., 1991; Zelenin et al., 1991) and because the gene transfer step takes less than a minute.

Thompson et al. (1993) and Yang et al. (1990) bombarded freshly isolated rat mammary ductal organoids before plating them in primary cultures. High level CMVβ-gal transgene activity was detected at the cellular level (Fig. 4C, Page 199), demonstrating efficient gene transfer into tissue clumps. Thompson et al. (1993) further demonstrated that gene transfer using the Accell bombardment method was 5- to 100-fold more efficient than calcium phosphate co-precipitation, lipofection, or electroporation in short-term primary cultures established from rat mammary epithelial cells.

Using a similar approach, Jiao et al. (1993) reported that particle bombardment can be effectively utilized for gene transfer into fetal rat brain cells prepared as freshly isolated tissue clumps or as single cells in suspension. Both neurons and glial cells showed similar transfection patterns. Even adult brain tissue clumps expressed significant levels of marker gene activity. These investigators also demonstrated that the Accell method resulted in a much higher transient gene expression efficiency (> 100-fold) in fetal rat brain tissues than that obtained from electroporation, calcium phosphate co-precipitation, or standard lipofectin methods. High efficiency transgenic β-gal expression in bombarded brain cells was detected at the cellular level (Fig. 4A, Page 199). Results obtained by Jiao et al. (1993) and Thompson et al. (1993) unambiguously showed that particle bombardment is a highly effective means for gene transfer into small tissue clumps and their derivative primary cultures. This should find utility in a variety of ex vivo gene transfer systems.

Jiao et al. (1993) also achieved relatively long-term transgene expression in fetal brain tissues transplanted into adult hosts. CMV-luc gene was bombarded into fetal rat brain tissue ex vivo, with expression lasting for up to two months after implantation into adult rat brains. In a similar experiment, they tested the tyrosine hydroxylase (TH) gene, a candidate therapeutic gene for Parkinson's disease. Significant ex vivo and in vivo expressions of the CMV-TH transgene were detected (Fig. 4B, Page 199).

Recently, Freed et al. (1992) and Spencer et al. (1992) demonstrated that transplantation of human fetal brain tissues into caudate tissue of patients with Parkinson's disease resulted in a significant reduction of patients' symptoms. By extension, if an introduced tyrosine hydroxylase gene can increase the production of L-dopa in fetal brain tissues, gene therapy may provide a more effective Parkinson's disease treatment with reduced requirement for fetal brain tissues.

Zelenin et al. (1991) also demonstrated ex vivo gene transfer by bombarding small pieces (~ 1 mm^3) of rodent liver, kidney, and mammary tissue explants. When bombarded tissues were plated for 24 hours in organ cultures, significant levels of CAT gene activity were detected. In a slightly different approach, we used tissue slices (~ 0.2 to 0.5 mm in thickness and 1 cm^2 in surface area) obtained by vibratome sectioning rat kidney, liver, spleen, and skin explants. Immediately after bombardment with CMV-luc DNA, tissue slices were incubated overnight in culture medium. From 4-16 hours post-bombardment, significant but variable levels of luc activity were detected (Yang et al., unpublished results). Because tissue slices can maintain certain infrastructures unique to a given organ, gene therapy and transplantation using tissue slices may have a number of advantages over the use of single cell samples.

Other primary cell culture systems also gave significant but variable transgenic luc expression after either Accell or Biolistic bombardment. These include rat kidney cells, rat myoblast cells, rat or rhesus monkey muscle cells, rat hepatocytes, human keratinocytes, mammary stromal fibroblasts, rat mesothelial cells, and rabbit blood vessel endothelial cells (Zelenin et al., 1991; Jiao et al., unpublished data; Cheng et al., unpublished data).

In addition to these attached tissue culture systems, suspension cell culture preparations, including human and rat peripheral blood lymphocytes, and mouse splenocytes, thymocytes, and peritoneal macrophages, also gave readily detectable transient gene expression after Accell bombardment (Burkholder et al., 1993). Using eight established mammalian cell culture lines, it was demonstrated that particle bombardment can be systematically used for gene transfection of a variety of different cell types in culture, including those derived from epithelium, endothelium, fibroblast, and lymphocyte origins (Yang et al., 1990). At the cellular level, 3 to 15% of bombarded monolayer cells in culture expressed high levels of transient β-gal activity. An example of CMVβ-gal expression in MCF-7 cells (a human mammary carcinoma cell line) is shown in Fig. 5 (Page 199), where gold microprojectiles delivered into the monolayer cells are readily observed at high magnification. Furthermore, we have shown that stable gene transfer events occurred at frequencies of 1.7×10^{-3} and 6×10^{-4} for CHO and MCF-7 cells, respectively (Yang et al., 1990). Similar transfection frequencies for cell culture lines have been obtained by Fitzpatrick-McElligott (1992) using the Biolistic bombardment method. These studies showed that particle bombardment can result in efficient gene transfer in bombarded cells in culture, with a frequency for stable transfection that compares favorably with those obtained by other direct gene transfer methods. It remains to be determined if in vivo selection of bombarded tissues can result in enrichment of stable transfectants in gene transfer experiments.

APPLICATION TO BASIC AND CLINICAL RESEARCH

In vitro expression of transgenes frequently does not reflect the regulatory controls found in vivo (Sharfmann et al., 1991; Miller, 1992). For effective evaluation of transgene expression levels and physiological effects in gene therapy research, an efficient in vivo gene transfer and assay system is needed.

The transgenic mouse system has been useful for evaluating transgene expression in vivo, most notably for analysis of tissue-specific promoter expression in various organs. This system, however, requires costly, highly specialized, and laborious techniques for the production of transgenic mice and does not lend itself to quick, convenient, and quantitative analysis. Furthermore, it was reported that, even within the same tissue type, highly variable levels (up to 10,000-fold) of reporter gene activity were found in different lines of transgenic mice generated using the same promoter-gene (e.g., CMV) construct (Furth et al., 1991). This was apparently the result of positional effects on transgene expression — the site of transgene integration on host chromosomes could dramatically affect expression levels (Isola and Gordon, 1991). Technically, methods for creating transgenic mice have not yet been systematically extended to other mammalian systems. These limitations make the transgenic mouse system impractical or impossible as a routine procedure for studying transgene expression in vivo in targeted somatic tissues of various experimental animal species.

Experimental results from studies using particle bombardment for in vivo gene transfer to date suggest that the method is useful in comparative studies of promoter strength and the expression of reporter, functional, as well as therapeutic genes in various mammalian somatic tissues. This method may be adapted as a routine laboratory assay for characterization and functional evaluation of marker or therapeutic gene constructs under in vivo conditions. A range of experimental animals, not just rodents, can be conveniently recruited for transgenic experiments. If proven clinically applicable, particle bombardment could even be used to evaluate and determine in vivo expression levels and physiological effects of therapeutic genes in targeted tissues of individual patients, providing a new tool for gene transfer and gene therapy studies.

To investigate some of these possibilities, in vivo expression levels from a number of commonly used viral and mammalian cellular promoters in five different rat somatic tissues were analyzed by using particle-mediated gene transfer (Cheng et al., 1993). In this study, tissue-type preferences in expression from several cellular promoters, including those derived from the mouse phosphoenolpyruvate carboxykinase (PEPCK), phosphoglycerate kinase (PGK), and metallothionein (mMT) genes, were measured in bombarded rat somatic tissues. The mMT and PGK promoters expressed very high levels of transgenic luc activity in rat epidermis and dermis, respectively. These levels were similar to or higher than the CMV-luc activity detected in the same tissues. In contrast, these two cellular promoters were much less active (~5- to 20-fold) than the CMV promoter in rat liver and pancreatic tissues. Apparent differences in expression of nominally constitutive viral promoters in different tissue types were also observed. For instance, the adenovirus major late promoter was as active as the CMV promoter in muscle tissue, but comparatively ineffective in rat skin or liver tissues. Cheng et al. (1993) further demonstrated that PEPCK and mMT promoter activity in liver can be readily stimulated in vivo by injection of the appropriate inducing agents at both 1 and 5 days post-bombardment. These results suggest that particle bombardment provides a convenient and effective technique for evaluating the in vivo regulation and induction of gene expression in many somatic tissues of different experimental mammalian species.

The effectiveness of particle bombardment in a wide range of experimental systems, including tissue clumps, tissue slices, cell aggregates, and single cell and primary cultures derived from these various tissue explant samples, provides a novel alternative for gene transfer studies. This strategy, when applied to nerve cell systems, could allow a new approach to study molecular neurophysiology at the cellular level. For example, fetal neurons or proliferative mature neurons in primary cultures may be bombarded with candidate functional genes to allow systematic evaluation of neuron degeneration, renewed growth, or synapsis formation in cell culture (Reynolds and Weiss, 1992). Similarly, mammary gland and muscle cells in primary cultures can also be bombarded to study the expression of genes involved in cellular differentiation and biochemical functions.

Particle bombardment has two major technical advantages over standard gene transfer methods. The high loading capacity of the microscopic gold particles means that large numbers of DNA molecules can be delivered to individual cells. The second advantage is the ability for particle bombardment to deliver large DNA molecules (Yang, 1992). These features may allow large quantities of genomic DNA fragments containing large size or clustered genes (cloned into cosmid or artificial chromosome vectors) to be transferred into mammalian cells. In basic research, this may allow the evaluation of coordinated expression of multiple genes under appropriate in vitro or in vivo experimental conditions. Li et al. (1993) and Thompson et al. (1991) have already demonstrated that the use of particle bombardment in gene-cotransfection experiments is very efficient for quantitative analysis of the effect of specific oncogenes in established cultured cell lines. These studies suggest that similar experiments can be performed in vivo or ex vivo in various somatic tissue systems.

Recent developments in molecular oncology suggest that in the future a range of cancerous diseases may be treated by using gene therapy approaches. An attractive strategy which is being evaluated by several laboratories, some in clinical trials, is the localized treatment of tumors by transferring therapeutic genes into affected tissue. Various lymphokine genes and "suicidal" thymidine kinase genes are being assessed for treatment of melanoma tumors and gliomas, respectively (Rosenberg et al., 1990; Anderson, 1992; Culver et al., 1992). Recently, tumor suppressor genes and antisense oncogenes or growth factors have also been reported to exhibit anti-tumor effects in animal experiments (Roth et al., 1992; Trojan et al., 1993). In vivo particle bombardment may find specific applications in gene therapy of solid tumors, such as the treatment of tissues surrounding surgically removed tumors. Also, in situations where surgical removal of multiple, small tumors is difficult, localized bombardment of tumors and their surrounding normal tissues with a therapeutic gene may be an attractive option.

Since DNA-coated microprojectiles can penetrate multiple cell layers of a target tissue, particle bombardment may enhance other gene transfer methods in in vivo gene therapy experiments. For example, bombardment of solid somatic tissues with relatively large beads (e.g., 5-7 μm microprojectiles) creates millions of microscopic "paths" through the tissue. Therefore, if transducing virus (e.g., retrovirus or adenovirus) preparations are spread onto or injected into target tissues (e.g., tumor tissues) immediately before bombardment, the paths generated by the gold beads may allow the virus to penetrate deeper into the target tissue resulting in more effective gene transfer. Similarly, liposomes or lipofectin methods may also benefit from deeper and more extensive penetration into targeted tissues. These combinations of gene transfer techniques may be more efficient than using a single method alone and may be especially attractive for gene therapy of solid tumors.

The use of the Biolistic bombardment method as a means for genetic immunization has been assessed by Tang et al. (1992). After bombardment of ear skin with hGH or human alpha-1-antitrypsin (hAAT) DNA, antibodies against these proteins were readily detected in sera of test mice. Skin is an excellent target since epidermal tissues contain competent antigen-presenting cells including Langerhan cells which are easily accessible for particle bombardment. In addition to antibody production, particle bombardment of skin tissue is also expected to elicit cytotoxic T lymphocyte-mediated cellular immune responses (Haynes et al., 1993) which are required for protection against viral or other pathogen infections. The combination of humoral and cellular immunities is crucial for the prevention or control of infectious disease. Studies on particle bombardment as a means for genetic immunization or vaccination are discussed in detail in another chapter.

As an emerging technology, the ballistic method of gene transfer currently has technical limitations. Unlike retrovirus vectors, in vivo gene transfer to most, but not all, somatic tissues using particle bombardment results in transgene expression lasting only from several days to 2 weeks. This probably results from the lack of stable gene integration in bombarded target cells. Episomal vectors or artificial chromosomes may be strategies for relatively long-term transgene expression using bombardment. Multiple and repeated bombardment regimes for certain tissues (e.g., epidermal skin tissues or exposed solid tumors), which would provide continuous transgene expression, may also be adequate to treat certain diseases. The in vitro stable gene transfection frequency of $\sim 10^{-4}$ (Yang et al., 1990) would be difficult to obtain in vivo unless methods for in vivo selection of stably transfected cells can be developed to enrich these cell populations.

Another current limitation of gene therapy via in vivo tissues is that although deep penetration can be achieved by using large size microprojectiles, transgene expression levels are often decreased. This is apparently related to the increased levels of cell damage observed in bombarded tissues. Modification of particle acceleration hardware designs, experimentation with gold particles of various forms and shapes, and optimization of bombardment parameters are being evaluated to upgrade this technology for in vivo gene transfer.

Safety is a key issue for any gene therapy protocol. To address this concern we are currently conducting studies to determine the distribution, physiological effects, and fate of gold particles in various rat somatic tissues, including skin and liver. A series of acute toxicity tests have not yet encountered any problems, nor have we observed any abnormal behavior or general health problems during 2 to 10 months following bombardment. Physiological levels of various index enzymes, proteins, and minerals in serum over one month showed no significant differences between test and control rats. Also, rats injected with relatively high doses of elemental gold into various organs have developed normally (Yang et al., unpublished data). Extensive studies, including GLP-certified toxicity studies, are being evaluated to clarify the safety issues involved in using particle bombardment for gene therapy protocols.

CONCLUDING REMARKS

Particle bombardment has been shown to be effective under various experimental conditions with in vivo, ex vivo, and in vitro mammalian gene transfer systems. For in vivo gene transfer into somatic tissues, this method is apparently applicable to all mammalian systems. As a physical means for ex vivo gene delivery into primary cultures of two tested systems (rat mammary and fetal brain tissues), Accell particle bombardment was found to be considerably more efficient than three other gene transfer techniques tested. It has demonstrated its utility in transfection of freshly isolated tissue explant samples, including tissue slices, tissue clumps, and cell aggregates, providing a new approach for gene transfer into surgically derived tissue samples.

Technological advances in particle bombardment have provided new tools for studying molecular and cellular biology in diverse experimental systems. For basic research, the particle bombardment method can be conveniently utilized to study transgene expression under various in vivo and ex vivo experimental conditions. Regulation of promoter activity and functional transgene expression as well as cell migration and turnover in various somatic tissues can be readily studied. For gene therapy research, this technology is useful in the verification and evaluation of in vivo expression and physiological effects of candidate therapeutic genes in targeted somatic tissues.

Particle bombardment-mediated gene delivery is a simple, fast, and versatile technique for gene transfer. With future modification and optimization, this evolving technology may serve as a generic approach for gene transfer and gene therapy experimentation.

ACKNOWLEDGMENTS

We are deeply grateful to J. Tuan, M. Allen, and R. De Luna for professional editing of the manuscript, and to P. Ziegelhoffer for collecting information.

REFERENCES

Anderson WF (1992): Human gene therapy. *Science* 256:808-813

Burkholder JK, Decker J, Yang N-S (1993): Transgene expression in lymphocyte and macrophage primary cultures after particle bombardment. *J Immunol Methods* (In Press)

Cheng L, Ziegelhoffer PR, Yang N-S (1993): A novel approach for studying in vivo transgene activity in mammalian systems. *Proc Natl Acad Sci USA* 90:4455-4459

Christou P, McCabe D, Martinell B, Swain W (1990): Soybean genetic engineering — commercial production of transgenic plants. *Trends Biotechnol* 8:145-151

Christou P, McCabe DE, Swain WF, Russell DR (1993): Legume transformation. In *Control of Plant Expression*, DPS Verma, ed., CRC Press, Boca Raton

Culver KW, Ram Z, Wallbridge S, Ishii H, Oldfield EH, Blaese RM (1992): In vivo gene transfer with retroviral vector-producer cells for treatment of experimental brain tumors. *Science* 255:434-440

Fitzpatrick-McElligott S (1992): Gene transfer to tumor-infiltrating lymphocytes and other mammalian somatic cells by microprojectile bombardment. *Bio/Technology* 10:1036-1040

Freed CP, Breeze RE, Rosenberg NL, Schneck SA, Kriek E, Qi J-X, Lone T, Zhang Y-B, Snyder JA, Wells TH, Ramig LO, Thompson L, Mazziota JC, Huang SC, Grafton ST, Brooks D, Sawle G, Schroter G, Ansari A (1992): Survival of implanted fetal dopamine cells and neurologic improvement 12 to 46 months after transplantation for Parkinson's disease. *N Engl J Med* 327:1549-1555

Furth LP, Hennighausen A, Baker C, Beatty B, Woychick R (1991): The variability in activity of the universally expressed human cytomegalovirus immediate early gene 1 enhancer/promoter in transgenic mice. *Nuc Acids Res* 19:6205-6208

Haynes J, Fuller D, Eisenbraun M (1993): Genetic immunization, In *Particle Bombardment Technology for Gene Transfer*, N-S Yang, P Christou, eds., W. H. Freeman, New York

Isola LM, Gordon JM (1991): Transgenic animals: A new era in developmental biology and medicine. In *Transgenic Animals*, NL First, FF Haseltine, eds., Butterworth, Heinemann, MA

Jiao S, Ascadi G, Jani A, Felgner PL, Wolff JA (1992): Persistence of plasmid DNA and expression in rat-brain cells in vivo. *Exp Neurol* 115:400-413

Jiao S, Cheng L, Wolff JA, Yang N-S (1993): Particle bombardment-mediated gene transfer and expression in rat brain tissues. *Bio/Technology* 11:497-502

Johnston SA, Riedy M, DeVit MJ, Sanford JC, McElligott S, Williams RS (1991): Biolistic transformation of animal tissue. *In Vitro Cell Dev Biol* 27P:11-14

Klein T, Wolf E, Wu R, Sanford J (1987): High-velocity microprojectiles for delivering nucleic acids into living cells. *Nature* 327:70-73

Li C-CH, Ruscetti FW, Rice NR, Chen E, Yang N-S, Mikovits J, Longo DL (1993): Differential expression of Rel family members in HTLV-I infected cells: Transcriptional activation of c-rel by Tax protein. *J Virol* (In Press)

McCabe D, Swain W, Martinell B, Christou P (1988): Stable transformation of soybean (*glycine max*) by particle acceleration. *Bio/Technology* 6:923-926

McCabe D, Martinell B (1992): Apparatus for genetic transformation. Patent #US 5149655

Miller AD (1992): Human gene therapy comes of age. *Nature* 357:455-460

Reynolds BA, Weiss S (1992): Generation of neurons and astrocytes from isolated cells of the adult mammalian central nervous system. *Science* 255:1707-1710

Rosenberg SA, Aebersold P, Cornetta K, Kasid A, Morgan RA, Moen RA, Karson EM, Lotze MT, Yang JC, Topalian SL, Merino MJ, Culver K, Miller AD, Blaese RM, Anderson WF (1990): Gene transfer into humans — immunotherapy of patients with advanced melanoma, using tumor-infiltrating lymphocytes modified by retroviral gene transduction. *N Engl J Med* 323:570-578

Roth JA, Mukhopadhyay T, Tainsky MA, Fang K, Casson AG, Schneider PM (1992): Molecular approaches to prevention and therapy of aerodigestive tract cancers. *Monogr Natl Cancer Inst* (13) 15-21

Sanford J (1988): The biolistic process. *Trends Biotechnol* 6:299-302

Sautter C, Waldner H, Neuhaus-Url G, Galli A, Neuhaus G, Potrykus I (1991): Micro-targeting: High efficiency gene transfer using a novel approach for the acceleration of micro-projectiles. *Bio/Technology* 9:1080-1085

Scharfmann R, Axelrod JH, Verma IM (1991): Long-term in vivo expression of retrovirus-mediated gene transfer in mouse fibroblast implants. *Proc Natl Acad Sci USA* 88:4626-4630

Spencer DD, Robbins RJ, Naftolin F, Marek KL, Vollmer T, Leranth C, Roth RH, Price LH, Gjedde A, Bunney BS, Sass KJ, Elsworth JD, Kier EL, Maruch R, Hoffer PB, Redmond DE (1992): Unilateral transplantation of human fetal mesencephalic tissue into the caudate nucleus of patients with Parkinson's Disease. *N Engl J Med* 327:1541-1548

Tang DC, DeVit M, Johnston SA (1992): Genetic immunization is a simple method for eliciting an immune response. *Nature* 356:152-154

Thompson TA, Burkholder J, Yang N-S, Gould MN (1991): Abstract: Qualitative differences in modulation of viral promoters by ras. *Proc Am Assoc Cancer Res* 32:294

Thompson TA, Gould MN, Burkholder JK, Yang N-S (1993): Transient promoter activity in primary rat mammary epithelial cells evaluated using particle bombardment gene transfer. *In Vitro Cell Dev Biol* 29A:165-170

Trojan J, Johnson TR, Rudin SD, Ilan J, Tykocinski ML, Ilan J (1993): Treatment and prevention of rat glioblastoma by immunogenic C6 cells expressing antisense insulin-like growth factor I RNA. *Science* 259:94-97

Williams RS, Johnston SA, Riedy M, DeVit MJ, McElligott SG, Sanford JC (1991): Introduction of foreign genes into tissues of living mice by DNA-coated microprojectiles. *Proc Natl Acad Sci USA* 88:2726-2730

Wolff JA, Malone RW, Williams P, Chong W, Acsadi G, Jani A, Felgner PL (1990): Direct gene transfer into mouse muscle in vivo. *Science* 247:1465-1468

Yang N-S (1993): Transgenic plants from legumes. In *Transgenic Plants*, S Kung, R Wu, eds., Academic Press, New York

Yang N-S (1992): Gene transfer into mammalian somatic cells in vivo. *CRC Crit Rev Biotechnol* 12:335-356

Yang N-S, Burkholder J, Roberts B, Martinell B, McCabe D (1990): In vivo and in vitro gene transfer to mammalian somatic cells by particle bombardment. *Proc Natl Acad Sci USA* 87:9568-9572

Zelenin AV, Alimov AA, Titomirov AV, Kazansky AV, Gorodetsky SI, Kolesnikov VA (1991): High-velocity mechanical DNA transfer of the chloramphenicolacetyl transferase gene into rodent liver, kidney and mammary gland cells in organ explants and in vivo. *FEBS Lett* 280(1):94-96

ELECTRICALLY-INDUCED DNA TRANSFER INTO CELLS. ELECTROTRANSFECTION IN VIVO

Sergei I. Sukharev, Alexander V. Titomirov, and Vadim A. Klenchin

INTRODUCTION

Electrotransfection, or transfection by electroporation (Neumann et al., 1982), is becoming more and more popular as a powerful tool for introduction of exogenous DNA into cells of virtually any origin (Potter et al., 1984, Fromm et al., 1985, Dower et al., 1988, Potter, 1988). In many cases, electroporation is the only method that works. Ultimately, it is because electrotransfection is to a great extent a physical rather than biological technique. In contrast to the traditional method of mammalian cell transformation by calcium phosphate-DNA coprecipitate (Graham and Van der Eb, 1973), which is efficient predominantly with fibroblastlike cells, practically all types of mammalian and other cells attempted are successfully transfected by electroporation (Potter, 1988). This is one of the reasons why electrotransfection is regarded as promising for human gene therapy.

There are two different strategies in electro-induced gene delivery into cells of the human organism. First is in vitro transfection of cells taken out of the organism with possible subsequent clone selection, followed by their reimplantation. This can be performed according to established electroporation protocols with blood and lymph cells, bone marrow and hematopoietic stem cells (Toneguzzo and Keating, 1986, Toneguzzo et al., 1986, 1988, Keating and Toneguzzo, 1990), primary skin fibroblasts (Fountain et al., 1988), and probably with some other reimplantable tissues. Electroporation can also be used in combination with techniques for targeted delivery of DNA to the surface of specific cells (Machy et al., 1988).

Another potential approach is transfection in vivo, which is not complicated with procedures of tissue isolation and reimplantation, but requires development of special surgical devices and procedures (Titomirov et al., 1991). In any event, the requirements for such applications must be exceptionally high: the technique must be reasonably efficient, it should not bring irreversible damage to tissue and DNA and should result in a minimum of side effects.

Historically, electrotransfection, as a field for investigation, laid on a crossroad between biophysical chemistry that studied the stability of cell and model

Gene Therapeutics: Methods and Applications of Direct Gene Transfer
Jon A. Wolff, Editor • ©1994 *Birkhäuser Boston*

membranes in an electric field, and molecular genetics. Many aspects of the problem are well reviewed in two detailed monographs issued during last three years: *Electroporation and Electrofusion in Cell Biology* (Neumann, Sowers, and Jordan, editors, Plenum, 1989) and *Guide to Electroporation and Electrofusion* (Chang et al., editors, Academic Press, 1992). Within these monographs, the phenomenologies, mechanisms and some applications of membrane poration by high-intensity electric field are overviewed (for example, see Tsong, 1989, Chernomordik, 1992, Weaver and Barnett, 1992). For a cellular and molecular-biological counterpart, see reviews by Potter (1989), Potter and Cooke (1992), and by Reid and Smithies (1992). In spite of an abundance of experimental observations and theoretical considerations, there is still a striking lack of information on the primary processes of DNA translocation into cells by the electric field.

The goals of this review are to shortly outline electroporation as a phenomenon, to summarize recent data on the mechanism of electrically induced DNA translocation through the plasma membrane of mammalian cells, and to describe the first in vivo electroporation technique that was developed especially for transformation of skin cells.

CELL IN AN ELECTRIC FIELD: MEMBRANE ELECTROPORATION

Electroporation, i.e. formation of hydrophilic pores in a cell membrane by the electric field, is the first and prerequisite of a sequence of events that leads to acquisition of exogenous DNA by cell. Since this phenomenon was previously reviewed in detail (Tsong, 1989,1992; Neumann, 1989; Chernomordik and Chizmadzhev, 1989; Deuticke and Schwister, 1989), we will briefly summarize the primary results and basic concepts.

A cell membrane is basically a thin insulating film that surrounds the conducting inner cell content. When a cell is placed in the chamber between two electrodes and an electric field, E, is turned on, ion movement inside the cell and movement of counterions in the outer medium will polarize the membrane, predominantly on the poles facing the electrodes (see Fig. 1A). Once the field is applied, the transmembrane voltage raises with the time constant $\tau = r \times C_m \times (\rho_{int} + \rho_{ext}/2)$, where r is the cell radius, C_m is specific membrane capacitance, and ρ_{int} and ρ_{ext} are conductivities of internal and external solutions, respectively. The maximal voltage across the membrane, V_m, induced by a DC-pulse of external electric field, E, on the poles of the spherical cell, can be calculated as $V_m = 1 \times 5 \times r \times E$ (Cole, 1972; Tsong, 1992). In the steady-state situation, when E is not too high, the electric field does not penetrate through the intact membrane and the field lines bypass the cell (Fig. 1A). When the field is high enough to induce V_m to 0.4-1 V, the ordered membrane structure is disturbed, leading to a dramatic increase in membrane conductance and non-specific permeability (electric membrane breakdown). As a result, the electric field pattern changes and the electric current flows through the permeabilized cell membrane (Fig. 1B). This phenomenon has been extensively studied by membrane permeability tests, mostly on hu-

FIGURE 1. Electric field and charge distribution around a cell placed between two parallel flat electrodes. (A) At low intensity the external field bypasses the cell with the intact membrane. (B) Higher electric field creates membrane pores which let the field and the current pass through the cell.

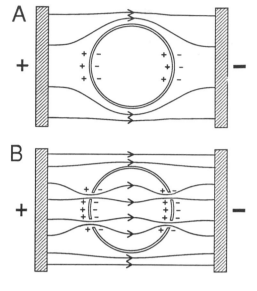

man erythrocytes (Kinosita and Tsong, 1977; Schwister and Deuticke, 1985), and also by direct electrical measurements on live cells (Zimmermann et al., 1976; Kinosita and Tsong, 1979; Sukharev et al., 1985; Chernomordik et al., 1987) and planar lipid bilayers (Abidor et al., 1979; Benz et al., 1979; Chernomordik et al., 1983, 1987). The events of membrane polarization and poration in an external electric field were visualized by using voltage-sensitive dyes (Kinosita et al., 1988). The results of these studies can be summarized as follows.

Pore formation and electric pulse parameters

The loss of barrier function of membrane in an intensive electric field is due to formation of local water-filled defects in membrane structure (electropores, pores). Similarity of the electroporation phenomena observed in cell and pure lipid membranes (Chernomordik et al., 1987) suggested that electropores are located primarily in the lipid matrix of membranes. Formation of a hydrophilic pore (Chernomordik and Chizmadzhev, 1989) is illustrated in Fig. 2. When the electric field is on, the local thermal fluctuation in bilayer structure creates the defect called a hydrophobic pore (Fig. 2A). This pore is immediately expanded by pressure of water, which is dielectrically drawn into the pore where the electric field intensity is maximal (Abidor et al., 1979). Upon reaching some critical radius (Leikin et al., 1986), such a short-living hydrophobic pore rapidly transforms into hydrophilic pore lined with polar lipid headgroups (Fig. 2B). Hydrophylic pores in a pure lipid bilayer are relatively stable; their lifetimes range from seconds to minutes. In cell membranes they may be further stabilized by involvement of proteins in the pore edge, forming so-called composite pore. (see Fig. 2C). The important observation that electroporation enhances flip-flop transitions of lipids in erythrocytes (Dressler

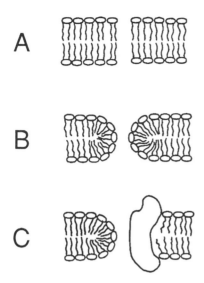

FIGURE 2. Schematic representation of the process of electropore formation. (A) A short-lived hydrophobic pore. (B) A hydrophilic (or 'inverted') pore. (C) A 'composite' pore stabilized by involvement of proteins in the pore edge. (Adapted with permission from Chernomordik, 1992.)

et al., 1983) strongly suggested that hydrophilic pores indeed may serve as "bridges" connecting inner and outer monolayers of the membrane.

The rate of electropore formation depends nonlinearly on V_m (Leikin et al., 1986, Glaser et al., 1988, reviewed by Chernomordik and Chizmadzhev, 1989). The rate is negligible at low V_m, but it steeply increases with voltage, giving the impression that electroporation is a threshold-like process (Zimmermann et al., 1976). At $V_m > 1$ V, for instance, the electropores appear within a microsecond in cell as well as in pure lipid membranes (Kinosita and Tsong, 1979, Benz et al., 1979). However, experiments have shown that there is no well defined critical "breakdown" voltage, V_m^*; the same raise in membrane conductance or permeability can be achieved either by a short high-intensity pulse, or by a longer pulse of lower amplitude (Sukharev et al., 1985, Chernomordik et al., 1987). This does not mean that pore populations in both cases will be the same. Because the electric field induces two distinct processes simultaneously, pore accumulation and pore expansion (Kinosita and Tsong, 1977b,1979; Chernomordik et al., 1983; Glaser et al., 1988), the pulse amplitude and duration may affect pore density in the plane of the membrane, as well as the mean pore size. Several theories of pore formation have been developed (Pastushenko et al., 1979; Sugar and Neumann, 1984; Leikin et al., 1986; Weaver and Barnett, 1992).

Processes associated with the electric current flow through the cells

According to theories, pore formation is predicted independent on pulse polarity. However electroporation of real cells assayed by entrapment or release of various dyes was found to be asymmetric. Entrapment of positively charged dyes was more pronounced on the pole facing the positive electrode (Mehrle et al., 1985), while extrusion of neutral dextrans from erythrocyte ghosts was directed mainly toward the negative electrode (Sowers and Lieber, 1986). Later, Dimitrov and Sowers (1990) showed that asymmetric release of fluorescent dextran from erythrocyte ghosts occurred due to electroosmotic water flux, which takes place near the charged pore edges during the pulse. The analysis of these data shows that the phenomena of electrodiffusion (electrophoresis) and electroosmosis must be regarded as important factors causing fast exchange of charged and neutral molecules between the cytoplasm and the cell exterior.

Electropore sizes and lifetimes

During the electric field pulse, and shortly after, electropores can be relatively wide - at least 8 nm in diameter as indicated by permeation of large dextrans (Sowers and Lieber, 1986) and monoclonal antibodies (Chakrabarti et al., 1989; Berglund et al., 1991). The longer the pulse, the wider the pores that may be created. Short pulses usually result in a more uniform population of smaller pores (Deuticke and Schwister, 1989).

Upon pulse termination, however, the electropores rapidly shrink (within 200 ms, Sowers and Lieber, 1986) to a smaller size, thus preventing, for instance, monoclonal antibodies penetration into cell if they were added after pulse application (Berglund et al., 1991). Such shrunk pores are long-lived lasting from minutes to hours depending on cell type and strength of electric treatment. Systematic permeability measurements on electrically treated erythrocytes using tracer molecules of different chemical nature gave pore radii about 0.5-1.0 nm (Kinosita and Tsong, 1977a,b; Schwister and Deuticke, 1985). Only after extremely intensive treatment (10 kV/cm, 40 μs, Schwister and Deuticke, 1985) were pores of r > 2 nm reported. Interestingly, the pore radius, r, predicted from the non-linear character of I(V)-relationship of electroporated lipid bilayer gave r = 0.6 nm (Chernomordik et al., 1987) consistent with experimental measurements.

If the field intensity and the pulse duration are not too high, membrane poration is reversible, i.e. electropores reseal. As previously mentioned, the first stage of after-pulse pore shrinkage is fast. The experiments with voltage-sensitive dyes (Kinosita et al., 1988) revealed that membrane conductance decreases even within a sub-millisecond upon pulse termination, this probably reflects a non-ohmic character of electropore's conductance (Chernomordik et al., 1987). Pore resealing in pure lipid bilayers observed by different techniques takes from milliseconds (Benz and Zimmermann, 1981) to seconds (Chernomordik et al., 1987). However resealing of small stable pores in cell membranes is a much slower process and is strongly temperature-dependent; in human erythrocytes it takes minutes at 37°C and days at 0°C (Kinosita and Tsong, 1977a; Deuticke and Schwister, 1989). Probably, small residual leaks could remain in the membrane indefinitely unless the cell repairs them by activating membrane turnover. In general, time constants of electropore resealing are cell-specific (Zimmermann, 1982; Knight and Scrutton, 1986) and are influenced by lipid composition of the membrane (Deuticke and Schwister, 1989).

The after-pulse cell viability is largely determined by the process of membrane resealing. Facilitated exchange by ions and small solutes between the cytoplasm and external medium through temporarily permeabilized membrane imposes some requirements on ionic composition of electric treatment medium. For example, millimolar calcium present in the electroporation medium will kill various types of fibroblastlike cells (Finaz et al.,1984; Sukharev et al., 1990), while, for some reason it does not harm lymphoid cells (Chakrabarti et al., 1989). Electroporation in the buffer simulating the ionic composition of intracellular medium was reported to be less damaging for some types of cells (Knight and Scrutton, 1986; van der Hoff et al., 1992).

Secondary pore evolution

The colloid-osmotic swelling of cells (Kinosita and Tsong, 1977a,b) induced by transient membrane electropermeabilization, results in increased membrane tension, which may lead to additional pore expansion. Formation and dynamics of such secondary pores of diameters up to 120 nm have been well documented by fast-freezing EM (Chang and Reese, 1990). If the cells are not osmotically protected by adding electropore-impermeant substances (Tsong, 1989), cell swelling prevents pore resealing and in some cases leads to cell lysis. Addition of high-molecular-weight compounds, such as polysaccharides (inulin or dextrans), polyethylene glycol, or serum proteins in the medium before or shortly after pulse treatment (Tsong, 1989; Herzog et al., 1986; Bahnson and Boggs, 1990) remarkably enhances membrane resealing and consequently increases cell viability. Besides osmotic balancing, the serum, containing partially hydrophobic proteins and lipoproteins, may have more specific effects on membrane resealing process.

Another possible source of membrane tension is cell deformation occurring in an intensive electric field (Bryant and Wolfe, 1987), especially if the cell is swollen in a hypoosmotic medium (V. Ph. Pastushenko, personal communication). Membrane stretch in this situation is more pronounced and also may expand the pores.

ELECTRICALLY-INDUCED DNA UPTAKE BY CELLS

The first observation that high-voltage pulses may lead to cellular uptake of exogenous nucleic acids was reported by Auer (Auer et al., 1976), however, the first genetic application of this phenomenon was not reported until six years later (Wong and Neumann, 1982; Neumann et al., 1982). Nowadays electrotransfection is widely used in molecular and cellular biology. However, the optimization of the electrotransfection procedure to every new system is highly empirical, mainly because the mechanism of this phenomenon is poorly understood. The only clear fact is that the extent of cell membrane poration determined by entrapment of low-molecular-weight dyes, and the transfection efficiency were highly correlated

(Presse et al., 1988; Sczakiel et al., 1989). The main problem in explaining of electrotransfection is a significant discrepancy between the apparent sizes of electropores and DNA. Typically, DNA is much larger than the pores, practically excluding the possibility of free DNA diffusing through them. Knutson and Yee (1987) reported cell transfection even with 150-kb fragments, which are predicted to form random coils of about 2,000 nm in diameter (Cantor and Shimmell, 1980). Several different hypothesis of DNA translocation were proposed. (a) DNA binds to the cell surface prior to translocation, then it approaches the pore and moves through the pore like a thread (Neumann et al., 1982; Xie et al., 1991). DNA also can be transferred (b) with the flow of water occurring due to the colloid-osmotic cell swelling following electropermeabilization (Stopper et al., 1987), or (c) with electroosmotic water flux that takes place near a charged cell surface in a high electric field (Dimitrov and Sowers, 1990). (d) The electrically induced DNA up-take by liposomes was shown to be mediated by a formation of membrane invaginations "swallowing" the DNA (Chernomordik et al., 1990), which led the authors to assume the same endocytosislike process in cells. (e) The possibility of electro-phoretic transfer of DNA as a polyanion was also considered (Winterbourne, 1988, Andreason and Evans, 1989), but only indirect evidence has been provided for this hypothesis. Here we present the recent data showing that the electrophoretic force plays a key role in electrotranslocation of DNA into cells in two aspects: it moves DNA toward and through the membrane electropore, and it adjusts pore size to allow this passage (Klenchin et al., 1991; Sukharev et al., 1992).

Experimental design

We electrotransfected simian Cos-1 cells with the plasmid pCH110, which contains a bacterial *lacZ* (β-galactosidase) as a reporter gene under the control of the SV40 early promoter, and also contains an SV40 *ori* providing for the plasmid amplification in Cos-1 cells. This construct served as a sensitive detection system for cell transformation. Experiments were carried out in a single or dual pulse mode. The sequences of two unequal pulses were delivered from two high-voltage laboratory-built generators, triggered by an electronic time delay. In most experiments, cell suspension was treated with electric pulses in the chamber with vertical stainless steel electrodes placed 2-4 mm apart. To electrotransfect cells grown as a monolayer on a porous cellophane film, the horizontal chamber (Sukharev et al., 1990) was used. In all sets, ten minutes after pulse application cells were resuspended in 5 ml of Dulbecco's modified Eagle's medium (DMEM) with 10% fetal calf serum, and plated on Petri dishes. Transfection efficiency (TE), determined as a specific b-galactosidase activity per viable cell, was assayed with a standard colorimetric technique (An et al., 1982) 48 h following transformation. The linear character of TE dependence on DNA concentration in the chamber confirmed that TE is a correct measure of the amount of DNA taken up by cells.

To study the in electric field-induced membrane permeability for molecules of different sizes, ethidium bromide, Lucifer Yellow, and fluorescein isothiocyanate

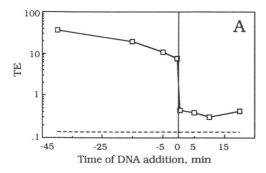

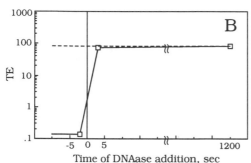

Time of DNAase addition, sec

FIGURE 3. The dependencies of transfection efficiency (TE) on time of addition of the plasmid (A) to the cell suspension and of the DNAase (B) to the cell suspension containing DNA. Time is shown relative to the moment of pulse application (indicated by vertical line). The 'negative' time indicates additions that were made prior to pulsation. The dashed line in (A) gives the level of spontaneous transfection without pulse. In (B), the DNAase and $MgCl_2$ were added to 5 mg/ml and 5 mM, respectively; the dashed line gives the TE level with only $MgCl_2$ added. Pulse: 3.5 kV/cm, 100 μs. (Adapted with permission of The Rockefeller University Press from Klenchin et al., 1991).

(FITC)-labeled dextrans with M_r of 4, 20, 40 and 70 kD (FD4-FD70) were used. Prior to experiments, all FDs were purified from free FITC using spin-column chromatography on Sephadex G-15. Aliquots of cell suspension (100 μl, $1-2\times10^6$ cells) were mixed with FD (to 0.5 mM), and in some cases with DNA, and subjected to electric pulse(s). The influence of three different kinds of DNA was studied: plasmid pCH110 (7.2 kb), phage λ DNA (48 kb) and sheared calf thymus DNA (mixture of fragments from 5 to 100 kb). After pulsation, cells were allowed to reseal, washed, and relative amounts of FD trapped in the cells were measured. (For detailed experimental information see Klenchin et al., 1991, and Sukharev et al., 1992).

Electrotransfection is a fast process

If DNA penetrates into the cell through long-lived pores some time after the pulse, then its addition to the cell suspension shortly after a pore-forming pulse should lead to significant transfection. On the other hand, the addition of DNAase to the cell-DNA mixture immediately after pulse application may lead to a significant decrease in TE since the transfecting plasmid will be inactivated by the enzyme before its delayed entering into the cell. In contrast to these predictions, we found that when the DNA was added 2 s following pulse application, TE dropped by two orders of magnitude when compared to pre-pulse DNA addition (Fig. 3A), while the membrane permeability to Lucifer Yellow, measured a few minutes later,

FIGURE 4. The system for studying the role of electric field direction on electrotransfection. Only the upper surface of cells grown on the porous film is accessible to DNA. Depending on polarity, the electric pulse causes DNA electrophoresis away from (A) or toward the cell (B). Numbers on the bottom show TE assay after transfection with single pulses (2.5 kV/cm, 100 µs) of each polarity. (Reprinted with permission of The Rockefeller University Press from Klenchin et al., 1991).

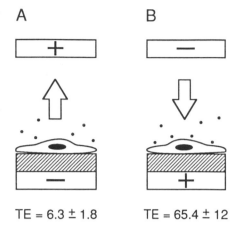

changed only slightly. When DNAase was introduced into the cell suspension with DNA 2 s prior to the pulse application, TE was reduced to a background level, whereas addition of DNAase 2 s after the pulse did not decrease TE as compared to the control (Fig. 3B). Similar results have recently been reported for bacteria (see review by Trevors et al., 1992). Thus, given the time resolution of the techniques used, we conclude that (a) to be efficiently translocated into cell, DNA must be present in the suspension during the pulse, and (b) shortly after the pulse all transfecting DNA is hidden from external DNAase. Apparently DNA is transferred into cells directly during the pulse.

We also tested the influence of the colloid-osmotic process on DNA penetration. Cells transfected in the presence of 20 mM inulin, which prevented cell swelling following electropermeabilization, showed no difference in TE as compared with the control (no inulin). Therefore, the water influx occurring due to colloid-osmotic cell swelling does not play the key role in DNA translocation.

DNA translocation is a vectorial process with the same direction as DNA electrophoresis

To elucidate the role of electric field direction, we transfected the cells grown as a confluent monolayer on a porous film (Fig. 4). In this system mainly the upper surface of cells was accessible to DNA. The electric field normal to the monolayer plane induced membrane poration and also DNA electrophoresis either toward or away from the cells, depending on pulse polarity used. The extent of cell poration, estimated by permeability for propidium iodide after the pulse, was the same at both pulse polarities. The results of the TE assay (Fig. 4, bottom) indicated that when DNA is driven electrophoretically toward the cells (bottom electrode positive), transfection efficiency was one order of magnitude higher than when a reverse polarity was used. Note, that the electroosmotic water flux through the electropores (Dimitrov and Sowers, 1990) has an opposite direction relative to DNA electrophoresis. Thus, we concluded that electroosmosis does not play any role in electrotransfection (Klenchin et al., 1991).

The velocity of electrophoretic DNA movement depends on medium viscosity and on the effective charge of the molecule. Indeed, increasing viscosity by adding the Ficoll-400 (up to 10% v/w), or partially neutralizing DNA charges by adding Mg^{2+} ions (up to 10 mM) in the electroporation medium reduces TE consistently. Since Mg^{2+} ions are also known as enhancers of DNA binding to the cell surface (Belyaev et al., 1988) and TE was remarkably lower in the presence of Mg^{2+}, binding of DNA to the membrane is apparently not necessary for electrotranslocation.

A low-intensity electric field following electroporation in the presence of DNA substantially increases the efficiency of DNA translocation

The first experiments that suggested the possibility of electrophoretic DNA transfer into cells were reported by Andreason and Evans (1989). We used a similar two-pulse protocol (Fig. 5A) to distinguish between two different effects of an electric field: electroporation and electrophoretic DNA translocation. The first pulse of 6 kV/cm and 10 μs provided efficient poration (98% of cells were stained with Lucifer Yellow), but was very weak in electrotransfection. The second pulse of 0.2 kV/cm and 10 ms, when applied alone, caused neither detectable poration nor transfection, but when applied immediately after the first pulse, enhanced TE by one order of magnitude. Reversing the order of the pulses gave the same result as the first (high-voltage) pulse alone. TE increased progressively with the second pulse duration (or, equivalently, with electric charge passed through the chamber during the pulse), as revealed in two-pulse experiments (Fig. 5B). TE declined with the increased time interval between the pulses, suggesting pore resealing between the pulses (Fig. 5C). The characteristic lifetime of pores that are permeable to DNA in conditions of low electric field in this experiment can be estimated as tens of seconds.

The two-pulse experiments demonstrated that an electric field provides for two different effects on cells and the nearby DNA: it creates electropores, and it induces DNA electrophoresis toward and then through the membrane. However, the existence of electropores in the membrane and the presence of a low-intensity electric field was not sufficient for effective DNA penetration. Introduction of DNA between the high-voltage and low-voltage pulses (which usually takes 5 s) gave a negligibly low level of TE, when compared with when the DNA was added prior to pulse treatment. This result indicates that the pores permeable to DNA (under conditions of low electric field) can be created by high-intensity electric field only in the presence of DNA. In other words, DNA itself influences electroporation. This interpretation is in good agreement with following results.

FIGURE 5. Transfection using the two-pulse protocol (A). The first pulse of 6 kV/cm, 10 μs was followed by second pulse of 0.2 kV/cm, and variable duration with the time interval Δt. (B) Transfection efficiency as a function of second pulse duration varied from 0 to 10 ms. The pulse duration is expressed in units of electric charge passed in the circuit during the second pulse. Δt = 100 μs. (C) The dependence of TE on the time gap between the two pulses.   The second pulse duration is 10 ms. (Reprinted with permission of The Rockefeller University Press from Sukharev et al., 1992).

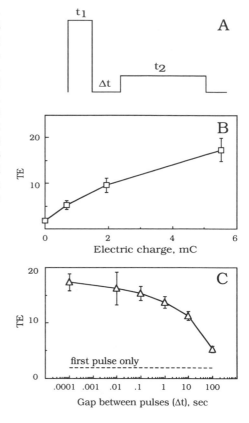

DNA present in the electrotreatment medium increases membrane permeability to indifferent dyes

The dependence of electrically- induced cellular FD4 uptake on the concentration of calf thymus DNA is shown in Fig. 6A. A reliable increase in cell fluorescence is observed beginning at 1 μg/ml of thymus DNA. The DNA-dependent increase in permeability is a long-lasting membrane alteration; it is seen if FD is added a minute after pulse application.

The FD entrapment was found to be dependent on sizes of both components, FD and DNA. The relative amounts of FDs of four different sizes, entrapped in cells by the action of equal pulses in the presence of thymus DNA, are plotted in Fig. 6B. The significant DNA-dependent increase in plasma membrane permeability is observed only for FD4 and FD20. DNA did not influence the entrapment of the larger dextrans FD40 and FD70. At the same time, the larger the DNA is, the higher the membrane permeability. The relative amounts of FD4 and FD20 taken up by cells in the presence of equimolar amounts of plasmid pCH110 and λ-phage

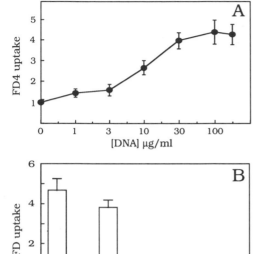

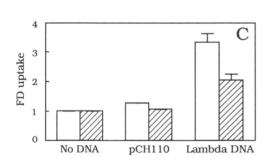

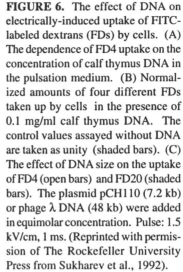

FIGURE 6. The effect of DNA on electrically-induced uptake of FITC-labeled dextrans (FDs) by cells. (A) The dependence of FD4 uptake on the concentration of calf thymus DNA in the pulsation medium. (B) Normalized amounts of four different FDs taken up by cells in the presence of 0.1 mg/ml calf thymus DNA. The control values assayed without DNA are taken as unity (shaded bars). (C) The effect of DNA size on the uptake of FD4 (open bars) and FD20 (shaded bars). The plasmid pCH110 (7.2 kb) or phage λ DNA (48 kb) were added in equimolar concentration. Pulse: 1.5 kV/cm, 1 ms. (Reprinted with permission of The Rockefeller University Press from Sukharev et al., 1992).

DNA are shown in Fig. 6C. The highest increase in permeability was observed for light dextran FD4 in the presence of λ-DNA, the larger DNA used.

It is important to note that in two-pulse experiments, the second low-voltage pulse applied in the presence of DNA increased the uptake of DNA as well FD4. Uptake of FD4 diminished with the time interval between pulses, and was highly correlated with TE (Sukharev et al., 1992). Thus, the effect of the FD uptake increase is not only because of the presence of DNA in the medium, but is apparently associated with DNA translocation through the plasma membrane.

To summarize the data described above, we may envision the process of electrically induced DNA translocation through the cell plasma membrane as follows: When the high electric field is applied to the suspension of cells with DNA, rapid electropore formation occurs, and electric field crosses cell membranes trough these conducting structures (primary pores). The lines of electric field are concentrated in the pores, so the intensity of electric field in the pore and in the nearby

FIGURE 7. Possible ways of DNA interaction with electroporated membrane in a high electric field. (A) DNA orients in an inhomogeneous electric field and squeezes through one pore. Passage of DNA coil can be initiated by penetration of one end of the thread, which then leads the whole molecule through the pore. (B) The DNA molecule may be involved in two (or more) pores and then cut 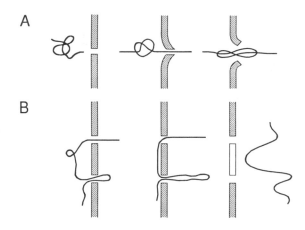 the membrane between these pores; the nonshaded block represents the slit opened between the two pores. (Reprinted with permission of The Rockefeller University Press from Sukharev et al., 1992).

vicinity should be higher than in the bulk (Fig. 1B). At appropriate field orientation, the polyanionic DNA experiences a strong attraction to the pore with simultaneous orientation and alignment due to the inhomogeneous character of field near the pore (Pastushenko and Chizmadzhev, 1992). Even if the size of the primary pore is smaller than the effective diameter of DNA, we suggest that the DNA can squeeze through the membrane because the pore, and also the DNA, are flexible. The mechanical interaction of DNA with the pore by the action of electric field may lead to pore expansion. The passage of the first DNA molecule should facilitate translocation of other molecules through the same pore. Even under conditions of relatively low electric field, DNA transport through these pores may occur due to the effect of field amplification (Cole 1972; Tsong, 1992): whole voltage across the cell actually drops inside the membranes, resulting in increased local field intensity in the pore. The tests for permeation of dextrans of different sizes allowed us to assess the effective size of pores passing the DNA. They showed that the membrane permeability grows with the size of DNA. However, even in the presence of long fragments, the resultant pore size is limited. Thymus DNA (fragments of 5-100 kb long) raised membrane permeability to FD4 and FD20, whereas the permeability to larger dextrans FD40 and FD70 remained unchanged. Taking into account effective diameters of these dextrans (Laurent and Granath, 1967), we can conclude that the resultant pore size is between 3.3 and 4.8 nm. Therefore, DNA likely crosses the pore not as a round globule, but as an elongated bundle.

There are several hypothetical modes of DNA interaction with porated membrane. (a) The DNA molecule squeezes through a single pore. If one of the ends of the DNA chain hangs loose from the globule, then it can be first pulled into the pore, and lead the whole globule through the membrane (Fig. 7A). (b) It is also possible that a single DNA thread enters two (or more) different pores. In this configuration (Fig. 7B), the electrophoretic force pulls DNA inside and the stretch of the molecule between the two pores is able to sever the connecting membrane between these pores, as a sharp thread cuts a block of cheese. Energetic estimates (Pastushenko and Chizmadzhev, 1992) show that electrophoretic pressure of DNA on membrane is high enough to cut the membrane. In this case the resultant pore is a narrow slit connecting two primary pores. (c) DNA pressing against the membrane forms membrane invagination, which later may bud off inside the cell. However, the results of two-pulse experiments, and also long-term alterations of membrane permeability found in experiments with FDs, contradict the hypothesis of endocytosis-like DNA entrapment induced by electric field (Chernomordik et al., 1990). They rather favor the above model of direct DNA passage through the plasma membrane pores, which is also consistent with the view that after electroporation DNA appears to be free (not surrounded with vesicular membrane) in the cytoplasm or nucleoplasm (Potter and Cooke, 1992).

The above model of electrically-induced DNA permeation into cells brings a new physical meaning to the parameters of applied pulses, and may raise some qualitative recommendations on optimization of electrotransfection procedure. The amplitude of the pulse should be high enough to efficiently create primary pores in the membrane (usually higher than 0.75 kV/cm), that can be tested by permeation of conventional dyes. Since the stage of electroporation is followed by a substantially slower stage of DNA electrodiffusion from the bulk to the membrane, and then through the membrane, the pulse should be sufficiently long, typically from 0.1 to 10 ms (Kubiniec et al., 1990). Assuming that the electrophoretic mobility of free DNA in the high field is the same as in the low field (about 1.5×10^{-4} cm^2 x V^{-1} x s^{-1}, see review by Stellwagen, 1987) and the pulse parameters are 1 kV/cm, 1 ms, the depth of the "reaction zone," i.e., the distance from which DNA molecule may reach the membrane, may be estimated as 1.5 μm. Once the pulse duration is chosen, the amplitude can be risen as far as cell viability remains acceptable. The appropriate combination of pulse amplitude and duration depends on the pulse shape used. Besides rectangular pulses, the exponentially decaying pulses also appear to be very suitable since they have a high peak providing for poration, and a long tail of relatively low amplitude, that is sufficient for effective DNA injection into cells. Optimization of membrane poration and DNA injection separately by using two-pulse protocols requires more sophisticated equipment, but may give almost 100% transfection of cells in a population (de Chasseval and de Villartay, 1992). Taking into account the vectorial character of DNA translocation, application of repetitive bipolar pulses (Tekle et al., 1991) should be also efficient because they eventually provide for DNA injection from both sides of the cell. The extent of membrane poration was found to be dependent on DNA concentration (Fig. 6A). Correspondingly, when the experimental conditions permit only low concentration of active plasmid, supplementing of pulsation medium with a nonspecific (carrier) DNA may improve TE (Chu et al., 1988). For the same reason DNA may be "toxic" to cells when present at very high concentration during pulse treatment (Winterbourne et al., 1988). However, the effect of carrier DNA on TE was found to be dependent on the source of the DNA (Chu et al., 1988), indicative of possible involvement of some biological factors.

When electroporation is used in combination with boosted expression of a reporter gene, the TE in optimal conditions may be close to 100%, whereas in the absence of booster the apparent TE is many fold lower (de Chasseval and de Villartay, 1992). This indicates that electrotransfection may readily deliver DNA into all cells in a treated population, but the resultant TE may be limited by subsequent processes of DNA acquisition by cell (i.e., transfer into nucleus, amplification, functioning of promoter). Even if the vector used is ideally compatible with transfected cells, it may be lost or damaged on its way through the cytoplasm to the nucleus. The manner of how the DNA injected into the cytoplasm penetrates into nucleus is unknown, and it is even hard to assess the efficiency of this process. It was reported that after electroporation the entry of plasmid DNA into the nucleus is rapid and the amount of transferred plasmid may reach 8% of the endogenous DNA content (Bertling et al., 1987). Supposingly, DNA may form complexes with some nuclear proteins (histones, for instance) that are synthesized in the cytoplasm. Since they contain the intrinsic nuclear localization sequences, the complexes should be actively transported into nucleus. Alternatively, DNA may penetrate into nucleus during mitosis, when nuclear envelope is dissolved. Studies of cytoplasmic transport of DNA may further improve efficiencies of laboratory and future clinical electrotransfection protocols.

Electroporation, when used for stable cell transformation, results in lower levels of mutations of transfected DNA and gives different patterns of chromosomal integration compared to traditional methods (see Toneguzzo et al., 1988, and review by Potter and Cooke, 1992). The procedure can be adjusted to yield low or high copy number of the inserted gene (Toneguzzo et al., 1986,1988) or large fragments of genomic DNA (Knutson and Yee, 1987; Jastreboff et al., 1987). Special approaches for selecting homologous recombinants after electrotransfection have been reviewed by Reid and Smithies (1992).

ELECTROTRANSFECTION IN VIVO: A FEASIBILITY EXPERIMENT

The temporary expression of foreign genes in several organs of mice and rats has been achieved using liposome-mediated DNA delivery (Nicolau et al., 1983) and by injecting of calcium phosphate-precipitated plasmid into liver, spleen, portal vein (Kaneda et al., 1989), or in peritoneal cavity (Benvenisty and Reshef, 1986). Even naked DNA was found to be expressed in the muscle tissue following direct injection (Wolff et al., 1990). The strategies and applications of non-retroviral gene delivery in mammalian bodies in vivo have been reviewed by Felgner and Rhodes (1991).

In this section we describe experiments aimed at electrical in vivo transformation of skin cells of mice, and the assaying of transfection efficiencies by isolating stably transformed cell clones from the treated tissue (Titomirov et al., 1991).

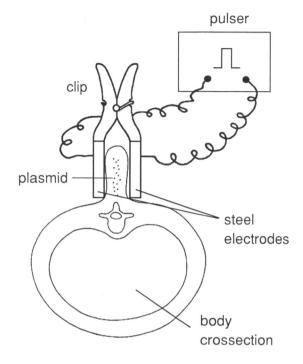

pulser

clip

plasmid

steel
electrodes

body
crossection

FIGURE 8. The scheme illustrating the experiment on *in vivo* electrotransfection. Two flat stainless steel electrodes were mounted on a plastic clip and connected to a pulse generator. Plasmid DNA was introduced subcutaneously and the pleat of skin was treated by two pulses of 400 V, 100-300 µs. (Adapted with permission of Elsevier Scientific Publishing Co. from Titomirov et al., 1991).

Experimental design

Two plasmids were used. First, a pSV3neo, contains a neomycin-resistance gene (NEO-R) under the transcriptional control of the SV40 early promoter and the gene coding the SV40 T-large antigen (Southern and Berg, 1982), which transforms primary rodent cells (Brockman, 1978). Second, a pHEB4, contains the E1A region of Adenovirus 2 frequently immortalizing primary rodent cells (Ruley, 1983). The plasmids were co-transfected to minimize the difficulties in determining expression of foreign DNA by colony phenotype. The mixture of the two supercoiled plasmids (usually, 5 µg of pSV3neo and 10 µg of pHEB4) was introduced subcutaneously to newborn CBA mice of 1-3 days age. 10-60 min later the pleat of skin was exposed to two high-voltage pulses (400 V, 100-300 µs) applied in opposite polarities using a special clip (see Fig. 8) with two stainless-steel electrodes of about 2 cm^2. Electric contact between electrodes and skin was facilitated by conductive grease (30% glycerol in 0.15 M NaCl). The samples of electroporated skin tissue were excised 24 to 168 h upon pulsation and treated by collagenase to prepare primary cultures. The antibiotic G418 was added 24-48 h following cell plating.

   After 2-3 weeks of selection on antibiotic G418, stable transformants were isolated. In four independent experiments we obtained 62 NEO-R colonies of fibroblast-like cells. Fourteen of them were isolated and their growth properties analyzed. All the clones grew in low serum medium and formed multilayer colonies indicating loss of contact inhibition. Stability of the NEO-R phenotype of all clones obtained was established by comparing the clone-forming efficiencies in the presence or absence of antibiotic G418. No significant differences were found. The plasmid DNA persisted in cells for at least 30 generations without selection. Although the cells obtained were immortal and showed altered phenotype as compared to the control primary cultures, no tumors were found in 18 mice during 3 months after in vivo electroporation of their skin using the mixture of the same plasmids.

To confirm that clones of transformants resulted from the foreign DNA incorporation, the total cellular DNA from six clones was analyzed by standard Southern blot method. The specific sequences for both plasmids were shown to be associated with non-digested high-molecular-weight DNA of all clones, indicative of their integration into chromosomes. Upon digestion of genomic DNA, all six clones were shown to contain the predicted 3.0 kb BamH1 fragment carrying SV40 early region and the SV40-specific 0.56 kb HindIII-PstI fragment. Four of these six clones contained also SV40-specific 1.25 kb HindIII-PstI fragment, which was lost as a result of a putative restriction site rearrangement in other two clones. Some of the clones shown to contain pSV3neo-specific fragments were also tested for the presence of pHEB4. Only one of four such clones was found positive for the presence of E1A gene. This analysis indicates a relatively low ratio of cotransformation compared to electrotransfection in vitro (Toneguzzo et al., 1988) and to the conventional calcium phosphate-DNA coprecipitate transfection. The Northern analysis of total RNA showed expression of a 2.6 kb fragment corresponding to the SV40 large T-antigene transcript in all six clones analyzed. Although these data show unambiguously the stable transformation of the clones obtained, we can not rule out the possibility that the plasmid DNA persisted in the skin cells in an extrachromosomal fashion and integrated into chromosomes only after plating cells to culture.

The electrical breakdown of frog skin tissue (Powell et al., 1989) was found to be fully reversible. In four independent experiments employing 6-8 animals each, we obtained 100% viability of mice, with little skin damage at given pulse parameters. Increasing the voltage to 600 V caused necrosis in the outer skin layers contacting the electrodes but was never lethal with the resulting wounds healing within two weeks. Transformation efficiency, i.e the number of NEO-R colonies relative to the total number of cell attached in primary culture, ranged between 0.2 and 7×10^{-4} (Titomirov et al., 1991).

The approach described above potentially could be used for treatment of pathologies resulting from the loss or malfunction of physiologically important genes and their products. Electrotransfection in vivo could also be applied to the investigation of multistep carcinogenesis of the skin. In some studies it could have advantage in creating small nests of cells with distinct genotype (and possibly phenotype) over a transgenic mice model in which all the cells contain the same set of genes.

CONCLUSIONS

Electrotransfection is an electrophoretic injection of DNA into cells through electric field-induced pores in the plasma membrane. Electroporation appears to be a biologically nonspecific phenomenon, and therefore electric transfection should work with any type of cells unless there is a strong steric hindrance for the access of DNA into the membrane. The process of DNA translocation is associated with limited pore expansion, but generally it does not lead to irreversible cell damage. Electrotransfection also appears to be non-damaging to transfecting DNA. The electrotransfection procedure is characterized with several well defined parameters such as peak intensity of electric field, pulse shape, and duration and number of pulses. Technically, all the parameters are 100 % reproducible and each has appropriate physical meaning for the translocation process. In practice, by optimizing the procedure, a substantial amount of DNA can be injected into all cells in a population, whereas the actual transfection efficiency may be dependent upon the compatibility of the vector with the cell type used. Electrotransfection is applicable in vivo. By contrast to chemical or virus-mediated transformation techniques, electrotransfection is intrinsically clean, fast, strictly local, and spatially directed. It allows many options in engineering of various devices for gene delivery and can be realized either in a small or relatively large volume, depending on requirements. We are rapidly approaching a time for detailed and rigorous investigation of the electrotransfection for in vivo applications.

ACKNOWLEDGMENT

We would like to thank our colleagues Leonid Chernomordik, Vassili Pastushenko, Yuri Chizmadzhev, and Alexander Zelenin for helpful discussions, and Paul Blount for critical reading of the manuscript.

REFERENCES

Abidor IG, Arakelyan VB, Chernomordik LV, Chizmadzhev YA, Pastushenko VF, Tarasevich MR (1979): Electric breakdown of bilayer lipid membrane. I. The main experimental facts and their qualitative discussions. *Bioelectrochem Bioenerg* 6:37-52

An G, Hidaka K, Siminovich L (1982): Expression of bacterial β-galactosidase in animal cells. *Mol Cell Biol* 2:1628-1632

Andreason GL, Evans GA (1989): Optimization of electro poration for transfection of mammalian cells. *Anal Biochem* 180:269-275

Auer D, Brander G, Bodemer W (1976): Dielectric breakdown of the red blood cell membrane and uptake of SV40 DNA and mammalian RNA. *Naturwissenschaften* 63:391-394

Bahnson AB, Boggs SS (1990): Addition of serum to electroporated cells enhances survival and transfection efficiency. *Biochem Biophys Res Commun*

171:752-757

Belyaev NV, Budker VG, Gorokhova OE, Sokolov AV (1988): Mg^{2+} dependent interaction of DNA with eukaryotic cells. *Mol Biologiya* 22:1667-1672

Benvenisty N, Reshef L (1986): Direct introduction of genes into rats and expression of the genes. *Proc Natl Acad Sci USA* 83:9551-9555

Benz R, Beckers F, Zimmermann U (1979): Reversible electrocal breakdown of lipid bilayer membranes: A charge-pulse relaxation study. *J Membrane Biol* 48:181-204

Benz R, Zimmermann U (1981): The resealing process of lipid bilayers after reversible electrical breakdown. *Biochim Biophys Acta* 640:169-178

Berglund DL, Starkey JR (1991): Introduction of antibody into viable cells using electroporation. *Cytometry* 12:64-67

Bertling W, Hunger-Bertling K, Cline MJ (1987): Intranuclear uptake and persistence of biologically active DNA after electroporation of mammalian cells. *J Biochem Biophys Methods* 14:223-232

Brockmann WW (1978): Transformation of BALB/c-3T3 cells by tsA mutants of simian virus 40: Temperature sensitivity of the transformed phenotype and retransformation by wild-type virus. *J Virol* 25:860-870

Bryant G, Wolfe J (1987): Electromechanical stresses produced in the plasma membranes of suspended cells by applied electric fields. *J Membrane Biol* 96:129-139

Cantor CR, Schimmel (1980): *Biophysical Chemistry*. Vol. III. San Francisco: W. H. Freeman and Company

Chakrabarti R, Wylie DE, Schuster SM (1989): Transfer of monoclonal antibodies into mammalian cells by electroporation. *J Biol Chem* 264: 15494-15500

Chang DC, Reese TS (1990): Changes in membrane structure induced by electroporation as revealed by rapid-freesing electron microscopy. *Biophys J* 58:1-12

de Chasseval R, de Villartay J-P (1992): High level transient gene expression in human lymphoid cells by SV40 large T antigen boost. *Nucl Acid Res* 20:245-250

Chernomordik LV, Sukharev SI, Abidor IG, Chizmadzhev YA (1983): Breakdown of lipid bilayer membranes in an electric field. *Biochim Biophys Acta* 640:169-178

Chernomordik LV, Sukharev SI, Popov SV, Pastushenko VF, Sokirko AV, Abidor IG, Chizmadzhev YA (1987): The electrical breakdown of cell and lipid membranes: The similarity of phenomenologies. *Biochim Biophys Acta* 902:360-373

Chernomordik LV, Chizmadzhev YA (1989): Electrical breakdown of lipid bilayer membranes. Phenomenology and mechanism. In: *Electroporation and Electrofusion in Cell biology*, Neumann E, Sowers AE, Jordan CA, eds. New York: Plenum Press

Chernomordik LV, Sokolov AV, Budker VG (1990): Electrostimulated uptake of DNA by liposomes. *Biochim Biophys Acta* 1024:179-183

Chernomordik LV (1992): Electropores in lipid bilayers and cell membranes. In:

Guide to Electroporation and Electrofusion, Chang DC, Chassy BM, Saunders JA, Sowers AE, eds. San Diego: Academic Press

Cole KS (1972): *Membranes, Ions and Impulses*. Berkeley: University of California Press.

Deuticke B, Schwister K (1989): Leaks induced by electrical breakdown in the erythrocyte membrane. In: *Electroporation and Electrofusion in Cell Biology*, Neumann E, Sowers AE, Jordan CA, eds. New York: Plenum Press

Dimitrov DS, Sowers AE (1990): Membrane electroporation - fast molecular exchange by electroosmosis. *Biochim Biophys Acta* 1022:381-392

Dower WJ, Miller JF, Ragsdale CW (1988): High efficiency transformation of E. coli by high voltage electroporation. *Nucl Acids Res* 16:6127-6145

Dressler V, Schwister K, Haest CVM, Deuticke B (1983): Dielectric breakdown of the erythrocyte membrane enhances transbilayer mobility of phospholipids. *Biochim Biophys Acta* 732:304-307

Finaz C, Lefevre A, Teissie J (1984): Electrofusion: A new, highly efficient technique for generating somatic cell hybrids. *Exp Cell Res* 150:477-482

Fountain JW, Lockwood WK, Collins FS (1988): Transfection of primary human fibroblasts by electroporation. *Gene* 68:167-172

Fromm ME, Taylor LP, Walbot V (1985): Expression of genes transferred into monocot and dicot plants by electroporation. *Proc Natl Acad Sci USA* 82:5824

Glaser RW, Leikin SL, Chernomordik LV, Pastushenko VF, Sokirko AI (1988): Reversible electrical breakdown of lipid bilayers: Formation and evolution of pores. *Biochim Biophys Acta* 940: 275-287

Graham F, van der Eb A (1973): A new technique for the assay of infectivity of human adenovirus 5 DNA. *Virology* 52:456-467

Herzog R, Muller-Wellensiek A, Voelter W (1986): Usefulness of Ficoll in electric field-mediated cell fusion. *Life Sci* 39:2279-2288

van der Hoff MJ, Moorman AF, Lamers WH (1992): Electroporation in 'intracellular' buffer increases cell survival. *Nucl Acid Res* 20:2902

Kinosita K, Tsong TY (1977a): Formation and resealing of pores of controlled sizes in human erythrocyte membrane. *Nature* 268:438-441

Kinosita K, Tsong TY (1977b): Voltage induced pore formation and hemolysis of human erythrocytes. *Biochim Biophys Acta* 471:227-242

Kinosita K, Tsong TY (1979): Voltage-induced conductance in human erythrocyte membranes. *Biochim Biophys Acta* 554:479-497

Kinosita K, Ashikawa I, Saita N, Yoshimura H, Itoh H, Nagayama K, Ikegami A (1988): Electroporation of cell membrane visualized under a pulsed-laser fluorescence microscope. *Biophys J* 53:1015-1019

Kaneda Y, Iwai K, Uchida T (1989): Increased expression of DNA cointroduced with nuclear protein in adult rat liver. *Science* 243:375-378

Keating A, Toneguzzo F (1990): Gene transfer by electroporation: a model for gene therapy. *Progress in Clinical and Biological Research* 333:491-498

Klenchin VA, Sukharev SI, Serov SM, Chernomordik LV, Chizmadzhev YA (1991): Electrically induced DNA uptake by cells is a fast process involving DNA electrophoresis. *Biophys J* 60:804-811

Knight DE, Scrutton MC (1986): Gaining access to the cytosol: The technique and some applications of electropermeabilization. *Biochem J* 234:497-506

Knutson JC, Yee D (1987): Electroporation: parameters affecting transfer of DNA into mammalian cells. *Anal Biochem* 164:44-52

Kubiniec RT, Liang H, Hui SW (1990): Effects of pulse length and pulse strength on transfection by electroporation. *Biotechniques* 8:16-20

Laurent CT, Granath KA (1967): Fractionation of dextran and ficoll by chromatography on Sephadex G-200. *Biochim Biophys Acta* 136:191-198

Leikin SL, Glaser RW, Chernomordik LV (1986): Mechanism of pore formation under electrical breakdown of membranes. *Biol Membr* 3: 944-951

Machy P, Lewis F, McMillan L, Jonak ZL (1988): Gene transfer from targeted liposomes to specific lymphoid cells by electroporation. *Proc Natl Acad Sci USA* 85:8027-8031

Mehrle W, Zimmermann U, Hampp R (1985): Evidence for asymmetrical uptake of fluorescent dyes through electropermeabilized membranes of Avena mesophyll protoplasts. *FEBS Lett* 185:89-94

Neumann E, Schafer-Rider M, Wang Y, Hofschneider PH (1982): Gene transfer to mouse lyoma cells by electroporation in high electric fields. *EMBO J* 1:841-845

Neumann E (1989): The relaxation hysteresis of membrane electropration In: *Electroporation and Electrofusion in Cell Biology*, Neumann E, Sowers AE, Jordan CA, eds. New York: Plenum Press

Nicolau C, Le Pape A, Soriano P, Fargette F, Juhel M-F (1983): In vivo expression of rat insulin after intravenous administration of the liposome-entrapped gene for rat insulin I. *Proc Natl Acad Sci USA* 80:1068-1072

Pastushenko, VF, Chizmadzhev YA, Arakelyan VB (1979): Electric breakdown of bilayer lipid membranes. II. Calculation of the membrane lifetime in the steady-state diffusion approximation. *Bioelectrochem Bioenerg* 6:53-63

Pastushenko VP, Chizmadzhev YA (1992): Energetic estimations of the deformation of the translocated DNA and cell membrane in the course of electrotransformation. *Biol Mem* 6:287-300

Potter H, Weir L, Leder P (1984): Enhancer-dependent expression of human k immunoglobulin genes introduced into mouse pre-B lymphocytes by electroporation. *Proc Natl Acad Sci USA* 81:7161-7165

Potter H (1988): Electroporation in biology: Methods, applications, and instumentation. *Anal Biochem* 174:361-373

Potter H (1989): Molecular genetic applications of electroporation In: *Electroporation and Electrofusion in Cell Biology*, Neumann E, Sowers AE, Jordan CA, eds. New York: Plenum Press

Potter H, Cooke SWF (1992): Gene transfer into adherent cells growing on microbeads. In: *Guide to Electroporation and Electrofusion*, Chang DC, Chassy BM, Saunders JA, Sowers AE, eds. San Diego: Academic Press

Powell KT, Morgenthaler AW, Weaver JC (1989): Tissue electro poration. Observation of reversible electrical breakdown in viable frog skin. *Biophys J*

56:1163-1171

Presse F, Quillet A, Mir L, Marchiol-Fournigault, Feunteun J, Fradelizi D (1988): An improved electrotransfection method using square shaped electric impulsions. *Biochem Biophys Res Commun* 151:982-990

Reid LH, Smithies O (1992): Gene targeting and electroporation. In: *Guide to Electroporation and Electrofusion*, Chang DC, Chassy BM, Saunders JA, Sowers AE, eds. San Diego: Academic Press

Ruley HE (1983): Adenovirus early region 1A enables viral and cellular transforming genes to transform primary cells in culture. *Nature* 304:602-606

Schwister K, Deuticke, B (1985): Formation and properties of aqueous leaks induced in human erythrocytes by electrical breakdown. *Biochim Biophys Acta* 816:332-348

Sczakiel G, Diffinger R, Pawlita M (1989): Testing for electrotransfection parameters by use of the fluorescent dye Lucifer Yellow CH. *Anal Biochem* 181:309-313

Southern PJ, Berg P (1982): Transformation of mammalian cells to antibiotic resistance with a bacterial gene under control of the SV40 early region promoter. *J Mol Appl Genet* 1:327-341

Sowers AE, Lieber MR (1986): Electropores in individual erythrocyte ghosts: diameters, lifetimes, numbers and locations. *FEBS Lett* 205:179-184

Stellwagen NC (1987): Electrophoresis of DNA in agarose and polyacrylamide gels. *Adv Electrophoresis* 1:179-228

Stopper H, Jones H, Zimmermann U (1987): Large-scale transfection of mouse L-cells by electropermeabilization. *Biochim Biophys Acta* 900:38-44

Sugar IP, Neumann E, (1984): Stochastic model for for electric field-induced membrane pores - electropration. *Biophys Chem* 19:211-225

Sukharev SI, Popov SV, Chernomordik LV, Abidor IG (1985): A patch-clamp study of electrical breakdown of cell membranes. *Biol Membr* 2:77-86

Sukharev SI, Bandrina IN, Barbul AI, Fedorova LI, Abidor IG, Zelenin AV (1990): Electrofusion of fibroblasts on the porous membrane. *Biochim Biophys Acta* 1034:125-131

Sukharev SI, Klenchin VA, Serov SM, Chernomordik LV, Chizmadzhev YA (1992): Electroporation and electrophoretic DNA transfer into cells. The effect of DNA interaction with electropores. *Biophys J* 63:1320-1327

Tekle E, Astumian RD, Chock PB (1991): Electroporation by using bipolar oscillating electric field: an improved method for DNA transfection of NIH 3T3 cells. *Proc Natl Acad Sci USA* 88:4230-4234

Titomirov AV, Sukharev S, Kistanova E (1991): In vivo electroporation and stable transformation of skin cells of newborn mice by plasmid DNA. *Biochim Biophys Acta* 1088:131-134

Toneguzzo F, Hayday AC, Keating A (1986): Electric field-mediated gene transfer: transient and stable gene expression in human and mouse lymphoid cells. *Mol Cell Biol* 6: 703-706

Toneguzzo F, Keating A (1986): Stable expression of selectable genes introduced into human hematopoietic stem cells by electric field-mediated gene transfer. *Proc Natl Acad Sci USA* 83:3496-3499

Toneguzzo F, Keating A, Lilly S, McDonald K (1988): Electric field-mediated gene transfer: Chatacterization of DNA transfer and patterns of integration in lymphoid cells. *Nucleic Acid Res* 16:5515-5532

Tsong TY (1989): Electroporation of cell membranes. Mechanisms and applications. In: *Electroporation and Electrofusion in Cell Biology*, Neumann E, Sowers AE, Jordan CA, eds. New York: Plenum Press

Tsong TY (1992): Time sequence of molecular events in electroporation. In: *Guide to Electroporation and Electrofusion*, Chang DC, Chassy BM, Saunders JA, Sowers AE, eds. San Diego: Academic Press

Weaver JC, Barnett A (1992): Progress toward a theoretical model for electroporation mechanism: Membrane electrical behavior and molecular transport. In: *Guide to Electroporation and Electrofusion*, Chang DC, Chassy BM, Saunders JA, Sowers AE, eds. San Diego: Academic Press

Wintrebourne DJ, Thomas S, Hermon-Taylor J, Hussain I, Johnstone AP (1988): Electric shock-mediated transfection of cells. Characterization and optimization of electrical parameters. *Biochem J* 251:427-434

Wolff, JA, Malone RW, Williams P, Chong W, Acsadi G, Jani A, Felgner PL (1990): Direct gene transfer into mouse muscle in vivo. *Science* 247:1465-1468

Wong TK, Neumann E (1982): Electric field mediated gene transfer. *Biochim Biophys Res Commun* 107:584-587

Xie T-D, Sun L, Tsong TY (1990): Study of mechanisms of electric field-induced DNA transfection I. DNA entry by surface binding and diffusion through membrane pores. *Biophys J* 58:13-19

Zimmermann U, Pilwat G, Beckers F, Riemann F (1976): Effects of external electric fields on cell membranes. *Bioeolectrochem Bioenerg* 3:58-83

Zimmermann U (1982): Electric field-mediated fusion and related electrical phenomena. *Biochim Biophys Acta* 694:227-277

Part III

APPLICATIONS

PHARMACOKINETIC CONSIDERATIONS IN THE USE OF GENES AS PHARMACEUTICALS

Fred D. Ledley

INTRODUCTION

Two paradigms for the clinical application of direct, somatic gene therapy can be distinguished. In one paradigm, genes are administered at a single point in time with the expectation that these genes will associate permanently with the target cell, producing therapeutic amounts of the gene product indefinitely. This requires the use of vectors which integrate their genetic material into the chromosomes of the host cell or persist in an episomal state through episomal replication or a latent phase. In the other paradigm, genes are administered like conventional pharmaceuticals with the knowledge that the gene will be eliminated from the cell after a finite and predictable period of time during which the therapeutic gene product is expressed. This can be achieved with the use of DNA-vectors which produce transient expression, or with the use of viral vectors which provide short-term expression but are incapable of persisting indefinitely in the target cell. This paradigm envisions the use of genes in a manner analogous to conventional medicines to treat acute diseases or to establish steady-state levels of the therapeutic product.

The use of genes as medicines may have several important clinical advantages. These include the ability to adjust the dose or schedule of administration to optimize therapy for individual patients and their changing therapeutic needs as well as the ability to stop therapy if adverse experiences are encountered. Various strategies for achieving long-term genetic or pharmacological regulation of genes which are permanently inserted into somatic cells have been described. Nevertheless, the flexibility inherent in being able to refine or stop administration of gene therapy may enhance the safety and efficacy of gene therapy as well as the acceptability of gene therapy products by physicians and patients.

The clinical application of genes as medicines will require methods for gene delivery which are safe for repetitive use over long periods of time, provide reproducible levels of the gene product, which are relatively non-invasive, and which are cost-effective. The use of genes as pharmaceuticals also raises unique issues of pharmacokinetics since, unlike a conventional drug, the administered material is not biologically active, and, unlike a conventional prodrug, the administered material is not consumed when the active product is formed. The pharmacokinetics of the gene product will be determined by many factors including the compart-

Gene Therapeutics: Methods and Applications of Direct Gene Transfer
Jon A. Wolff, Editor • ©1994 *Birkhäuser Boston*

mentalization, trafficking, degradation, and processing of the administered gene, the rate of transcription and stability of its mRNA, and the rate of translation, processing, and elimination of the gene product itself.

This chapter describes preliminary data on the feasibility and pharmacokinetics of using genes as pharmaceuticals in two experimental models. The first involves the use of asialo-orosomucoid-polylysine-DNA complexes to deliver genes to the liver. The second involves direct injection of genes into the thyroid, an organ which, like muscle, has been observed to take up recombinant genes and express recombinant gene products after interstitial injection of plasmid DNA.

MODEL 1: ASIALO-OROSOMUCOID-POLYLYSINE-DNA MEDIATED GENE DELIVERY TO THE LIVER

We have performed a series of studies aimed at developing methods for somatic gene therapy of methylmalonic acidemia (MMA). This disease is an often-fatal inborn error of metabolism caused by deficiency of the enzyme methylmalonyl CoA mutase (Ledley, 1990). There is considerable individual variability in the clinical phenotype with some individuals suffering from fulminant neonatal acidosis and others having benign organic aciduria. There is also considerable temporal variability, and even the most severely affected individuals will have long periods of stability on dietary therapy interrupted by episodes of acute-life threatening acidosis. In part because of this variability, high risk therapies such as hepatic transplantation have never been attempted (Ledley, 1992). MMA represents a prototype for a genetic disease which might be treated using genes as medicines to express the enzyme transiently in the liver (Ledley, 1990; Wilkemeyer et al., in press; Stankovics et al., submitted). Two clinical strategies may be envisioned. The first would involve administering the gene to treat the acute, life-threatening episodes of acidosis. The second would involve administering the gene regularly to constitute steady state levels of the gene product.

Studies have been performed in collaboration with Drs. George and Catherine Wu to assess whether current strategies for asialoglycoprotein-mediated gene delivery to the liver (Wu and Wu, 1987; 1988a; 1988b; Wu et al., 1989; Wu et al., 1991; Wilson et al., 1989; 1992) could be applicable to therapy of MMA (Stankovics et al. submitted). In these studies, mice were injected with a vector expressing human MCM from a cytomegalovirus immediate early promoter was complexed with covalently coupled asialo-orosomucoid and polylysine. The complex was administered by bolus intravenous injection and vector sequences were identified by semiquantitative PCR in the serum or DNA purified from tissues (Stankovics et al., submitted). Semiquantitation was achieved using a set of standards containing 10^{-9} to 10^{-15} g of the vector mixed with mouse DNA or mouse serum amplified contemporaneously with each experiment under identical conditions. Reaction products were visualized by bidirectional Southern blotting and quantified using a Betascope 603 Blot Analyzer (Betagen Corp., Waltham, MA). The half life ($t_{1/2}$) of vector sequences (S) as a function of time (t) was calculated from the rate constant for elimination (k_e) where $k_e = -\log[S]/t * 2.3$ and $t_{1/2} = 0.693/k_e$ (Goldstein et al. 1974).

These experiments demonstrated that MCM could be overexpressed at levels 30-50% higher than (normal) endogenous mouse MCM 6-24 hours after injection. By 48 hours after injection enzyme activity in the liver had returned to baseline (Figure 1A). Pharmacokinetic studies demonstrated that the vector could be detected in blood drawn immediately after injection and decreased rapidly thereafter. First order kinetics were apparent from the log-linear relationship between time and the log of the concentration of vector sequences (R^2=0.98) with the half life $t_{1/2}$ = 2.5 minutes (Figure 1B). The vector was taken up primarily by the liver, though sequences could be amplified as well from the spleen and lung. The highest concentrations of vector were observed in the liver at the earliest time point studied (one hour) with approximately 10^6 copies of the PCR template/cell. Vector sequences were eliminated by first order kinetics during the first 24 hours after injection as evidenced by the log-linear relationship between time and the log of the concentration of vector sequences (R^2= 0.78-0.92) with a calculated half life $t_{1/2}$=1.0-1.3 hours (Figure 1C). Significantly, vector sequences were never completely eliminated from the liver and could be identified using 35 cycles of PCR as late as 30 days after administration at levels representing approximately <1 copy/10^2-10^3 cells. These sequences maintained the bacterial pattern of methylation (*Sau*3A sensitive/*Dpn*I sensitive/*Mbo*I resistant) suggesting that they were not replicated or integrated into the host cells genes.

To assess the feasibility of repetitive administration of the asialo-orosomucoid-polylysine-DNA complexes several mice were injected at four different times over a period of 8 months with the asialo-orosomucoid-polylysine-DNA complex. One animal died of respiratory distress within minutes of the last injection. To investigate whether antibodies were formed against the asialo-orosomucoid-polylysine-DNA complex, the remaining animals were sacrificed 10 days after the last injection. Complete autopsies were performed which were unremarkable and serum was assayed for antibodies against the asialo-orosomucoid-polylysine-DNA complex. Serum from all animals precipitated [^{125}I]-asialo-orosomucoid-polylysine-DNA complexes at dilutions of >1:1000. This precipitation could be competitively inhibited by 10-100 fold molar excess of unlabeled asialo-orosomucoid or a mixture of asialo-orosomucoid + polylysine + DNA in proportions identical to those in the asialo-orosomucoid-polylysine-DNA complex (Figure 2, left). Precipitation could be partially inhibited by polylysine but not by DNA. The antiserum from injected animals did not precipitate [^{32}P]-DNA (Figure 2, right) and tests for antinuclear antibody were negative.

MODEL 2: DIRECT GENE DELIVERY TO THE THYROID

We have injected various organs in the rabbit and assessed their ability to express recombinant genes after direct injection of plasmid DNA. We observed that the thyroid, like muscle (Wolf et al., 1990), is capable of taking up plasmid after inter-

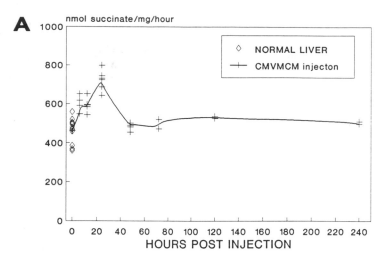

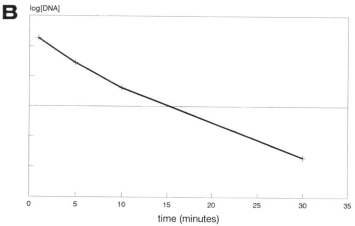

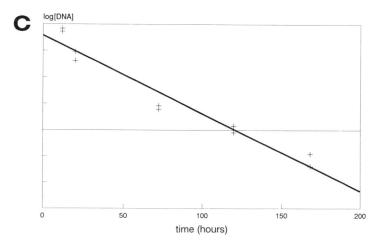

stitial injection, and that recombinant gene products will be expressed at levels equivalent to those seen in muscle after intramuscular injection (Sikes et al., submitted). Histochemical studies using a β-galactosidase reporter gene demonstrate expression of β-gal in cells with the morphology and position of follicular cells as well as within disrupted tissue and collapsed follicles along the track of injection (Sikes et al., submitted).

The level of DNA and activity of a reporter gene (chloramphenicol-acetyltransferase) was assayed in thyroid tissue at various intervals after injection of plasmid DNA. The injected DNA was eliminated from the injected tissue by first order kinetics as evidenced by the log-linear relationship between time and the log of the concentration of vector sequences ($R^2=0.95$) with the half life $t_{1/2} =$ 10 hours (Figure 3A). The level of CAT activity remained high for three days and exhibited first order elimination kinetics from 24-480 hours after injection with a log-linear relationship between time and the log of CAT activity ($R^2=0.93$) and a calculated $t_{1/2} = 46-48$ hours (Figure 3B).

While most of the injected DNA was eliminated from the thyroid, small amounts of DNA representing <1 copy/100 cells was detectable by PCR up to 20-34 days after injection. This DNA exhibited the bacterial pattern of methylation suggesting that it was not replicated (DpnI sensitive/MboI resistant).

ISSUES IN THE CLINICAL APPLICATION OF DIRECT GENE DELIVERY

The design of somatic gene therapy requires attention to a wide range of issues pertaining to the feasibility of gene transfer, the adequacy of gene expression, the activity of the recombinant gene product, and the ability of cells transformed with the recombinant gene to alter the systemic phenotype of the disease being treated (Ledley, 1990b; Ledley, 1991). It is also necessary to demonstrate that the vectors and procedures which are used for gene therapy are safe. The development of genes as pharmaceuticals will raise additional issues of pharmacokinetics and the ability to achieve reproducible delivery of the recombinant gene and expression of the gene product. The two model systems described in this report differ substantially in their methodology and state of development. Nevertheless, these experiments illustrate certain common issues that need to be addressed in the preclinical assessment of direct gene delivery.

Our studies with the asialo-orosomucoid-polylysine-DNA mediated delivery to the liver (Stankovics et al., submitted) confirms the results of others who have

FIGURE 1. Asialo-orosomucoid-polylysine-DNA mediated gene transfer of human methylmalonyl CoA mutase. (A) Overexpression of MCM in the liver of mice after administration of asialo-orosomucoid-polylysine-DNA complex. (B) Rate of elimination of complex from the blood plotted as the log of the concentration of vector sequences in the blood versus time. The linear approximation of first order kinetics is shown. (C) Rate of elimination of complex from the liver plotted as the log of the concentration of vector sequences in the liver versus time. The linear approximation of first order kinetics is shown.

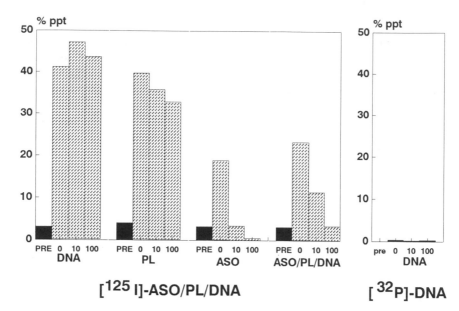

FIGURE 2. Formation of antibodies against asialo-orosomucoid-polylysine-DNA complex. LEFT: Competition of [^{125}I-asialo-orosomucoid-polylysine-DNA precipitation with unlabeled asialo-orosomucoid, polylysine, DNA, or a mixture of all three materials. RIGHT: Absence of precipitation of [32-DNA.

demonstrated the feasibility of expressing CAT (Wu et al., 1988; 1989), LDL-receptor (Wilson et al., 1989), or albumin (Wu et al., 1991) from hepatocytes after administration of asialo-orosomucoid-polylysine-DNA complexes. Our data confirms the rapid clearance of the complex from the blood and demonstrates that this clearance exhibits first order kinetics as expected. The demonstrated half-life of the vector sequences within the liver is somewhat shorter than expected from previous data on the duration of expression of various gene products. The apparent duration of expression is defined, however, by several processes including the rate of elimination of DNA in the cell, the stability of mRNA (not examined in these studies), or the rate of elimination of the gene product. It is likely that the longer duration of hepatic gene expression after asialoglycoprotein-polylysine-DNA mediated gene transfer reflects a longer half-life of the transcribed mRNA sequences or, more likely, the longer half-life of the recombinant gene products. Future studies will need to describe the kinetics of each of the processes that determine the level of the gene product. In fact, considerably more fundamental knowledge will be required about the trafficking and fate of DNA administered to cells to understand the factors which affect the metabolism, compartmentalization, and clearance of DNA vectors. Computer simulations of the pharmacokinetics of gene pharmaceuticals which take into account these processes (Ledley and Ledley, in preparation) may assist in the assessment of gene transfer methods as well as the optimization of delivery strategies, doses, and schedules.

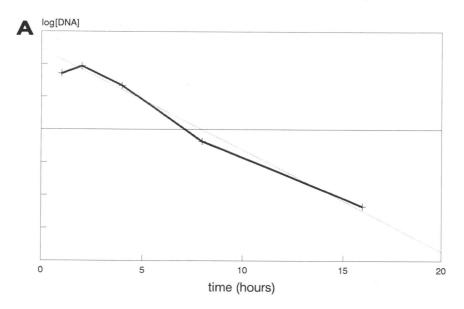

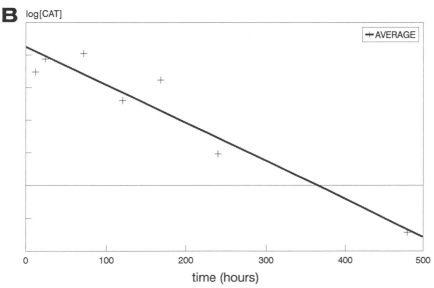

FIGURE 3. Pharmacokinetics of DNA and chloramphenicol acetyltransferase in the thyroid after direct injection of DNA encoding this marker gene. (A) Rate of elimination of DNA from whole thyroid tissue plotted as the log of the concentration of vector sequences in the blood versus time. The linear approximation of first order kinetics is shown. (B) Rate of elimination of chloramphenicol acetyltransferase enzyme activity plotted as the log of the concentration of vector sequences int he liver versus time. The linear approximation of first order kinetics is shown.

Our data demonstrates an order of magnitude difference in the rate of DNA clearance from the liver after receptor mediated gene transfer (1-1.3 hours) and thyroid after direct injection (10 hours). A considerably longer half life is evident after direct injection of DNA into muscle where DNA and gene expression can persist for months (Wolf et al., 1990). The reasons for this variance are not immediately apparent. This variability could reflect differences in the trafficking or compartmentalization of DNA after different modes of gene delivery. Alternatively, this variability could reflect tissue specific patterns of metabolism or intracellular compartmentalization of DNA. It has been demonstrated that the replicative state of cells may alter intracellular compartmentalization. Wilson et al., (1992) demonstrated that subtotal hepatectomy performed in conjunction with asialo-orosomucoid-polylysine-DNA mediated delivery alters the compartmentalization of the DNA leading to persistence of the recombinant sequences and gene expression (Wilson et al., 1992).

One disturbing issue which is raised in both of our experimental systems is the persistence of very small amounts of DNA for long periods of time after administration. The safety of genes as pharmaceuticals would be enhanced if the administered genes were completely eliminated from the target tissue. While much of this material is apparently not integrated into the host cell chromosomes, the sensitivity of current methods may not be sufficient to identify isolated integrants in $<10^{-5}$-10^{-6} cells. Further studies will be required to assess the compartmentalization and fate of this residual material.

The last observation is that repetitive administration of the asialo-orosomucoid-polylysine-DNA complex led to the production of high titers of antibody against the asialo-glycoprotein/polylysine complex. There was no evidence of antibodies against DNA and no evidence of anti-nuclear antibodies. We have not yet assessed whether these antibodies compromise the activity of the asialo-orosomucoid-polylysine-DNA complex. It should be noted that many biological products are associated with seroconversion in clinical use, though the presence of antibodies can complicate the dose response and can cause immunologically mediated Adverse Experiences.

This observation demonstrates the importance of considering carriers which may be used for delivery of genetic pharmaceuticals as independent elements. It is not surprising that covalent modification of orosomucoid with polylysine may render this molecule antigenic. Several strategies can be considered to avoid seroconversion including the use of steroids or other immune suppressants in conjunction with gene delivery. Alternatively, it may be possible to develop of methods for targeting using natural, unmodified ligands as vehicles for gene therapy (Stankovics and Ledley, unpublished data) or small molecule ligands or synthetic molecules which are analogues for surface receptors may be developed (Woo and Smith, unpublished data) which are less likely to be antigenic. Any material which is used as a carrier for gene transfer will have to be studied in the same detail as the DNA vector and the therapeutic product itself. It will be necessary to characterize the distribution, metabolism, elimination, antigenicity, and biological activities of the compound and its metabolites to ensure that there are no untoward biological effects.

CONCLUSION

The use of genes as medicines holds great promise for the treatment of both genetic and non genetic diseases. The two methods described in this report may be used for a variety of clinical applications. Methods for hepatic gene targeting may enable treatment not only of metabolic diseases but also hepatitis, cirrhosis, hemophilia, and atherosclerosis. Methods for thyroid gene targeting may be used not only to treat inherited or acquired thyroid disease, but to secrete circulating serum proteins, hormones, or neurotropic peptides from thyroid cells which exhibit a large protein synthetic capacity and susceptibility to various regulatory agents.

As we move beyond assessing the technical ability to transfer genes into various organs, the applicability of genes as medicines will increasingly be defined not by the elegance of the molecular biology, but by conventional pharmacological issues. These include having a clinically acceptable mode and frequency of administration, achieving an appropriate therapeutic dose, having an adequate therapeutic index, and offering a significant benefit in cost and risk. In these issues, the use of genes as pharmaceuticals will ultimately be judged against conventional approaches to treating the same diseases using small molecular drugs, natural products, or biological products.

ACKNOWLEDGEMENTS

I would like to acknowledge the members of my laboratory who performed the studies described in this report as post doctoral fellows (Jozsef Stankovics, M.D., Bert O'Malley, Jr., M.D., and Elizabeth Andrews, Ph.D.) or graduate students (Michael Sikes and R. Mark Adams) as well as the collaboration of Dr. George Wu, Dr. Catherine Wu, and Dr. Milton Finegold. This work was supported in part by NIH grant R29 HD-24186, by a grant from the Mathers Foundation, by residency research funds from the Department of Otorhinolaryngology, and by the ACTA Foundation. Dr. Ledley has equity interest in GeneMedicine, Inc.

REFERENCES

Andrews E, Jansen, R, Crane AM, Wilkemeyer MF, MacDonall D, Ledley FD (1993): Activity of a recombinant human methylmalonyl CoA mutase primary fibroblasts and Saccharomyces cerevisiae. *Biochem Med Met Biol* (In press)

Goldstein A, Aronow L, Kalman SM (1974): *Principles of Drug Action*, second edition. John Wiley and Sons: New York, pp 854

Ledley FD (1990a): Perspectives on methylmalonic acidemia resulting from molecular cloning of methylmalonyl CoA mutase. *Bioessays* 12:335-340

Ledley FD (1990b): Clinical application of somatic gene therapy in inborn errors of metabolism. *J Inher Met Dise* 13:597-616

Ledley FD (1991): Clinical considerations in the design of protocols for somatic gene therapy. *Hum Gene Ther* 2:77-84

Ledley F (1992a): Transplantation in Genetic Disease. *Curr Op Pediatr* 4:972-997

Ledley FD (1992b): Somatic gene therapy in gastroenterology: approaches and applications. *Pediatr Gast Nutr* 14:328-337

Ledley TS, Ledley FD: A multicompartment computer model for the pharmokinetics of in vivo gene therapy with DNA vectors. (In Preparation)

Sikes M, O'Malley Jr. BW, Finegold MJ, Ledley FD: In vivo gene transfer into rabbit thyroid by direct DNA injection: a novel strategy for gene therapy. (Submitted)

Stankovics J, Andrews E, Wu CH, Wu CY, Ledley FD: Overexpression of human methylmalonyl CoA mutase in mice after in vivo gene transfer with asialoglycoprotein/polylysine/plasmid complexes. (Submitted)

Wu GY, Wu CH (1987): Receptor-mediated in vitro gene transformation by a soluble DNA carrier system. *J Biol Chem* 262:4429-4432

Wu GY, Wu CH (1988): Evidence for targeted gene delivery to hepG2 hepatoma cells in vitro. *Biochem* 27:887-892

Wu GY, Wu CH (1988): Receptor-mediated gene delivery and expression in vivo. *J Biol Chem* 263:14621-14624

Wu GY, Wilson JM, Wu CH (1989): Targeting genes: delivery and persistent expression of a foreign gene driven by mammalian regulatory elements in vivo. *J Biol Chem* 264:16985-16987

Wu GY, Wilson JM, Shalaby F, Grossman M, Shafritz DA, Wu CH (1991): Receptor-mediated gene delivery in vivo. Partial correction of genetic analbuminemia in Nagase rats. *J Biol Chem* 266:14338-14342

Wilkemeyer MF, Stankovics J, Foy T, Ledley FD (1993): Propionate metabolism in cultured human cells after overexpression of recombinant methylmalonyl CoA mutase:Implications for somatic gene therapy. *Som Cel Mol Genet* (In Press)

Wilson JM, Grossman M, Cabrera JA, Wu CH, Wu GY (1992): A novel mechanism for achieving transgene persistence in vivo after somatic gene transfer into hepatocytes. *J Biol Chem* 267:11483-11489

Wilson JM, Wu CH, Wu GY (1989): Targeting genes: delivery and persistent expression of a foreign gene driven by mammalian regulatory elements in vivo. *J Biol Chem* 264:16985-16987

Wolff JA, Malone RW, Williams P et al., (1990): Direct gene transfer into mouse muscle in vivo. *Science* 247:1465-1468

VIRUS-MEDIATED GENETIC TREATMENT OF RODENT GLIOMAS

E. Antonio Chiocca, Julie K. Andersen, Yoshiaki Takamiya, Robert L. Martuza, and Xandra O. Breakefield

CHARACTERISTICS OF GLIOMAS

The most common primary central nervous system neoplasm in adults is the malignant glioma. Approximately 5,000 new cases are diagnosed annually in the United States. This tumor has proven to be extremely refractory to currently available therapeutic modalities. A combination of aggressive surgical excision, radiation therapy, and chemotherapy has increased the life expectancy of patients suffering from this illness by only a few months (Schoenberg, 1983; Salcman, 1985; Kornblith et al., 1985). Sometimes the aggressive pursuit of these therapeutic modalities results in considerable neurologic dysfunction.

Several factors contribute to the failure of current therapies: 1) tumor recurrences can arise from migrating glioma cells that have escaped surgical excision and focal radiation (Hochberg and Pruitt, 1980; Goldberg et al., 1991); 2) many chemotherapeutic agents are not effective due to poor penetration of the blood-brain barrier and reduced diffusion within the tumor (Clifford et al., 1985); 3) the blood-brain barrier and poor antigen presentation limit immune responses to glioma cells (Hewitt et al., 1976; Trojan et al., 1993); 4) clonally derived tumor cells become phenotypically heterogeneous during their expansion, limiting the efficacy of treatments targeted against a specific phenotype; 5) radiation and chemical therapies target tumor cells in the S phase of the cell cycle, yet only a small percentage of glioma cells are in this phase at any one time (Yoshii et al., 1986).

Virus vectors have the potential to circumvent the limitations of current therapeutic approaches to gliomas. To date both retrovirus and herpes simplex virus type 1 (HSV) have been employed experimentally. Other types of viruses (such as adenoviruses [Rosenfeld et al., 1991] and adeno-associated viruses [Samulski et al., 1991]) and non-virus vectors (such as various ligand-polylysine-DNA complexes [Wagner et al., 1992]) could also be used to achieve destruction of gliomatous tumors, but have not been tested to date. Vectors successful in the destruction of gliomas might also be able to mediate regression or destruction of other types of brain tumors (such as lymphomas, meningiomas, medulloblastomas, cerebral metastases). An advantage inherent to tumor-gene therapy is that it is probably not

Gene Therapeutics: Methods and Applications of Direct Gene Transfer
Jon A. Wolff, Editor • ©1994 *Birkhäuser Boston*

necessary to achieve long term expression of a peptide product to effect cell death. In fact transient expression of a toxic molecule may be sufficient to destroy a glioma cell. Therefore, difficulties obtaining long term expression of a gene product (which have plagued investigators in gene therapy for other illnesses) may not be an issue to the genetic treatment of brain tumors.

Many features of virus vectors make them attractive experimental candidates for the selective killing of gliomas. Since retrovirus and HSV have different characteristics, we will first briefly describe aspects of each of these viruses pertaining specifically to tumor killing. We will also discuss issues concerning the selectivity of these vectors for tumor cells versus normal neurons and glia, their safety, and the efficiency of gene delivery to tumor cells.

HSV IN GLIOMA TUMOR THERAPY

Characteristics of HSV

HSV is a double-stranded DNA virus of 150 kb that contains approximately 72 genes (Roizman and Sears, 1990). Genetic manipulation of the HSV genome can be rather extensive (Roizman and Jenkins, 1985). Many viral genes can be disrupted and deleted without affecting the ability of the virus to be propagated in some cells. The HSV1 genome can be altered either by addition of foreign genes (up to 8 kb) or by replacing viral genes with foreign genes. It is estimated that at least 30 kb of the HSV genome can be replaced in this latter manner with minimal effects on viral packaging, replication and infectivity. This virus appears to be an ideal vehicle for gene transfer in the central nervous system since it efficiently infects neural cells (for a more extensive review, see Breakefield and DeLuca, 1991).

Two types of HSV vectors have been utilized for gene transfer to cells: 1) plasmid-derived vectors known as "amplicons" (Spaete and Frankel, 1985), and 2) recombinant HSV1 vectors. Figure 1 illustrates examples of each of these vectors. *Amplicons* consist of a plasmid that contains an HSV origin of replication and packaging signal (Geller and Breakefield, 1988). To produce an infectious particle, the amplicon is transfected into a permissive host cell which is then infected with "helper" HSV (Geller, 1991). This leads to replication and packaging of the amplicon as a concatenate in HSV capsids which, upon release from the cell, can be used to infect target cells. Progeny particles from the permissive host cell consist of a mixture of amplicons packaged into HSV capsids (vector) and "helper" virus. "Helper" HSV is usually attenuated through a conditional mutation, such as temperature-sensitivity of thymidine kinase (TK) needed for viral DNA replication, or a deletion in a critical gene, such as that encoding ICP4 [Shepard et al., 1989]). *Recombinant vectors* are engineered by direct alteration of the viral genome (e.g. Roizman and Jenkins, 1985; Glorioso et al., 1992). This is usually performed by homologous recombination between HSV DNA and a plasmid that contains a transgene flanked by HSV DNA sequences in permissive cells.

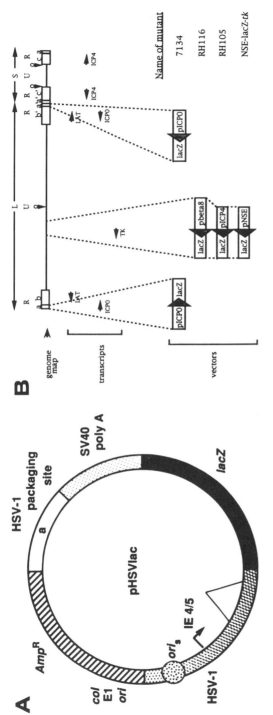

FIGURE 1. Two types of herpes virus vectors. A. Amplicon (plasmid) vector pHSV lac. The clear region contains the HSV-1 a segment, nucleotides 127 - 1132, containing the HSV packaging site. The stipled region symbolizes the HSV-1 c region, nucleotides 47 to 1066, containing the HSV ori and the E4/5 HSV early promoter region. The vector contains lacZ and SV40 polyadenylation sequences following the promoter, as well as a gene for ampicillin resistance for growth in bacteria. [Reproduced with permission from Geller and Breakefield, 1988.] B. Recombinant virus vectors. NSE-lacZ-tk, RH105, and RH116 (latter two from Ho and Mocarski, 1988) are recombinant viruses that contain a promoter-driven lacZ gene cassette inserted into the HSV-TK locus, which is located within the unique region (U) of the long arm of the HSV-1 genome (L). The 7134 recombinant (Cai and Schaffer, 1989) contains a ICP0 promoter-lacZ cassette inserted into both of the ICP0 sites located within the terminal repeats in the long arm of the virus. RH105 and 7134 contain immediate early HSV promoter elements, while RH116 contains a early HSV promoter. The promoter for neuron-specific enolase (NSE) drives expression of lacZ in NSE-lacZ-tk. S, Short arm of HSV-1 genome; R, HSV-1 repeat element; o, origin of replication; smaller-case letters are repeat elements where a = a', b = b', and c = c'. Plain arrows indicate transcripts and boxed arrow indicate vector insertion. ICP4, infected cell polypeptide 4; ICP0, infected cell polypeptide 0; LAT, latency-associated transcripts; tk, thymidine kinase (modified from Roizman and Batterson, 1985). Reprinted with permission of Mary Ann Liebert, Inc. from Andersen et al., 1992.

Toxicity of HSV to cells results from two phenomena: virus-induced disruption of host cell macromolecular synthesis and viral replication resulting in production of progeny virions (for review see Roizman and Sears, 1990). Numerous genes participate in both these processes. Once the virus enters a target cell, viral DNA is transferred into the nucleus where a capsid protein, VP16, interacts with cellular transcription factors, such as Oct-1 (Stern et al., 1989). This complex binds to a specific DNA sequence found upstream of the five viral "immediate-early" genes, leading to their transcription. These encode for viral transcription factors that regulate the expression of the second set of transcribed genes: the "early" genes, which encode for enzymes involved primarily in viral DNA replication. They include genes for the HSV thymidine kinase (TK), ribonucleotide reductase (RR) and dUTPase. Transcription of a third set of genes (the "late" genes) occurs later during viral infection and these gene products participate in assembly of virus particles. Host cell death occurs during virus replication partly because of extensive chromosomal damage (Peat and Stanley, 1986; Johnson et al., 1992). Host cell toxicity also results from the "shut-down" of cellular macromolecular synthesis mediated by the HSV protein UL41 (Read and Frenkel, 1983; Kwong et al., 1989) and other viral proteins (for a review, see Roizman and Sears, 1990). In addition, expression of immediate-early proteins, such as ICP4 and ICP27, can contribute to cell toxicity (Johnson et al., 1992).

Numerous amplicon-based and recombinant-based HSV vectors have been constructed for gene transfer to neurons. Most systems contain disruptions of one or more immediate-early or early viral genes rendering the "helper" virus (in the amplicon-based system) or the recombinant virus vector replication-defective or - compromised so as to reduce pathogenicity to the host. Additional features in some constructs involve the elimination of cytotoxic genes such as UL41. Herpes vectors can also be used to deliver transgenes encoding genes that confer toxicity on tumor cells (see below). The future challenge for gene delivery to the nervous system rests on the creation of HSV vectors that can efficiently deliver transgenes of interest without harming the integrity of normal host cells.

Destruction of glioma tumors with herpes virus mutants

Some of the earliest published experiments of viral genetic treatment of tumors in patients were made in the sixties and seventies. For instance Wheelock and Dingle wrote in 1964 that "...viruses could be used to modify the disease (leukemia) in man by a direct oncolytic effect..." and proceeded to treat a man suffering from leukemia with repeated inoculations of six types of animal viruses, albeit without success. Since then a few reports of treatments of tumors in man or rodents with wild type viruses have appeared (Taylor et al., 1971; Cassel et al., 1983). These historical vignettes illustrate the rather old hypothesis that viruses might be useful oncolytic agents either by delivery of their own toxic genes or by inducing a host cell response against the cell harboring the virus. The host cell toxicity and death mediated by HSV provides the theoretical framework for using the virus in tumor cell destruction. In this case, the HSV vector retains its cytotoxicity for tumor cells, while at the same time it loses its ability to damage other cell types, in particular, neurons. An initial approach to the achievement of this goal takes advantage of the fact that actively proliferating cells, such as tumor cells, possess high levels of several enzymes involved in host cell DNA synthesis. Conversely nonproliferating cells, such as neurons and glia, have low levels of these enzymes. Some of these cellular enzymes, such as TK, ribonucleotide reductase, DNA polymerase, dUTPase, are analogous to HSV enzymes that catalyze reactions in viral DNA synthesis (Lipson et al., 1989). Therefore, the replication deficiency of HSV with mutations in the genes encoding these enzymes can be complemented in tumor cells but not in neurons or glia.

To explore this tumor-killing scheme, pathologic effects of three different HSV mutants were assessed in rat brains (Chiocca et al., 1990). These mutants possessed insertions of the *E. coli* lacZ gene in the coding regions of the HSV immediate-early ICP0 gene (mutant name, 7134; Cai and Schaffer, 1989), the HSV TK gene (RH105; Ho and Mocarski, 1988), and the HSV immediate-early ICP4 gene (GAL4; Shepard et al., 1989). The lacZ gene, which encodes beta-galactosidase, served as a marker of immediate-early and early virus gene expression. Expression of this enzyme confers blue cytoplasmic staining upon addition of the substrate, 5-bromo-4-chloro-3-indolyl, beta-D-galactoside (X-gal) (Price et al., 1987). No pathologic behavioral effects (seizure-like activity, lack of feeding and drinking, and ultimately death) were observed in six of seven rats inoculated with the ICP0 mutant (200,000 plaque forming units, pfus) into the right caudate nucleus. Histological staining of these brains for lacZ expression, showed that the ICP0 mutant had spread in a limited and concentric fashion three days after the injection (Fig. 2). The one animal that displayed pathologic behavior demonstrated extensive viral spread of the ICP0 mutant virus throughout the cortex. A long term follow-up of rats inoculated with this mutant showed that the injected caudate nuclei decreased in size over two months probably due to a "smoldering" infection (Huang et al., 1992). In contrast, inoculation of the TK mutant or of the ICP4 mutant into the right caudate nucleus did not cause animal deaths or pathologic behavior. In these cases, histochemical staining of inoculated rat brains for lacZ expression 3 and 14 days after injection, did not reveal evidence of virus spread beyond those few cells that had been initially infected. Furthermore there were no long term neuropathologic consequences of infection with these vectors (Huang et al., 1992). This indicated that HSV TK and ICP4 mutants did not cause marked neuronal damage.

One of the authors (Martuza et al., 1991) assessed the capacity of an HSV TK mutant virus to destroy human glioma cells both in culture and in animals. He employed a mutant HSV1 (named dlsptk) that possessed a 360 base pair deletion in the TK coding region (Coen et al., 1989). To assess whether inoculation of the TK mutant could inhibit tumor growth, human U87 gliomas were established intracranially in nude mice and then injected stereotactically with the TK mutant (or

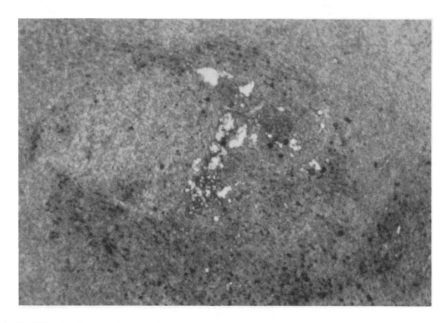

FIGURE 2. Gene delivery to rat brain using recombinant virus vectors. Coronal section illustrating beta-galactosidase expression in cells in the frontal area of the brain after inoculation with 7134. Rat brains were removed after perfusing animals with 4% paraformaldehyde. Brains were then placed in a solution containing 30% sucrose and 4% paraformaldehyde for 24 hours prior to sectioning on a cryostat. Forty micron sections were placed in phosphate buffered saline. Sections were then placed overnight in a solution containing 0.1% X-gal, 2 mM magnesium chloride, 35 mM potassium ferrocyanide, 35 mM potassium ferricyanide, 0.1% sodium deoxycholate, and 0.1% Nonidet P-40 (Turner and Cepko, 1987). After washing in phosphate buffered saline, the sections were mounted on glass slides without further counterstaining and examined by light microscopy. The presence of β-galactosidase enzyme in a cell will cause a blue stain in the presence of the substrate X-gal (5-bromo-4-chloro-3-indolyl-beta-D-galactoside). The inoculation in this area was carried out in the frontal/caudate area and the blue stain is located both in glia and in neurons with extravasation of X-gal product in the extracellular space. This gives the appearance of a "halo" around the zone of tissue loss where damage from the injection needle occurred (Chiocca et al., 1990). The black spots represent artifacts from tissue processing. Reprinted with permission of W. B. Saunders Co. from Chiocca et al., 1990.

control medium alone). Control rodents succumbed to their tumors within 6-8 weeks (Fig. 3). In contrast, one third of animals treated with the TK mutant survived five months before sacrifice. Histologic analysis of brains revealed no surviving tumor cells. However, foci of inflammatory infiltrates were noted. Some of the early deaths in the treated animals may have been due to a virus-induced panencephalitic process resulting from low level viral replication in normal brain cells, possibly in reactive glia or endothelial cells. However the LD_{50} (dose that was lethal to 50% nude mice) for the TK mutant was approximately 10^6 pfu com-

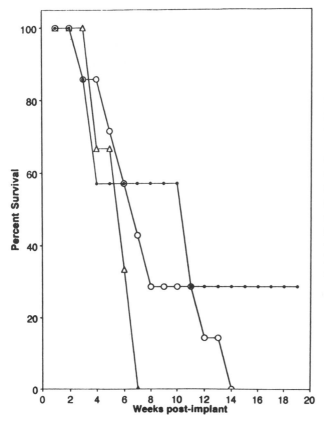

FIGURE 3. Animal survival following treatment of tumors with TK⁻ herpes virus. Ten days after intracerebral injection of 1.6×10^5 U87 human glioma cells into 20 nude mice, the tumors were treated with either 10^3 pfu *dl*sptk (open circles), 10^5 pfu *dl*sptk (solid circles), or with medium (DME)+ (triangles). Percent animal survival was followed over time. Reprinted with permission from Martuza et al., 1991. ©1991 AAAS.

pared to about 10^3 pfu for the wild type virus. Therefore, the TK mutant displays an encouraging pattern of rather selective tumor cell destruction, but its genetic structure needs to be refined further in order to achieve a greater degree of rodent survival and a reduction of pathologic effects to normal brain cells.

Current experimental avenues have focused on the creation of HSV vectors that undergo productive infection in tumor cells and spare normal brain cells. Several mutants appear promising in this respect including those with mutations in the viral DNA polymerase, γ34.5, and ribonucleotide reductase genes (Markert et al., 1993; Kaplitt et al. ,1992). In the future, HSV vectors that possess mutations in two or more of these genes might provide additional safety features.

RETROVIRUS VECTORS IN GLIOMA THERAPY

Characteristics of retrovirus vectors

The most important advantage of retrovirus-mediated gene therapy of brain tumors is the selectivity of the virus for proliferating cells. In fact, the retrovirus DNA will integrate into the host cell's genome (and thus be transcribed and expressed) only during DNA synthesis (Cepko, 1988). Neurons are terminally differentiated cells and do not divide in the adult brain. Glial cells only proliferate if there has been an injury. Thus the only proliferating cells in an adult brain that contains a tumor are glioma cells themselves, as well as some endothelial cells associated with tumor-induced neovascularization, and some astrocytes involved in the process of reactive astrocytosis. Retrovirus-mediated destruction of glioma cells and tumor-associated endothelial cells would be a desirable feature, and destruction of astrocytes proliferating in the gliotic process would not necessarily be detrimental.

The low efficiency of retrovirus-mediated gene transfer to tumor cells has been one of the major concerns of this therapeutic scheme. Direct inoculation of the retrovirus is not very efficient at gene delivery to tumor cells in the brain (Short et al., 1990; Yamada et al., 1992). Gene delivery is more efficient (10-70% tumor cells) by direct intratumoral grafting of a packaging cell line (Short et al., 1990; Ram et al., 1993). This procedure provides the continuous release of retrovirus vector that can infect proliferating tumor cells over a period of several days. These results emphasize the difficulty in infecting all tumor cells even in the primary mass. Therefore transfer of a gene which has to be expressed in every tumor cell to cause tumor destruction is not a feasible means of therapy.

To circumvent this limitation, one needs to transfer into glioma cells a gene able to generate a toxic product that can be transferred to other tumor cells or a gene that can enhance specific immune responses to the tumor. At least four types of genetic approaches appear to fulfill these criteria. The first approach includes transfer of genes encoding enzymes that, when expressed in the tumor cell, can transform a prodrug into an active analog that is toxic to tumor cells. For example, expression of the HSV1 TK enzyme will convert the nucleoside analog, ganciclovir, into a toxic phosphorylated derivative. The second approach includes transfer of a gene whose products elicit a specific immune response against the tumor. For example expression of a foreign MHC-1 molecule on the surface of tumor cells enhances their rejection and that of adjacent tumor cells by MHC-1-mediated enhancement of immune response against tumor cell antigens (Itaya et al., 1987). The third approach includes soluble toxins or immune response modifiers, such as diptheria toxin (Maxwell et al., 1986 and 1991), interleukin-2 (Fearon et al., 1990) and interleukin-4 (Tepper et al., 1989). Another example is the recent finding that antiglioma CD8 + T-cell immune responses were enhanced by introduction of an antisense cDNA to insulinlike growth factor I (IGF-1) (Trojan et al., 1993). A fourth approach has been to introduce tumor suppressor genes (like p53 or the retinoblastoma gene, RB) into tumor cells to allow the resumption of normal growth characteristics (Chang et al., 1992; Huang et al., 1988). However, this may not be ideal for tumor therapy since these genes would have to be expressed in all tumor cells and might only slow growth of transfected cells until a new mutation occurred that enhanced the transformed phenotype.

Preliminary findings suggest that retrovirus-based genetic therapy may hold distinct theoretical advantages compared to traditional therapy (such as radio- and chemotherapies and neurosurgery) for brain tumors. Transfer of oncolytic products from infected to noninfected tumor cells may spread toxic effects throughout the tumor. Addition of replication-competent retrovirus may also allow the transgene to spread thoughout the tumor by generation of vector in vivo and migration of infected tumor cells, as well as enhancing the immune response against retrovirus antigens expressed on the surface of infected cells. These theoretical considerations have not been documented but illustrate the potential "expansive" power of retrovirus-based gene therapy. Further this new therapy can be combined with more traditional ones to achieve multi-faceted and complementary therapeutic strategies.

Safety issues in retrovirus-based therapies have been addressed by many investigators. In fact human clinical trials using these vectors are underway for many illnesses. We have found that a mouse packaging line injected into the rat cerebrum is rejected by 5 days (Short et al., 1990). The lack of permanence of the packaging line in the brain minimizes the risk of recombinatorial events leading to the creation of a wild-type retrovirus or a new type of retrovirus. We have also used packaging lines that secrete replication-competent retroviruses into nude mice and have not seen evidence of retrovirus-induced pathology (Takamiya et al., 1992 and 1993). Careful long-term follow-up studies of multiple tissues from these rodents will need to be analyzed, however, before the relative risk can be assessed.

Retrovirus-mediated destruction of rodent gliomas with the HSV TK gene

Retrovirus-mediated delivery of a foreign gene into intracerebral rat gliomas in vivo is limited by the low efficiency of gene transduction. Short et al. (1990) found that direct intratumoral injection of a retroviral vector bearing the *E. coli* lacZ marker gene introduced the transgene into only about 0.1% of tumor cells. However, intratumoral grafting of the retroviral packaging line that released the lacZ-bearing retrovirus dramatically increased the efficiency of gene transfer to approximately 10% (Fig. 4). The majority of infected cells were located in the periphery of the tumor where active cell proliferation usually occurs. The grafted mouse cell did not survive more than a week probably due to immune rejection.

In order to exploit gene transfer as a possible therapeutic approach to gliomas, the HSV TK gene was chosen. This therapeutic paradigm for tumors was first developed by Moolten (1986 and 1990). The HSV TK enzyme will phosphorylate nucleoside analogs, such as ganciclovir and acyclovir, thereby leading to their incorporation into replicating DNA. The incorporated analogs will cause strand breaks and ultimately lead to cell death. A rat glioma C6 derived cell line (C6VIK) was engineered in culture to express HSV TK (Ezzeddine et al., 1991). These cells exhibited increased chemosensitivity to ganciclovir compared to parental cells. When injected subcutaneously into the flanks of nude mice, they rapidly formed tumors. If the mice were treated with daily intraperitoneal injections of ganciclovir (or with ganciclovir delivered as a continuous infusion), complete inhibition of

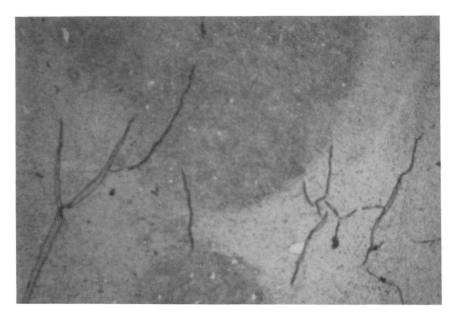

FIGURE 4. Delivery of lacZ gene to tumor cells in rat brain by co-grafting of psi 2-BAG (Price et al., 1987) packaging cells. Coronal sections of brain from a rat, which was initially implanted with C6 cells in the right frontal lobe, and then received a graft of psi 2-BAG cells (5 x 10⁵ cells) into the same site 3 days later, and was sacrificed 7 days after the second graft. Coronal section was stained for beta-galactosidase activity (as described in figure 2). The tumor is readily visible as a discrete mass within the parenchyma X25. The long dark wavy lines are artifacts from folding of tissue slices on slides. Reprinted with permission of Dr. M. Priscilla Short.

tumor growth was evident. These results indicated that in vivo inhibition of glioma growth could be achieved with the HSV TK/ganciclovir therapy.

An important observation that enhances the HSV TK/ganciclovir therapeutic paradigm concerns the process first described by Moolten (1990) and then also by others, termed the "bystander effect" (Freeman et al., 1991; Culver et al., 1992). The following set of published experiments illustrates this effect (Takamiya et al., 1992). A C6 glioma cell line (C6BAG) constitutively expressing the lacZ gene was engineered in order to permit the identification of these tumor cells (Shimohama et al., 1989). These cells were cocultured with C6VIK cells (that express the HSV TK gene) in a ratio of 1:100 for 7 days. Cells were then incubated with varying concentrations of ganciclovir for 14 days after which the number of surviving lacZ-positive colonies was assayed. Figure 5a shows that, at ganciclovir concentrations above 2 uM, C6BAG colony survival was dramatically decreased when cocultured with C6VIK, whereas C6BAG colony survival in the presence of parental C6BU1 cells was not affected by ganciclovir doses as high as 500 uM. The decreased survival exhibited by C6BAG cells cocultured with C6VIK did not ap-

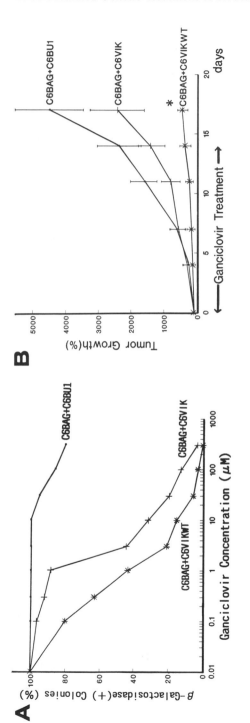

FIGURE 5. "Bystander effect" whereby tumor cells with the HSV TK gene can effect death of other non-transfected tumor cells in the presence of ganciclovir. A. Ganciclovir sensitivity of C6BAG glioma cells after simultaneous co-culture with other C6-derived lines. Simultaneous co-culture experiment with C6BAG cells as recipients and C6VIK and C6VIKWT cells as donors (1:100). Ganciclovir treatment was begun 7 days after plating and continued for 14 days. Only beta-galactosidase-positive colonies were counted. Colony numbers are expressed as a percentage of those seen for parallel cultures without ganciclovir. Studies were done in triplicate with less than 0.5% variability. Legends: C6BU1= Rat C6 glioma cells that lack endogenous (mammalian) thymidine kinase activity; C6BAG= Rat C6BU1 glioma cells that express beta-galactosidase (by infection and G418 selection of cells infected with the BAG retrovirus that contains both a beta-galactosidase gene and a neomycin resistance gene); C6VIK= Rat C6BU1 cells that express herpes simplex virus type 1 thymidine kinase (by infection and G418/HAT selection of cells infected with a retrovirus that bears both the HSV thymidine kinase gene and the neomycin resistance gene); C6VIKWT= Rat C6VIK cells that have been superinfected with a wild-type murine Moloney leukemia retrovirus and that produce both the wild-type retrovirus and the retrovirus that bears the HSV thymidine kinase gene. B. Tumor cells were inoculated into the flanks of nude mice in different combinations in a ratio of 1:10 [recipient (C6BAG) to donor cells: C6BU1 (n=9), C6BVIK (n=9), or C6BVIKWT (n=7), where n=number of animals in each group]. After tumors reached 1 cm in diameter animals were treated with 50 mg/kg/day ganciclovir for 14 days (*p<0.01). Bars indicate standard error of the mean. Reprinted with permission of Alan R. Liss, Inc. from Takamiya et al., 1992.

pear to be due to a diffusible product, because conditioned medium from C6VIK treated with ganciclovir did not decrease the cloning efficiency of C6BAG cells. This suggested that cell-to-cell contact with passage either of toxic ganciclovir metabolites or of the virus TK enzyme itself from the C6VIK "donor" cells to the C6BAG "naive" cells, possibly through gap junctions, was necessary for this "bystander effect." The presence of wild type retrovirus (WT) in this assay increased killing of C6BAG cells either by generation of vector in culture and secondary infection of C6BAG cells or by interference of the virus with host cell metabolism. Animal studies confirm the finding that C6BAG glioma cells that are combined with C6VIK glioma cells exhibit decreased growth rates upon treatment of animals with ganciclovir and again this effect is enhanced by the presence of wild type virus (Fig. 5b).

In order to achieve in vivo transfer of the TK transgene, a retrovirus packaging line (psi2STK), with and without wild type retrovirus, was cografted with C6 glioma cells (in a ratio of 1 packaging cell to 1 tumor cells) subcutaneously into nude mice (Takamiya et al., 1993). Retrovirus-mediated gene transfer was allowed to occur over several days (3-7) before beginning a 14 day treatment with ganciclovir (given as an intraperitoneal injection of 25 mg/kg/day). Figure 6a shows that these tumors regressed, while tumors cografted with psi2 cells did not.

Another group has also demonstrated inhibition of growth of a syngeneic 9L gliosarcoma tumor in rat brains by grafting of a packaging cell line releasing a HSV TK retrovirus vector without wild type virus (Culver et al., 1992; Ram et al., 1993). These investigators applied an experimental procedure similar to those described above. Potentially relevant differences between the two set of experiments involve the type of animal model (rat brain vs. subcutaneous flank of nude mice), the retrovirus packaging cell line used (PA317 vs. psi2), the promoter used to regulate expression of HSV TK (cytomegalovirus versus SV40), and the ratio of packaging cells to tumor cells (10:1 versus 1:1). Ganciclovir-induced regression of intracerebral tumors was also reported by these investigators. Since they used an immunocompetent animal, the combination of HSV TK/ganciclovir therapy coupled to an immune response to mouse fibroblast antigens, retrovirus glycoproteins displayed on the surface of the intratumoral packaging cells, and possibly HSV TK may have contributed to tumor regression in their study.

A modified packaging cell line was also created by infecting psi2STK cells with "helper" wild-type retrovirus (Takamiya et al., 1993). This new line (psi2STK-WT) displayed a marked increase of TK gene transfer to C6 gliomas both in culture and in vivo. In fact, after ganciclovir treatment was stopped, C6 glioma tumors treated with psi2STK cells often recurred, while those treated with psi2STK-WT did not (Fig. 6b). Our current hypothesis is that some C6 glioma cells were infected by both TK-bearing defective retrovirus and "helper" wild-type retrovirus. The wild-type retrovirus sequences allowed the infected C6 glioma cells to package vector sequences. Further C6 glioma cells might be able to migrate and deliver TK-bearing defective-retrovirus (and "helper" retrovirus) throughout the tumor. While the use of wild type virus cannot be advocated in the present format for

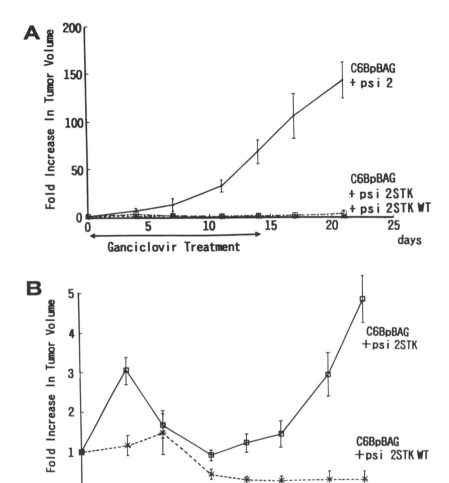

FIGURE 6. Gene transfer and drug treatment of C6BU1pBAG tumor in vivo. Mixtures of 10[6] recipient C6BU1pBAG, and 10[6] donor cells: psi 2 (.), psi 2STK ([]), or psi 2STKWT (*), were injected subcutaneously into nude mice, 20 for each group. When tumors reached 1 cm³ in diameter animals were treated with 25 mg/kg/day ganciclovir for 14 days. Tumor growth was calculated as the fold increase compared to the volume at the time treatment started. Bars indicate the standard error of the mean. A. Fold increase scale 0-200; B. Fold increase scale 0-5. Legends: Psi2= parental mouse producer cell line; psi2STK= mouse fibroblast producer cells that package the retrovirus bearing the HSV thymidine kinase gene; Psi2STKWT= Psi2STK cells superinfected with a wild-type Moloney murine leukemia virus (thereby producing both wild-type and thymidine kinase bearing retroviruses). Reprinted with permission of the American Association of Neurological Surgeons from Takamiya,1993.

human therapies, it could provide an experimental framework for the construction of retrovirus-producer cells that are able to migrate in the tumor bed and in the brain. This would permit the delivery of transgenes and gene products at a distance from the primary graft site of the packaging cells. This should greatly increase the therapeutic effectiveness of focal grafting of murine packaging cells into glioma tumors. Our results suggest that this might lead to longer lasting regression (and possibly a cure) of rodent gliomas compared to use of replication-incompetent retroviruses. Construction of autologous packaging cell lines would also enhance therapeutic effectiveness by increasing the length of survival of packaging cells in vivo and increasing the time during which viral release and infection can occur. The autologous packaging cells would be screened for toxicity and tumorigenicity prior to implantation. The retroviral TK gene present in the autologous implants would permit their ganciclovir-mediated elimination (assuming that the implanted cells were capable of some cell division) and thereby reduce the chance of long-term release of retroviruses that might lead to harmful recombinatorial events.

In conclusion, we believe that the next few years will witness an expansion of the unprecedented collaboration between the molecular biologist/virologist and the neurosurgeon/neurooncologist, perhaps similar to the one between the immunologist and the transplant surgeon that occurred over the past decade. This can only lead to the refinement of the ideas and methodologies necessary for the genetic treatment of human central nervous system disorders.

REFERENCES

Andersen JK, Garber DA, Meaney CA, Breakefield XO (1992): Gene transfer into mammalian central nervous system using herpes virus vectors: extended expression of bacterial *lacZ* in neurons using the neuron-specific enolase promoter. *Hum Gene Ther* 3:487-499

Breakefield XO, DeLuca NA (1991): Herpes simplex virus for gene delivery to neurons. *The New Biologist* 3:203-218

Cai W, Schaffer PA (1989): Herpes simplex virus type 1 ICP0 plays a critical role in the de novo synthesis of infectious virus following transfection of viral DNA. *J Virol* 63:4579-4589

Cassel W, Murrary DR, Phillips H (1983): A phase II study on the postsurgical management of stage II malignant melanoma with a Newcastle disease virus oncolysate. *Cancer* 52:856-860

Cepko C (1988): Retroviral vectors and their applications in neurobiology. *Neuron* 1:345-353

Chang T, Yee J-K, Yeargin T, Friedman T, Haas M (1992): Suppression of acute lymphoblastic leukemia by the human p53 gene. *Cancer Res* 52:222-226

Chiocca EA, Choi BB, Weizhong C, DeLuca NA, Schaffer PA, DiFiglia M, Breakefield XO, Martuza RL (1990): Transfer and expression of the lacZ gene in rat brain neurons mediated by herpes simplex virus mutants. *New Biologist*

2:739-746

Clifford S, Schold JR, Gregory Carncross, Bullard DE (1985): Chemotherapy of primary brain tumors. In: *Neurosurgery*, New York: McGraw-Hill Co. pp 1143-1152

Coen DM, Kosz-Vnenchak M, Jacobson JG, Leib DA, Bogard CL, Schaffer PA, Tyler KL, Knipe DM (1989): Thymidine kinase-negative herpes simplex virus mutants establish latency in mouse trigeminal ganglia but do not reactivate. *Proc Natl Acad Sci USA* 86:4736-4740

Culver KW, Ram X, Waebridge S, Ishii H, Oldfield EH, Blaese RM (1992): In vivo gene transfer with retroviral vector-producer cells for treatment of experimental brain tumors. *Science* 256:1550-1552

Ezzeddine ZD, Martuza RL, Short MP, Platika D, Malick A, Choi B, Breakefield XO (1991): Selective killing of glioma cells in culture and in vivo following retrovirus transfer of the herpes simplex virus thymidine kinase gene. *New Biologist* 3:1-7

Fearon ER, Pardoll DM, Itaya T, Golumbek P, Levitsky HI, Simons JW, Karasuyama H, Vogelstein B, Frost P (1990): Interleukin-2 production by tumor cells bypasses T helper function in the generation of an antitumor response. *Cell* 60:397-403

Freeman SM, Whartenby KA, Koeplin DS, et al. (1992): Tumor regression when a fraction of the tumor mass contains the HSV-TK gene. *J Cell Biol* 168:47

Geller AI (1991): A system, using neural cell lines, to characterize HSV-1 vectors containing genes which affect neuronal physiology, or neuronal promoters. *J Neurosci Methods* 36:91-103

Geller AI, Breakefield XO (1988): A defective HSV-1 vector expresses *E. coli* beta-galactosidase in cultured rat peripheral neurons. *Science* 241:1667-1669

Glorioso JC, Sternberg IR, Groins WF, Fink DJ (1992): Development of herpes simplex virus as a gene transfer vector for the central nervous system. In: *Gene Transfer and Therapy in the Nervous System*, Gage F, Christen Y eds. New York: Springer-Verlag, pp 133-145

Goldberg WJ, Laws ER, Bernstein JJ (1991): Individual C6 glioma cells migrate in adult rat brain after neural homografting. *J Neuroscience* 9:427-437

Hewitt HB, Blake ER, Walder AS (1976): A critique of the evidence for active host defence against cancer, based on personal studies of 27 murine tumors of spontaneous origin. *Br J Cancer* 33:241-259

Ho DY, Mocarski ES (1988): Beta-galactosidase as a market in the peripheral and neural tissues of the herpes simplex virus-infected mouse. *Virol* 167:279-283

Hochberg FH, Pruitt A (1980): Assumptions in the radiotherapy of glioblastoma. *Neurology* 30:907-911

Huang J-S, Yee J-K, Shew J-Y, Chen P-L, Bookstein R, Friedmann T, Lee EY, Lee W-H (1988): Suppression of the neoplastic phenotype by replacement of the RB genetic human cancer cells. *Science* 242:1563-1566

Huang Q, Vonsattel J-P, Schaffer PA, Martuza RL, Breakefield XO, DiFiglia M (1992): Introduction of a foreign gene (*Escherichia coli lacZ*) into rat neuostriatal neurons using herpes simplex virus mutants: A light and electron microscopic study. *Exp Neurol* 115:303-316

Itaya T, Yamagiwa S, Okada S, Oikawa F, Kuzumaki N, Takeichi N, Hosokawa M, Kobayashi H (1987): Xenogenization of a mouse lung carcinoma (3LL) by transfection with an allogeneic class I major histocompatibility complex gene. *Cancer Res* 47:3136-3140

Johnson PA, Miyanohara A, Levine F, Cahill T, Friedmann T (1992): Cytotoxicity of a replication-defective mutant of herpes simplex virus type 1. *J Virol* 66:2952-2965

Kaplitt M, Tjuvajev J, Berk J, Rabkin SD, Posner JB, Pfaff DW, Blasberg RG (1992): Treatment of W256 tumors in immunocompetent rats using herpes simplex virus mutants (Abstract). In: *Gene Therapy*, Anderson UF, Friedmann T, Mulligan R, eds New York: Cold Spring Harbor Labs., p 81

Kornblith PL, Walker MD, Cassady RJ (1985): Neoplasms of the central nervous system. In: *Principles and Practice of Oncology*, Helmann S, Rosenberg SA, eds. Philadelphia: J.B. Lipincott Co., pp 1437-1511

Kwong AD, Kruper JA, Frenkel N (1989): HSV virion host shutoff function. *J Virol* 62:912-921

Lipson KE, Chen ST, Koniecki J, Ku DH, Baserga R (1989): S-phase-specific regulation by deletion mutants of the human thymidine kinase promoter. *Proc Natl Acad Sci USA* 89:6848-6852

Markert JM, Malick A, Coen DM, Martuza RL (1993): Reduction and elimination of encephalitis in an experimental glioma therapy model with attenuated herpes simplex mutants that retain susceptibility to acyclovir. *Neurosurgery* 32: 597-603

Martuza RL, Malick A, Markert JM, Ruggner KL, Coen DM (1991): Experimental therapy of human glioma by means of a genetically engineered virus mutant. *Science* 252:854-856

Maxwell IH, Maxwell F, Globe LM (1986): Regulated expression of diphteria toxin A-chain gene transfected into human cells: a possible strategy for inducing cancer cell suicide. *Can Res* 46:4660-4664

Maxwell IH, Globe LM, Maxwell F (1991): Expression of the diptheria toxin A chain coding sequence under the control of promoters and enhancers from immunoglobulin genes as a means of directing toxicity to B-lymphoid cells. *Cancer Res* 51:4299-4304

Moolten FL (1986): Tumor chemosensitivity conferred by inserted thymidine kinase genes: paradigm for a prospective cancer control strategy. *Cancer Res* 46:5276-5281

Moolten FL (1990): Mosaicism induced by gene insertion as a means of improving chemotheraeutic selectivity. *Critical Rev Immunol* 10:203-233

Peat DS, Stanley MA (1986): Chromosome damage induced by herpes simplex virus type 1 in early infection. *J Gen Virol* 67:2273-2277

Price J, Turner D, Cepko C (1987):Lineage analysis in the vertebrate nervous system by retrovirus-mediated gene transfer. *Proc Natl Acad Sci USA* 84:156-160

Ram Z, Culver KW, Walbridge S, Blaese RM, Oldfield EH (1993): In situ retroviral-mediated gene transfer for the treatment of brain tumors in rats. *Cancer Res* 53:83-88

Read GS and Frenkel N (1983): Herpes simplex virus mutants defective in the virion-associated shutoff of host polypeptide synthesis and exhibiting abnormal synthesis of alpha (immediate-early) viral polypeptides. *J Virol* 46:498-512

Roizman B, Batterson W (1985): Herpes viruses and their replication. In: *Virology*, Fields BN ed. New York: Raven Press, p 497-526

Roizman B, Jenkins FJ (1985): Genetic engineering of novel genomies of large DNA viruses. *Science* 229:1208-1214

Roizman B, Sears AE (1990): Herpes simplex viruses and their replication. In: *Virology* (2nd ed) Fields BN, Knipe DM eds. Raven Press, pp 1795-1842

Rosenfeld MA, Siegfried W, Yoshimura K, Yoneyama K, Fukayama M, Stier LE, Paakko PK, Gilardi P, Stratford-Perricaudet LD, Perricaudet M, Jallat S, Pavirani A, Lecocq J-P, Crystal RG (1991): Adenovirus-mediated transfer of a recombinant alpha1-antitrypsin gene to the lung epithelium in vivo. *Science* 252:431-434

Salcman M (1985): Supratentorial gliomas. In: *Neurosurgery*, Wilkins RH, Rengachary SS, eds. New York: McGraw-Hill Book Co., pp 579-581

Samulski RJ, Zhu X, Xiao X, Brook JD, Housman DE, Epstein N, Hunter LA (1991): Targeted integration of adeno-associated virus (AAV) into human chromosome 19. *EMBO Journal* 10:3941-3950

Schoenberg BS (1983): The epidemiology of nervous system tumors. In: *Oncology of the Nervous System*, Walker MD ed. Boston: Martinus Nijhoff

Shepard AA, Imbalzano AN, DeLuca NA (1989): Separation of primary structural components conferring autoregulation, transactivation, and DNA-binding properties to the herpes simplex virus transcriptional regulatory protein ICP4. *J Virol* 63:3714-3728

Shimohama S, Rosenberg MB, Fagan AM, Wolff JA, Short MP, Breakefield XO, Gage FH (1989): Grafting geneticially modified cells into the rat brain: Characteristics of *E. coli* β-galactosidase as a reporter gene. *Mol Brain Res* 5:271-278

Short MP, Choi B, Lee J, Malick A, Breakefield XO, Martuza RL (1990): Gene delivery to glioma cells in rat brain by grafting of a retrovirus packaging cell line. *J Neurosci Res* 27:427-433

Spaet RR, Frankel N (1985): The herpes simplex virus amplicon: Analyses of cis-acting replication functions. *Proc Natl Acad Sci USA* 82:694-698

Stern S, Masafumi T, Herr W (1989): The Oct-1 homoeodomain directs formation of a multiprotein-DNA complex with the HSV transactivator VP16. *Nature* 341:624-630

Takamiya Y, Short MP, Ezzedine ZD, Moolten FL, Breakefield XO, Martuza RL (1992): Gene therapy of malignant brain tumors: A rat glioma line bearing the herpes simplex virus type 1-thymidine kinase gene and wild type retrovirus kills other tumor cells. *J Neuroscience Res* 33:493-503

Takamiya Y, Short MP, Moolten FL, Fleet C, Mineta T, Breakefield XO, Martuza RL (1993): An experimental model of retrovirus gene therapy for malignant brain tumors. *J Neurosurgery* 79: 104-110

Taylor MW, Cordell B, Souhrada M, Prather S (1971): Viruses as an aid to cancer therapy: Regression of solid and ascites tumors in rodents after treatment with bovine enterovirus. *Proc Natl Acad Sci USA* 68:836-840.

Tepper RJ, Pattengale PK, Leder P (1989): Murine interleukin-4 displays potent anti-tumor activity in vivo. *Cell* 57:503-512

Trojan J, Johnson TR, Rudin SD, Ilan J, Tykocinski ML, Ilan J (1993): Treatment and prevention of rat glioblastoma by immunogenic C6 cells expressing antisense insulin-like growth factor I RNA. *Science* 259:94-97

Turner DL and Cepko CL (1987) A common progenitor for neurons and glia persists in rat retina late in development. *Nature* 328: 131-136

Wagner E, Plank C, Zatloukal K, Cotten M, Birnstiel ML (1992): Influenza virus hemagglutinin HA-2 N-terminal fusogenic peptides augment gene transfer by transferrin-polylysine-DNA complexes: Toward a synthetic virus-like gene-transfer vehicle. *Proc Natl Acad Sci USA* 89:7934-7938

Wheelock EF, Dingle JH (1964): Observations on the repeated administration of viruses to a patient with acute leukemia. *New Eng J Med* 271:645-651

Yamada M, Shimizu K, Miyao Y, Hayakawa T, Ikenaka K, Nakahira K, Nakajima K, Kagawa T, Mikoshiba K (1992): Retrovirus-mediated gene transfer targeted to malignant glioma cells in murine brain. *Japan J Cancer Res* 83:1244-1247

Yoshii Y, Maki Y, Tsuboi K, Tomono Y, Nakagawa K, Hoshino T (1986): Estimation of growth fraction with bromodeoxyuridine in human central nervous system tumors. *J Neurosurg* 65:659-663

GENE THERAPY FOR ADENOSINE DEAMINASE DEFICIENCY AND MALIGNANT SOLID TUMORS

Kenneth W. Culver and R. Michael Blaese

INTRODUCTION

Gene therapy may be considered the ultimate treatment for genetic diseases (Anderson, 1984). The possibility of reversing genetic defects by replacing the defective gene instead of merely treating symptoms is very appealing. Significant progress in the development of clinical applications of gene therapy has occurred. More than 40 human gene transfer and therapy experiments have been initiated since the introduction of this approach in 1989 (Anderson, 1992; Miller, 1992).

The development of gene therapy first requires the identification and cloning of the normal gene(s). More than 3,000 of the more than 100,000 genes thought to reside in the human genome have been identified. Once a gene has been isolated and its function understood, the newly isolated gene may then be used for treatment by either inserting the normal gene into the cells whose function is dependent upon that gene (such as in the treatment T-cells in patients with adenosine deaminase deficiency) or by transferring a new activity to a cell which can be exploited therapeutically (such as transfer of the Herpes simplex-thymidine kinase (HS-tk) gene transfer into tumor cells to confer a selective sensitivity to ganciclovir). Once the strategy is established, the cellular targets of gene transfer and the method for gene transfer must be decided. The gene transfer method must deliver the corrective gene to the proper cells and result in gene expression at a level sufficient to restore normal function. Highly efficient gene transfer may be required in order to prevent residual, defective "non-corrected" cells from limiting the effectiveness of the "corrected cells" or in the case of cancer, prevent the regrowth of malignant cells. Optimally, the gene delivery procedure should be simple and safe. In addition, it should avoid the introduction of genes into the patient's reproductive tissues to prevent germline transmission of the introduced trait.

These basic requirements have posed very significant obstacles to the development of gene therapy for many inherited and non-inherited diseases. Lack of efficient, clinically available gene transfer methods and an inability to closely regulate gene expression limits attempts at gene therapy for most of the more than 4000 known inherited diseases. The best early candidates for gene therapy are diseases that involve a relatively simple "housekeeping" gene defect that does not

Gene Therapeutics: Methods and Applications of Direct Gene Transfer
Jon A. Wolff, Editor • ©1994 *Birkhäuser Boston*

require tight regulation and whose function is not absolutely critical to the initial differentiation and development of the affected cell lineage. Once a candidate disorder is identified, the next step is the development of in vitro and in vivo models for the study of gene transfer.

GENE TRANSFER TECHNIQUES

A number of methods have been developed for the introduction of genes into living cells. These include chemical methods (e.g. calcium-phosphate transfection), physical techniques (e.g. electroporation, microinjection, particle bombardment), fusion (e.g. liposomes), receptor-mediated endocytosis (e.g. DNA-protein complexes, viral envelope/capsid-DNA complexes) and recombinant viruses (e.g. Herpes Simplex, Adenovirus, Adeno-Associated Virus[AAV], and Moloney Murine Leukemia Virus [MoMLV]). Each technique has its own theoretical advantages and disadvantages (Culver and Blaese, 1992). For example, if a corrective gene is to be inserted into the lymphohematopoietic stem cell, a process which will give highly efficient stable integration and expression of the inserted gene must be utilized. Otherwise, as the stem cell proliferates and differentiates, the inserted gene could be progressively diluted out and eventually lost from, or unevenly distributed in, the mature erythroid, myeloid and lymphoid lineages. By contrast, gene insertion into a terminally differentiated non-proliferative tissue such as skeletal muscle or liver might not require gene integration. For tumor cell treatment, the requirement for integration is less definite since the duration of gene expression depends upon the strategy to obtain tumor destruction. In circumstances where the tumor is altered ex vivo or the transduced tumor cells are required to grow in vivo for a period of time, stable gene integration may be required.

The MoMLV-based retroviral vectors have the advantage of high integration efficiency into proliferating tissues like hematopoietic cells and tumor cells (Miller, 1992). These vectors stably integrate into the chromosomes of the target-cell and are passed along to all cell progeny during normal cell division. The efficiency of murine retroviral vector gene transfer approaches 95% in some cell types in vitro. One potential disadvantage of retroviral vectors is that they randomly integrate into the host cell genome. Random integration can lead to highly variable levels of gene expression between cells because of the influence of local chromatin structure at each unique integration site (Kantoff et al., 1986). Random integration may also lead to an integration event that could disable a crucial gene required for normal cell function or survival. In such a case, the transduced cell might be killed. With millions of cells being treated, the loss of an occasional cell would probably be of little consequence. A more worrisome theoretical problem with random integration is insertional mutagenesis where an oncogene is activated or a tumor suppressor gene is inactivated. This could contribute to the eventual transformation of that cell to a malignant phenotype. While this is of theoretical concern, the use of replication incompetent retroviral vectors has not been reported to result in malignant transformation in any *in vivo* system (Cornetta et al., 1990; Rosenberg et al.,

1990; Anderson, 1992). Finally, retroviral vectors only integrate their genes into cells that are actively proliferating and synthesizing DNA. This feature may limit gene transfer into some candidate tissues like skeletal muscle. However, it can also be exploited to target genes directly into tumor cells since tumor cells may be proliferating at a significantly greater rate compared to surrounding normal tissues. This results in preferential delivery of genes to tumor cells in vivo.

GENE THERAPY FOR ADENOSINE DEAMINASE DEFICIENCY

Genetics

Adenosine deaminase (ADA) deficiency (EC 3.5.4.4) is inherited as an autosomal recessive disorder with a frequency of less than 1 in 100,000 births. A defect in the ADA gene leads to absent or diminished ADA enzyme activity in all tissues of the body, but the only consistent clinical consequence is immune system dysfunction resulting in severe combined immunodeficiency (SCID). ADA(-)SCID is a heterogeneous disorder with clinical presentations ranging from mild (repeated infections with diagnosis after several years of age) to severe (the development of severe infections within several days of birth) (Hirschhorn, 1983). ADA catalyzes the conversion of adenosine and 2'-deoxyadenosine (dAdo) to inosine and 2'-deoxyinosine in the normal pathway of purine catabolism and salvage (Figure 1). In the absence of ADA, dAdo accumulates to high levels in the tissues and body fluids of these patients. Subsequently the dAdo becomes phosphorylated to deoxyATP which acts to inhibit DNA synthesis resulting in cell death. T-cells are the primary site of the toxic effects of ADA deficiency although B cells may also be severely reduced in number and function (Ammann et al., 1989).

Current therapies for ADA(-)SCID

The current treatment of choice for ADA(-)SCID is an HLA-matched sibling bone marrow transplant. This therapy can be curative for those 20-30% of children fortunate enough to have an HLA-identical sibling donor, and the best results are achieved if the transplant can be performed before the child acquires severe opportunistic infections (O'Reilly, et al., 1989). For children without an HLA-matched sibling donor, treatment with ADA enzyme replacement has been attempted. In 1985, enzyme replacement was initiated with parenteral injections of bovine ADA conjugated to polyethylene glycol (PEG-ADA; Adagen) (Hershfield et al., 1987). Children receive this drug as an intramuscular injection once or twice weekly, resulting in a substantial increase in plasma levels of ADA activity and a marked decrease in 2'-dAdo levels. Most, but not all, children derive some clinical benefit from PEG-ADA, with a few of the children demonstrating near normalization of immunologic functioning. Other patients have responded less well to the enzyme replacement even though their levels of dAdo are as effectively decreased as in

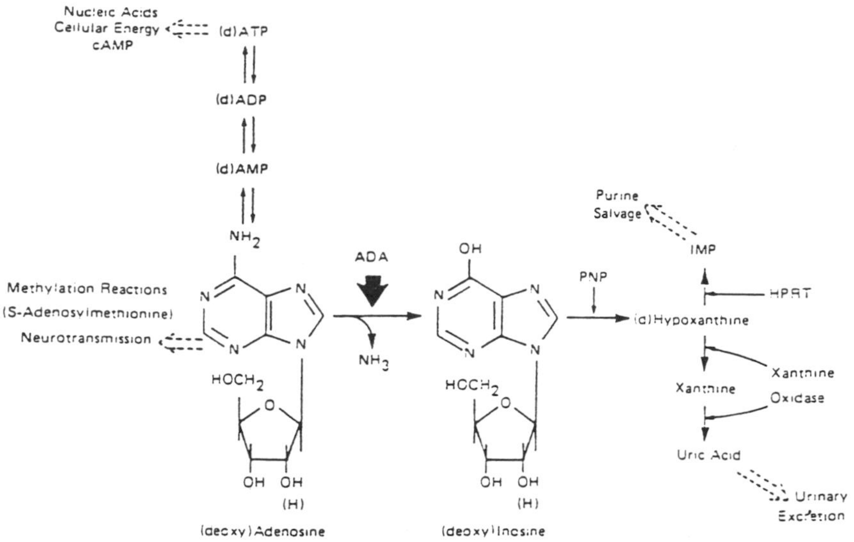

FIGURE 1. *Adenosine nucleoside metabolism.* Adenosine (Ado) or deoxyadenosine (dAdo) may be irreversibly deaminated by adenosine deaminase (ADA) to inosine or deoxyinosine, respectively. These serve as substrates for nucleic acid synthesis or may be used in cellular metabolism. Immature intrathymic lymphocytes are especially rich in adenosine kinases and, in the absence of ADA, tend to rapidly convert Ado and dAdo to their triphosphate forms. dATP is thought to be the primary mediator of lymphocyte toxicity.

those patients who experience greater immune reconstitution. The reasons under-lying this differential response remain unexplained.

Gene therapy for ADA(-)SCID

ADA deficiency has a number of characteristics that made it an attractive initial candidate for gene therapy. The gene was isolated independently by 3 groups in 1983 (Orkin et al., 1983; Valerio et al., 1983; Wiginton et al., 1983), and over the ensuing decade, much has been learned about the gene, its function and regulation. HLA-matched sibling bone marrow transplantation in children with ADA(-)SCID may be curative. Therefore, gene-correction of an autologous population of mar-row stem cells might be expected to also cure the disease. Third, the ADA gene behaves somewhat like a "housekeeping" gene that is constitutively expressed in cells but does not appear to require stringent regulation of its expression. ADA levels in immunologically normal individuals have been shown to vary over a very broad range. Heterozygote carriers and rare other individuals have been re-ported with as little as 10% of the normal mean ADA level in their blood cells and yet their immune system function is intact (Daddona et al., 1983) At the other extreme, individuals with 50 times the normal mean ADA concentration have been described with mild hemolytic anemia but no immune abnormality (Valentine et al., 1977). Potentially there is a 500 fold range of enzyme concentration which might help these patient's T-cells survive without causing significant side effects. Since retroviral-mediated gene transfer can result in a wide variability of gene expression between cells (Kantoff et al, 1986), the broad range of ADA expression seen in normal persons provides a very forgiving system for its clinical application. Further, the experience with allogeneic bone marrow transplantation suggests that ADA normal cells have a selective growth advantage over the uncorrected ADA(-) cells; therefore, gene transfer into only a fraction of the bone marrow stem cell population may be sufficient to successfully reconstitute the immune system without the need to eliminate the uncorrected stem cells by ablative treatment.

Although ADA gene transfer into totipotent bone marrow stem cells would be theoretically curative, the inability to achieve stable long term expression of genes transplanted into non-human primate bone marrow led us to begin to explore the possibility of using T-lymphocytes as the cellular vehicle. T-cells seemed a rational choice for this approach for several reasons (Table 1). Some ADA(-)SCID patients were found to have engrafted donor T-cells alone with full immune reconstitution following allogeneic bone marrow transplantation. This suggested that the genetic correction of autologous T-cells may have a similar growth advantage and that correction of the T-cells alone might be sufficient to reconstitute their immune function. In 1987, we knew that the insertion of a normal ADA gene with retroviral vectors could completely correct the metabolic defect in ADA(-) T-cells (Kantoff et al., 1986) so we reasoned that the delivery of the corrective gene to the T-cells might be useful even if bone marrow gene transfer had not yet been solved. Finally, cultured T-cells were being employed successfully in the treatment of cancer so that this new approach to cellular therapy had some precedent.

TABLE 1. Advantages of T-lymphocytes as cellular vehicles for gene therapy.

---

1. Lymphocytes grow rapidly as single cells in suspension culture allowing for in vitro expansion and selection of the transduced population.

2. T-lymphocytes are terminally differentiated which should decrease the risk of down regulation of the exogenous gene as the cells differentiate from stem cells.

3. The transduced cells can be tested for stability of gene expression, growth characteristics and safety considerations such as virus shedding prior to reintroduction into the host.

4. The use of antigen responsive cells could theoretically permit specific expansion of the reintroduced lymphocyte population by booster immunization of the recipient or "homing" to deposits of antigen in vivo.

Pre-clinical experiments in mice and monkeys demonstrated prolonged survival of genetically-altered T-cells with continued expression of the inserted genes in vivo (Culver et al., 1991 and 1991b). Primary ADA(-) T-cell cultures were established from 3 ADA(-)SCID patients. A portion of each culture was genetically-corrected following retroviral-mediated transduction with the LASN vector. LASN is a Moloney murine leukemia-based vector which contains a hADA gene promoted by the 5'-LTR and an internal SV40 early promoter/enhancer-NeoR gene segment, downstream of the hADA gene (Osborne et al, 1990). Parallel growth of these LASN-transduced and non-transduced cultures noted that all of the non-transduced cultures reached senescence and died within a few weeks of the beginning of the culture, while the genetically-corrected cells continued to grow for months and continued to express the introduced ADA genes. These observations suggested that production of ADA in an intracellular location provided a survival advantage to the cells in vitro. Ferrari and colleagues (Ferrari et al., 1991) extended these observations one step further by transferring ADA(-)SCID T-cells from a child receiving PEG-ADA into immunodeficient BNX mice +/- transduction with a hADA gene vector. Despite the fact that these animals are ADA normal and thus do not have elevated tissue or body fluid levels of dAdo, only the BNX mice receiving ADA gene-corrected cells had evidence of survival of the patient's T-cells. In addition, these studies demonstrated that the surviving human T-cells were also capable of mediating some T-cell effecter functions *in vivo*. Taken together, these in vitro and in vivo findings suggested that the insertion of a normal ADA gene into the cell, confers a survival and functional advantage to those cells beyond that obtained by surrounding the cells with ADA enzyme in the extracellular medium or body fluids.

Based upon these pre-clinical studies, we proposed a human clinical trial involving the genetic correction of autologous human T-cells with the LASN vector. For children to be eligible, they must not have an available matched sibling bone marrow donor and they must have been receiving PEG-ADA for a minimum of 9 months with persistent evidence of immunodeficiency. We have continued PEG-ADA injections throughout the course of the study since we did not feel justified in removing therapy which may be beneficial to these children during the early phases of the experiment. T-cells from 5 different children with ADA(-)SCID were evaluated for their in vitro growth to a variety of mitogens and their expression of functional human ADA.

On September 14, 1990, the first of two children, a 4 year old girl was enrolled in the protocol (Culver et al, 1992a). Each child (now 7 and 12 years old) had been treated with regular injections of PEG-ADA for at least 22 months and had documented persistent immunodeficiency. Once enrolled, the children underwent apheresis to obtain peripheral blood mononuclear cells (PBMC's) every 6-8 weeks (Figure 2). The PBMC's were placed in culture with OKT3 and rIL-2 which stimulated vigorous T-cell proliferation. 24 hours after initiation of culture, the proliferating cells were exposed twice daily to LASN retroviral vector supernate for a total of 4-6 exposures. Using this supernate transduction procedure, an esti-

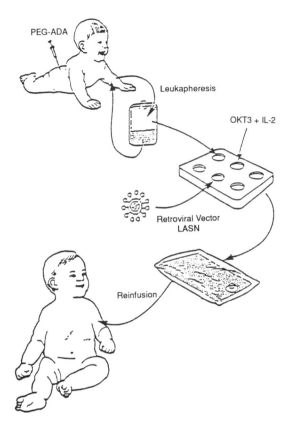

FIGURE 2. *Schema of lymphocyte gene therapy for ADA (-)SCID.* The children have been maintained on weekly injections of PEG-ADA for at least 9 months. During the first year, the children underwent a leukapheresis every 4-6 weeks. The mononuclear cells are then placed in culture with the monoclonal antibody OKT3 and rIL-2 (interleukin-2) which induce vigorous T-cell proliferation. Beginning on the second day, LASN retroviral vector supernate is added twice daily for 4-6 exposures. The cells continue to expand in number and are then reinfused after 9-13 days in culture.

mated 1 to 10% of the cultured ADA(-) T-cells acquire and express the human ADA gene. The T-cells were expanded 50 to 100 fold in number in culture and then reinfused IV. This short term culture process was used to minimize any tendency of the cultured T-cells to develop the oligoclonality known to occur with long term in vitro culture. No in vitro selection for gene-expressing cells was used.

In the first child treated, there has been a substantial increase in the number of circulating T-cells ($<600/\mu l$ pre-gene therapy vs. a mean of $2100/\mu l$ on gene therapy) with gene therapy infusions every 6-8 weeks for the first year and then every 3-6 months thereafter. The ADA activity in peripheral blood T-cells isolated from the blood has increased from <1% prior to gene therapy to 25% of normal levels. This is quite significant in light of the fact that her parents have completely normal immune functioning with heterozygous levels of ADA activity. Persistence of ADA gene-corrected T-lymphocytes as measured by PCR and vector gene protein expression *in vivo* has been documented in both children even during the discontinuation of T-cell infusions for more than 11 months in one child. This suggests that the re-infused ADA gene-corrected T-cells may survive for many months and that the survival advantage seen *in vitro*, *in vivo* in mice and in human bone marrow transplantation is also true for these gene-corrected T-cells.

TABLE 2. Measures of Humoral Immunity in Patient 1 Treated with Gene Therapy

Characteristic	Before Gene Therapy	After 10 months
Total blood B-cells (per µl)	85	89
Tonsils	None	Present
Isohemagglutinins	<1:16	1:16
Serum IgA (mg/dl)	25	41

Normal values: B-cells (>88//ml); Isohemaglutinins (≥1:16); Serum IgA (>42mg/dl)

Both children have also developed persistent evidence of *in vivo* humoral and cellular immune functions not present with PEG-ADA treatment alone. The humoral-mediated immune status of patient 1 before and 10 months after beginning treatment is characterized in Table 2. There had been no low or absent spontaneous production of isohemagglutinins on PEG-ADA prior to gene therapy by either child. However, repeated infusions of gene-corrected T-cells has resulted in normal levels of isohemagglutinins and the growth of tonsils in both children. These findings suggest that the gene-corrected T-cells can provide the T-helper cell function necessary to promote normal spontaneous antibody production.

Table 3 depicts the cell-mediated immune status of patient 1 before and 10 months after beginning treatment with infusions of ADA gene-corrected autologous T cells. She had received weekly injections of PEG-ADA for 22 months prior to the initiation of lymphocyte gene therapy. Prior to gene therapy, she was anergic, but now has positive skin tests to Tetanus, Candida, and Diphtheria. These results confirm that the gene-corrected T-cells can perform normal immune functions such as delayed type hypersensitivity reactions (DTH). We can conclude that: 1) rIL-2 expanded autologous ADA gene-corrected T-lymphocytes will survive and function *in vivo* and 2) regular infusions of ADA gene-corrected T-cells can provide meaningful immune reconstitution beyond that achieved with enzyme replacement alone.

In May, 1993 we initiated an attempt to genetically correct the peripheral blood stem cells (PBSC) of one of these 2 children. Until recently, the efficiency of trans-

TABLE 3. Measures of Cellular Immunity in Patient 1 Treated with Gene Therapy

Characteristic	Before Gene Therapy	After 10 months
Total CD3$^+$ cells (per µl)	571	1995
PHA response (cpm)	18,500	48,200
OKT3 response (cpm)	700	29,000
Number of Positive Skin Tests	0/8	3/8

duction of stem cells has been too low for consideration of a clinical trial for immunodeficiency. However, the growth of totipotent stem cells with combinations of colony stimulating factors has resulted in an increased efficiency of transduction to 10-20% in non-human primate stem cells (Dunbar, 1992). Transplantation of CSF-driven, vector-transduced CD34 enriched stem cells into irradiated primates has resulted in engraftment of all lineages with 5-10% of the PBMC's having the vector. The selective growth advantage for ADA gene-corrected T-cells *in vivo* has suggested that the genetic correction of a few totipotent stem cells may be sufficient for improvement in the combined immunodeficiency. Claudio Bordingnon and colleagues in Italy have recently initiated a protocol using the combination of gene-corrected T-cells and bone marrow for 2 children with ADA deficiency.

Our first use of stem cell gene therapy involved an attempt to genetically correct peripheral blood stem cells. The patient was given subcutaneous injections of G-CSF, which mobilized stem cells from the marrow into the peripheral blood. These stem cells were then harvested by apheresis, cultured in retroviral vector supernate with 3 different growth factors (IL-3, IL-6 and SCF) and reinfused IV 72 hours later. A different ADA retroviral construct was used that will allow distinction of the T-cells altered in the T-cell protocol versus those that would have matured from a corrected PBSC.

IN VIVO GENE TRANSFER FOR THE TREATMENT OF SOLID TUMORS

In our approach to the gene therapy of solid tumors, the gene transfer would be carried out in vivo. The ability to directly gene-modify a growing tumor in situ to confer new drug sensitivity, to induce anti-tumor immunity or restore normal cellular growth control would be a significant advance in cancer therapy (Short et al., 1990). We have focused on an in vivo gene delivery system based upon the direct injection of retroviral vector-producer cells (VPC) into growing tumors, where the VPC would continuously produce retroviral vectors capable of transferring the vector genes into the surrounding tumor cells as they proliferate.

Initial experiments were designed to determine if retroviral-mediated gene transfer would occur in vivo after implantation of mixtures of tumor cells with VPC (genetically engineered NIH 3T3 cells; PA317). These experiments demonstrated that genes could be transferred to tumor cells in vivo with an efficiency of ~60%. We then evaluated the use of the Herpes Simplex- thymidine kinase (HS-tk) gene as a "sensitivity" gene for destroying tumors in vivo. HS-tk confers sensitivity to the anti-herpes drugs acyclovir and ganciclovir (DHPG ; GCV; Faulds and Heel, 1990), that could result in the ability to selectively destroy growing tumors in situ without significant damage to surrounding normal tissues. A number of investigators have demonstrated that the insertion of HS-tk into mammalian cells and treatment with acyclovir or ganciclovir would result in destruction of transduced normal or malignant cells in vitro and in vivo (Elion, 1980; Moolten, 1986; Heyman et al, 1989; Ezzedine et al., 1991). To determine if the in vivo HS-tk gene-transfer system would be capable of eliminating tumors, mice were injected subcutaneously with mixtures of tumor cells and non-producer HS-tk-containing fibroblasts (controls) or HS-tk VPC. The growing tumors were allowed to become palpable before GCV treatment. Tumors in animals injected with mixtures of tumor and control HS-tk cells showed a modest slowing of growth suggesting a mild anti-tumor effect. By contrast, the animals carrying tumors derived from a mixture of tumor cells and HS-tk VPC regressed rapidly and completely with GCV treatment and the animals remained tumor free. Since the efficiency of this in vivo gene transfer system is less than 100%, we postulated that there must be a "bystander" effect that is responsible for the destruction of surrounding non-transduced tumor cells.

To further explore this "bystander" effect, normal mice were injected SQ with wild-type tumor cells mixed at various ratios with tumor cells that had been transduced and were expressing the HS-tk gene. GCV treatment produced complete tumor regression in nearly all animals with 50:50 tumor mixtures and in >50% of mice bearing tumor mixtures consisting of only 10% HS-tk expressing cells (Culver et al, 1992b). The mechanism mediating this "bystander" tumor killing is not fully understood. The ability to destroy tumors in vivo in mice with the HS-tk/GCV system occurred without evidence of damage to surrounding normal tissues.

GENE THERAPY FOR THE TREATMENT OF MALIGNANT BRAIN TUMORS

The treatment of brain tumors by the use of this retroviral-mediated in vivo HS-tk gene delivery system has a number of attractive features for the initial application of this technology (Table 4). First, these retroviral vectors can only integrate and express their genes in dividing tissues. Neurons and most other cellular elements in the brain are not actively synthesizing DNA. Thus, within the brain, the principal mitotically active cells will be within the tumor. Second, brain tumors are locally invasive and rarely metastasize, but are difficult to surgically excise because

---

TABLE 4. Reasons why brain tumors were chosen as the first use of in vivo VPC injection.

---

1. This gene transfer method utilizes murine retroviral vectors which can only integrate and express their genes in proliferating tissues. The majority of the normal brain tissue is non-proliferative. This feature serves as a targeting strategy.

2. The brain is an immunologically-privileged site and the murine VPC should not be rapidly destroyed.

3. GCV is known to cross the blood-brain barrier in humans.

4. Experimentation in rats demonstrated complete destruction of growing brain tumors using this technique.

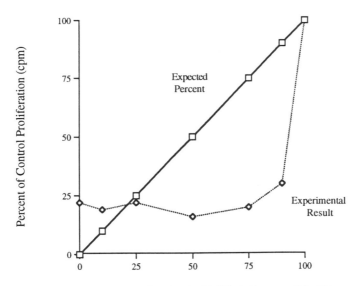

Percent of Wild-type Tumor cells mixed with HS-tk Gene-modified Tumor cells

FIGURE 3. *In vitro Bystander killing by the 9L Gliosarcoma.* Mixture of wild-type and HS-tk containing 9L cells were cultured in 96 well plates at 10,000 cells per well. GCV was added at 5.1 µg/ml. 44 hours later, tritiated thymidine was added to each of the well and harvested 4 hours later. The results are expressed as a percent of the proliferation of triplicate wells that contained no GCV. "Expected" represents the expected decrease in proliferation if there was no bystander killing. For example, a 1:1 mixture would be expected to result in a 50% decrease in proliferation. However, a 1:1 mixture actually decreases the proliferation greater than 80%.

of their location and relationship to adjacent critical structures. Therefore, the ability to directly inject the tumor without the need for surgical resection would be advantageous. Another advantage of the brain for this technique is that the brain is a relatively immunologically privileged site and could permit a longer survival of xenogeneic VPC which would expose the tumor cells to potential transduction for a significant interval without immunologic rejection.

Prior to establishing an animal brain tumor model for study, we evaluated the rat 9L gliosarcoma for the presence of an in vitro bystander effect (Figure 3). HS-tk positive and negative 9L tumor cells were cultured at various dilutions to determine if the degree of tumor cell proliferation was directly proportional to the percent of HS-tk transduced tumor cells. These studies demonstrated a 70% decrease in proliferation if as few as 10% of the cells in the culture were HS-tk positive. This finding confirmed a bystander effect similar to the murine tumors in vivo. Similar studies have also been conducted with human cell lines (Figure 4). While there is variability in the degree of bystander killing, each of the cell lines evaluated dem-

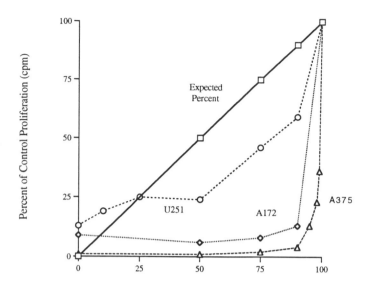

Percent of Wild-type Tumor cells mixed with HS-tk Gene-modified Tumor cells

FIGURE 4. *In vitro Bystander killing Human Tumor Cell Lines.* Mixtures of wild-type and HS-tk containing tumor cells were cultured as noted in the legend for figure 3. The U251 glioblastoma demonstrated a 40% decrease in proliferation with 10% HS-tk positive cells while 90% and 98% decreases were seen with the A172 glioblastoma and A375 melanoma respectively.

onstrated bystander killing. While significant bystander killing occurs with as few as 10% of the cells containing HS-tk in most lines, other tumor cell types such as the A375 melanoma appear to have significantly greater bystander effect in vitro.

We then established a Fisher 344 rat brain tumor model using the syngeneic 9L rat gliosarcoma cell line (Weisacker et al, 1981). 9L tumor cells were stereotaxically implanted in the right cerebral hemisphere. 5 days later, the animals were subjected to an intratumoral injection of HS-tk VPC by stereotaxic guidance. After 5 days to allow time for the VPC to transduce the neighboring proliferating glioma cells, GCV was administered IP to the tumor-bearing rats twice daily for 5 days. Controls receiving VPC without GCV treatment had large tumors that rapidly progressed in size and grew out of the brain along the needle tract. In striking contrast, 11 of 14 of the GCV-treated rats demonstrated complete macroscopic and microscopic tumor regression. In 3 rats, microscopic examination showed residual tumor composed of viable and necrotic malignant cells without evidence of residual VPC. Adjacent brain tissue, which should not integrate the retroviral vector or express the HS-tk enzyme, was not detectably harmed (Ram et al, 1993).

We observed no toxicity in the brain related to the VPC injection or evidence of wide spread systemic HS-tk gene transfer in the animals that received this treat-

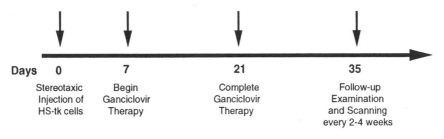

Denotes the timing of an MRI or CT scan.

FIGURE 5. *Schema of brain tumor gene therapy.* Patients with *recurrent* primary (i.e. glioblastoma multiforme) or metastatic (i.e. lung, breast, melanoma, renal cell carcinoma) cancer in the brain may be eligible. Under general anesthesia, the patient undergoes direct injection of VPC into various areas of the growing tumor using an MRI-guided stereotaxic injection technique (day 0). The VPC are allowed to effect in vivo gene transfer within the tumor for 1 week. GCV is then administered IV for 14 days. The GCV is expected to destroy all VPC and transduced tumor cells. Response to therapy is monitored by MRI and PET scanning.

ment protocol during the 30 day observation period. In control experiments, other bodily tissues containing rapidly proliferating cells, such as the intestinal epithelium, thymus, and bone marrow were unaffected in GCV-treated animals that had previously been injected IV or IP with the HS-tk VPC. On December 7, 1992 the first human brain tumor patient was treated with the stereotaxic injection of HS-tk VPC into their growing malignancy at the National Institutes of Health (Figure 5) (Oldfield et al, 1993). As of June, 1993, 8 patients have been treated without evidence of acute toxicity related to the implantation of the producer cells or treatment with GCV. Five of 8 patients have demonstrated an anti-tumor effect.

With this gene delivery system, the HS-tk gene transfer efficiency and the bystander effect may be limited by scarring and necrosis within the tumors. The effects of previous therapies may impede the ability of the transduced tumor cells to migrate within the tumor, an important aspect in maximizing the bystander effect. Therefore, repeated injections of VPC may be required. Another potential limiting factor of this gene delivery system is the heterogeneous mitotic rate within many tumors. One possible strategy to improve gene delivery within glioblastomas, where a substantial proportion of the tumor cells are not actively synthesizing DNA, is to administer a tumor growth factor (e.g. epidermal growth factor) for several days after the VPC injection to stimulate tumor cell division to facilitate gene delivery and integration. Other gene constructs such as anti-sense IGF-1 (insulin-like growth factor type 1) or a tumor suppressor gene (e.g WT p53) may also be delivered directly with VPC. Gene constructs that augment immune responsiveness to the tumor such as the down-regulation of IGF-1 secretion (Trojan et al, 1993) may be less affected by local effects such as scarring.

GENE THERAPY FOR THE TREATMENT OF NON-CNS SOLID TUMORS

The direct implantation of PA317/HS-tk VPC into growing tumors is designed to transduce cells in the local area of injection and the bystander effect appears to be a local phenomenon. Therefore, the successful use of this technique is probably limited to localized tumor nodules. There are several human tumors that are likely to be localized at the time of diagnosis and may be candidates for this HS-tk VPC in vivo gene transfer technique (Table 5).

For those cancers that have usually spread into the locoregional area (e.g. pancreas, lung, esophageal) at the time of diagnosis, HS-tk gene transfer is not expected to be efficacious alone. There are several potential methods of increasing gene delivery to a locoregional area or augmenting the anti-tumor immune response (Table 6). First, the VPC cell type can be optimized for survival within the tumor such as using an autologous tumor cell. We have demonstrated in vivo that HS-tk-containing tumor cells provide more effective bystander effect than HS-tk-containing NIH 3T3 cells. Second, one might chose a VPC cell type that can migrate through the tissues. If this requires an allogeneic or xenogeneic cell type, then transient immunosuppression to allow migration and gene transfer might be indicated. Third, VPC that produce replication-competent vector particles containing the genes of interest might be the most efficient gene delivery method. Construction of vectors with HS-tk would allow the elimination of the infection once there had been sufficient time for the vector to spread through the tumor. Obviously, this approach will require long term in vivo animal studies to determine the likelihood of potential adverse side effects. Another method for increasing the effects of HS-tk, is to combine several different genes. The insertion of immune-enhancing genes (e.g. interleukins, anti-sense IGF-1), might boost the immune responsiveness to the residual microscopic tumor while the bulk of the primary tumor is destroyed with HS-tk. In the brain a number of cytokines are toxic (e.g. IL-2), but outside of the CNS, delivery of these cytokines alone or in combination with HS-tk, may have a synergistic effect when the full potential of

---

TABLE 5. Tumors that may be suitable for treatment by direct injection of VPC

Brain (e.g. glioblastoma, metastases from breast, lung, kidney, skin)

Peritoneal carcinomatosis (e.g. stage III ovarian carcinoma, colorectal cancer)

Meningeal carcinomatosis (e.g. metastatic colorectal, lung, and breast cancer)

Pleural carcinomatosis (e.g. lung adenocarcinoma, mesothelioma)

Liver (e.g. hepatoma, metastases such as melanoma and colorectal cancer)

Head/Neck (e.g. squamous cell carcinoma)

Bladder (e.g. transitional cell carcinoma)

TABLE 6. Potential methods for improving the anti-tumor efficacy of direct VPC Injection.

Production of vector producer cell lines form tumor cells
  •May have the ability to proliferate within the tumor
  •May metastasize with tumor cells allowing transduction in metastatic deposits
  •Allogeneic or xenogeneic antigens can be removed to enhance in vivo survival
  •Motile cell lines can be used

Production of replication-competent retroviral vectors
  •Use of a "sensitivity" gene(s) could allow destruction of the infection in situ
  •Use of tumor-specific promoters could limit spread and vector gene expression

the immune system is available. There is some evidence that systemic immunity can be increased in certain tumor models with the implantation of gene-altered syngeneic tumors expressing an anti-sense IGF-1 vector in high IGF-1 producing tumors (Trojan et al, 1993) or with IL-4 (Golumbek et al., 1991).

We have begun preliminary experiments using in vivo gene transfer for the treatment of localized malignancies such as liver tumors. There may be an increased risk of damage to surrounding normal liver cells as compared to the brain since a greater proportion of liver cells are proliferating than in the brain. We have demonstrated that murine HS-tk VPC directly injected into rat liver will survive for 7 days without immunosuppression. Rejection of the xenogeneic murine cells occurs during the second week. GCV treatment did not demonstrate any evidence of damage to the normal surrounding liver tissue. A preliminary experiment with a mixture of tumor and VPC has shown that the tumors can be destroyed within the liver with GCV without evidence of hepatic cell necrosis. These findings suggest that the implantation of VPC into the liver can result in tumor eradication without significant general hepatic injury. Investigators in France have also implanted mixtures of tumor and VPC within the liver of rats with similar efficacious, non-toxic findings (Panis et al., 1992).

Tumor that is located within a body cavity such as the the pleural or peritoneal cavities or the subarachnoid space may be particularly amenable to this therapy. We have conducted several preliminary experiments in a model of peritoneal carcinomatosis which have demonstrated elimination of transplanted tumor cells with an IP injection of VPC followed by GCV injections (preliminary observations). Taken together, these findings suggest that the direct injection of VPC can result in sufficient gene transfer to allow in situ destruction of solid tumors and tumors within the peritoneal cavity. Despite the fact, that the VPC are allogeneic or xenogeneic in these tumor models, the VPC survive long enough to result in complete tumor eradication. In none of these experiments have we noted toxicity to surrounding normal tissues.

CONCLUSIONS

Novel, new therapies for the treatment of primary immunodeficiency diseases have had a significant impact upon medicine and science. Allogeneic bone marrow transplantation, enzyme replacement therapy and the first application of human gene therapy were successfully introduced into clinical practice as a treatment for severe combined immunodeficiency. The new information generated from the T-lymphocyte gene therapy experiment for ADA(-)SCID, may provide the basis for the application of gene therapy to HIV infection. We are hopeful that the upcoming stem cell gene therapy experiment for ADA(-)SCID will prove successful in genetically modifying the totipotent stem cell. Such a method, if successful, will allow the application of gene therapy to many genetic, autoimmune, oncologic and infectious diseases. As our understanding of the molecular basis of the immunodeficiency diseases accumulates along with parallel progress in basic cell biology and gene transfer modalities, prospects are that gene therapy can be applied successfully to an ever enlarging number of human diseases.

The optimal form of gene therapy for the treatment of genetic diseases and cancer alike would be the direct injection of the curative gene into the body. In this ideal delivery system, the gene would "home" to the desired tissue, enter the desired cells and restore normal cellular functions. To target specific cell types in vivo, one would need to define a specific cell surface structure (e.g. CD34 for stem cells or unique galactose receptors on hepatocytes). The use of the natural specific tropism of different viruses is another strategy for targeting gene delivery (e.g. rabies virus for brain, hepatitis virus for liver). Another strategy for specific expression of the desired gene is to place it under the control of a specific cellular or tissue-specific promoter (e.g. a-fetoprotein for hepatoma cells). The rapid advancement of gene transfer as a therapeutic modality for the treatment of cancer holds a great promise for selective, non-toxic therapies that will profoundly change the practice of medicine over the next decade.

REFERENCES

Ammann AJ, Hong R (1989): Disorders of the T-cell system. In Immunologic Disorders of Infants and Children, Steihm ER, ed. Philadelphia. 3rd edition, WB Saunders Co. pgs. 257-315

Anderson WF (1984): Prospects for human gene therapy. *Science* 226:401-409

Anderson WF (1992): Human gene therapy. *Science* 256:808-813

Cornetta K, Moen RC, Culver K, et al. (1990): Amphotropic murine leukemia virus is not an acute pathogen for primates. *Human Gene Ther* 1:15-30

Culver K, Cornetta K, Morgan R, et al. (1991a): Lymphocytes as cellular vehicles for gene therapy in mouse and man. *Proc Natl Acad Sci USA* 88:3155-3159

Culver KW, Anderson WF, Blaese RM (1991b): Lymphocyte gene therapy. *Human Gene Ther* 2:107-109

Culver KW, Blaese RM (1992): Gene therapy for immunodeficiency disease. In

New Concepts in Immunodeficiency Diseases. Gupta S and Griscelli C (eds). Sussex, UK, Wiley & Sons. pgs. 427-456

Culver KW, Berger M, Miller AD, Anderson WF, Blaese RM (1992a): Lymphocyte gene therapy for adenosine deaminase deficiency. *Ped Res* 31:149A

Culver KW, Ram Z, Walbridge S, et al. (1992b): In vivo gene transfer with retroviral vector producer cells for treatment of experimental brain tumors. *Science* 256:1550-1552

Daddona PE, Mitchell BS, Meuwissen HJ, et al. (1983): Adenosine deaminase deficiency with normal immune function. J Clin Invest 72:483-492

Dunbar C (1992): Personal communication

Elion GB (1980): The chemotherapeutic exploration of virus-specified enzymes. *Adv Enz Regulation* 18:53

Ezzedine ZD, Martuza RL, Platika D, et al. (1991): Selective killing of glioma cells in culture and in vivo by retrovirus transfer of the herpes simplex virus thymidine kinase gene. *New Biologist* 3:608-614

Faulds D, Heel RC (1990): Ganciclovir. *Drugs* 39:596-638

Ferrari G, Rossini S, Giavazzi R, et al. (1991): An in vivo model of somatic cell gene therapy for human severe combined immunodeficiency. *Science* 251:1363-1366

Golumbek PT et al. (1991): Treatment of established renal cancer by tumor cells engineered to secrete interleukin-4. *Science* 254: 713-716

Hershfield MS, Buckley RH, Greenberg ML, et al. (1987): Treatment of adenosine deaminase deficiency with polyethylene glycol-modified adenosine deaminase. *N Engl J Med* 16:589-596

Heyman RA, Borrelli E, Lesley J, et al. (1989) Thymidine kinase obliteration: creation of transgenic mice with controlled immunodeficiency. *Proc Natl Acad Sci USA* 86:2698-2702

Hirschhorn R (1983): Genetic deficiencies of adenosine deaminase and purine nucleoside phosphorylase: overview, genetic heterogeneity and therapy. *Birth Defect* 19:73-81

Kantoff PW, Kohn DB Mitsuya H, et al. (1986): Correction of adenosine deaminase deficiency in cultured human T and B cells by retrovirus-mediated gene transfer. *Proc Natl Acad Sci USA* 83:6563-6567

Miller AD (1992): Human gene therapy comes of age. *Nature* 357:455-460

Moolten FL (1986) Tumor chemosensitivity conferred by inserted herpes thymidine kinase genes: Paradigm for a prospective cancer control strategy. *Cancer Res* 46:5276-5281

Oldfield EH, Culver KW, Ram Z, Blaese RM (1993): A clinical protocol: Gene therapy for the treatment of brain tumors using intra-tumoral transduction with the thymidine kinase gene and intravenous ganciclovir. *Hum Gene Ther* 4:39-69

O'Reilly RJ, Keever CA, Small TN, Brochstein J (1989): The use of HLA-nonidentical T-cell-depleted marrow transplants for the correction of severe combined immunodeficiency disease. *Immunodeficiency Rev* 1:273-309

Orkin SH, Daddona PE, Shewach DS, et al. (1983): Molecular cloning of human adenosine deaminase gene sequences. *J Biol Chem* 158:12753-12756

Osborne WRA, Hock RA, Kaleko M, Miller AD (1990): Long-term expression of human adenosine deaminase in mice after transplantation of bone marrow infected with amphotropic retroviral vectors. *Human Gene Ther* 1:31-41

Panis Y, Caruso M, Houssin D, et al (1992): Treatment of experimental hepatic tumors with in vivo transfer of a suicide gene in the rat. *C R Acad Sci Paris* 315:541-544

Ram Z, Culver KW, Walbridge S, Blaese RM, Oldfield, EH (1993): In Situ Retroviral-mediated Gene Transfer for the Treatment of Brain Tumors in Rats. *Cancer Res* 53:83-88

Rosenberg SA, Aebersold P, Cornetta K, et al. (1990): Gene transfer into humans-Immunotherapy of patients with advanced melanoma, using tumor-infiltrating lymphocytes modified by retroviral gene transduction. *N Engl J Med* 323:570-578

Short MP, Choi, JK, Lee A, et al. (1990): Gene delivery to glioma cells in rat brain by grafting of a retrovirus packaging cell line. *J Neuroscience Res* 27:427-433

Trojan J, Johnson TR, Rudin SD, Ilan J, Tykocinski ML, Ilan J (1993): Treatment and prevention of rat glioblastoma by immunogenic C6 cells expressing antisense insulin-like growth factor 1 RNA. *Science* 259:94-97

Valentine WN, Paglia DE, Tartaglia AP, Gilsanz F (1977): Hereditary hemolytic anemia with increased adenosine deaminase (45-70 fold) and decreased adenosine triphosphates. *Science* 195:783

Valerio D, Duyvesteyn MGC, Meera Khan P, et al. (1983): Isolation of cDNA clones for human adenosine deaminase. *Gene* 25:231-240

Wiginton DA, Adrian GS, Friedman RL, et al. (1983): Cloning of cDNA sequences of human adenosine deaminase. *Proc Natl Acad Sci USA* 80:7481-7485

Weisacker M, Deen DF, Rosenblum ML, Hoshino T, Gutin PH, Barker M (1981): The 9L rat brain tumor model: Description and application of the model. *J Neurol* 224:183-192

DEVELOPMENT OF HERPES SIMPLEX VIRUS VECTORS FOR GENE TRANSFER TO THE CENTRAL NERVOUS SYSTEM

Joseph C. Glorioso, Neal A. DeLuca, William F. Goins, and David J. Fink

INTRODUCTION

Advances in understanding the molecular basis of human disease in the past decade have led to the identification and cloning of genes responsible for certain heritable diseases of the central nervous system (CNS) as well as many of those encoding neurotransmitters, receptors, and growth factors which influence brain function. For example, the genes responsible for the neurodegenerative diseases amyotrophic lateral sclerosis (Rosen et al., 1993) and Huntington's chorea (Goldberg, et al., 1993; Mac Donald et al., 1993) have recently been identified. Ongoing research promises to identify the genes primarily responsible for other more complex neurodegenerative disorders such as Alzheimer's and Parkinson's disease. Currently, many neurodegnrative diseases are not treatable. Even in cases where therapies exist, drugs which control symptoms may ultimately fail in the late stages of neurological disease in a considerable percentage of affected patients. For example, the administration of L-DOPA to Parkinson's patients may even accelerate the decline in dopamine producing neurons. Other difficulties with traditional therapies are that the blood-brain barrier limits the delivery of systemically administered drugs into the brain parenchyma, and even drugs delivered by intraventricular injection penetrate poorly from the ventricular surface into the substance of the brain. Empediments to drug delivery and bioavailability are further complicated by the regional and cellular specialization that is characteristic of the brain. Direct targeting of the therapeutic product to specific brain regions or to cells within those regions may be required to overcome these limitations.

As an alternative to targeted drug delivery, neurodegenerative diseases may be treated by gene therapy, where direct gene transfer to the affected brain region will accomplish local therapeutic gene product synthesis. Recessive metabolic diseases of the nervous system caused by defects in single genes potentially could be cured by replacement of the defective gene with a correct gene. Multifactorial neurodegenerative conditions might be ameliorated by the production of therapeutic products from transferred genes. In addition, animal models of human disease like Alzheimer's might be produced by transgene overexpression of potentially pathogenic proteins such as normal or mutant forms of the amyloid precursor pro-

Gene Therapeutics: Methods and Applications of Direct Gene Transfer
Jon A. Wolff, Editor • ©1994 *Birkhäuser Boston*

tein. Such animals could be used both to explore the role of those substances in the pathogenesis of the disease, as well as to test the effects of potential therapeutic agents. Finally, gene transfer holds considerable promise for the treatment of acquired disease processes affecting the nervous system such as autoimmune degeneration of white matter, cancer and brain scaring due to injury.

The same features that make the brain a desirable target for gene transfer, though, also serve as constraints on the accomplishment of these objectives. The brain and spinal cord are physically inaccessible. Nervous system cells cannot be removed from brain in order to be transduced and subsequently transplanted. Alternatively, allogeneic fetal or differentiated brain cells or fibroblasts of nonneuronal origin which are transduced to express therapeutic gene products may have utility in restoring functions to damaged brain. This approach is not without drawbacks since implantation of transformed cells requires the surgical creation of space within the brain to contain the transplant which in turn can result in iatrogenic focal neurologic deficits. Moreover, the relationship of the transplanted cells to the resident brain cells is unpredictable, and the long-term behavior of these grafts remains to be established.

Direct gene transfer using virus vectors may prove to represent an important alternative approach to cell transplantation. Retroviral vectors, which have been successfully exploited in the transfer of genes to bone marrow-derived cells, fibroblasts, and neoplastic cells, cannot be used to transfer genes directly into the brain because these vectors require cell division for the incorporation of the therapeutic recombinant vector into the cellular genome, and neurons are postmitotic. Recent reports describing the use of replication compromised adenovirus vectors to express reporter genes following direct inoculation of animal brains appear promising (Akli et al., 1993; Bajocchi et al., 1993; Davidson et al., 1993; LeGal LaSalle et al., 1993). It is not yet clear, however, whether these viruses can express foreign genes in the brain without continued expression of viral genes and limited viral DNA synthesis. These reports also show that adenovirus is toxic for brain tissue in doses required for high levels of foreign gene expression.

In search of an appropriate gene transfer system for the CNS, we have focused on the development of modified herpes simplex virus type 1 (HSV-1) as a potential vector. This herpesvirus is transmitted by direct contact and replicates in the skin or mucous membranes before invading the peripheral nervous system. Following retrograde axonal transport of the virus capsid to neuronal cell nuclei, and viral genome entry into the nucleus, one of several viral gene expression pathways may ensue. In some cells, the virus may express lytic functions, replicate and destroy the infected cell (see Fig. 1). In others, the virus may enter a latent state in which latency genes rather than lytic genes are expressed and the virus does not replicate. The viral genome can persist in this state for the life of the host or may be reactivated to reenter the lytic cycle and cause a secondary infection usually at the primary site. Although the molecular basis of latency and reactivation is still poorly understood despite the research efforts of many laboratories, it is nonetheless clear that if the virus can be manipulated in a manner to force it into the latent

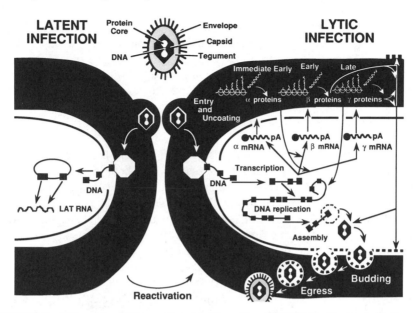

FIGURE 1. Life cycle of Herpes Simplex Virus Type 1 (HSV-1). During infection of neurons, the virus can proceed through either the lytic phase ultimately leading to the death of the nerve cell or the viral genome can persist within the nucleus of neurons in a latent state in which the latency-associated transcripts (LATs) are the sole viral RNAs transcribed. Reprinted with permission of Academic Press from Glorioso et al., 1992.

state without the possibility for reactivation, we should be able to exploit the latent genome for targeted gene expression in neurons. Thus, our rationale for choosing HSV as a gene transfer vector for brain is predicated on the highly evolved mechanism for establishing life long latency in neurons without harming the host cell.

In addition to the phenomenon of latency, HSV possesses a number of other attractive features as a gene transfer vector. First, the virus is capable of accommodating large amounts of foreign DNA and can be readily manipulated since the vast majority of viral genes are continuous (lacking intervening introns) and the genome is highly recombinogenic easing the introduction of foreign DNA in the virus backbone. Second, the virus can be forced into "latency" in any cell type by the removal of immediate early lytic gene functions. As described below, such defective HSV vectors can be propagated on cell lines which express the deleted essential functions in trans. These complementing cell lines are capable of producing defective virus to high titers without wild type recombinants which highlights the safety of these defective vectors. Third, latent viral genomes exhibit a characteristic and restricted pattern of expression of RNA transcripts implying that latency active promoters exist and can be exploited to express foreign genes from the latent viral genome.

Taking these features into consideration, the creation of an HSV vector would require engineering the virus in a manner to make it : (1) noncytotoxic for nerve cells and defective for carrying out the lytic cycle (2) capable of establishing latency and, (3) able to produce persistent and appropriate levels of therapeutic gene expression from the latent viral genome through the activity of suitable promoter/ regulator elements. The experimental approaches taken to achieve these objectives, by our laboratory and others, are described below.

CONSTRUCTION OF A NONCYTOTOXIC HSV VECTOR

HSV-1 is a large, enveloped, double-stranded DNA virus that is composed of approximately 152 kb (McGeoch et al., 1986) encoding about 75 genes. These genes specify sets of proteins that regulate transcription and gene expression, DNA replication, membrane mediated functions, components of the icosahedral nucleocapsid and core, and possibly functions involved in replication in neurons. During lytic infection, many of the functions specified by HSV augment, or usurp, the existing host cell metabolic machinery, or are configured to mimic processes found in healthy cells in order to ensure the synthesis of progeny virions.

Viruses that infect eukaryotic cells often specify regulatory proteins to ensure the appropriate expression of genes during the viral life cycle. HSV encodes several proteins that directly modulate viral and cellular gene expression and mediate the complex temporal cascade exhibited by the 75 different transcription units in the HSV genome. This cascade unfolds in three phases of coordinated gene expression—immediate early (IE or α), early (E or β), and late (L or γ) (Honess and Roizman, 1974). In the context of viral infection, late gene expression also requires viral DNA synthesis (Holland et al., 1980).

One IE protein, ICP4, is required for viral infection to proceed past the IE phase of transcription (Dixon and Schaffer, 1980; Preston, 1979; Watson and Clements, 1978) and is therefore absolutely essential for virus growth. ICP4 activates transcription of many promoters in the viral genome and in transient assays (Everett et al., 1984; DeLuca and Schaffer, 1985; O'Hare and Hayward, 1985; Quinlan and Knipe, 1985) and is also autoregulatory (Dixon and Schafer, 1980), repressing transcription of its own promoter (DeLuca and Schaffer, 1985; O'Hare and Hayward, 1985). ICP4 function can be eliminated by genetically altering the two copies of the ICP4 gene in the viral genome. The isolation and propagation of such mutants in cell culture requires that complementing levels of the ICP4 protein are provided in trans. This can be accomplished through the use of cell lines stably transformed with the ICP4 gene, which have been engineered to express the ICP4 gene product under the conditions of infection (DeLuca et al., 1985). Mutants deficient in ICP4 show efficient transcription from only the four other IE genes in standard cell lines used to propagate wild-type HSV. These represent the most compromised single mutants with respect to the expression of HSV gene products. Mutants in ICP4 have been used in several studies evaluating HSV as a vehicle for gene transfer (Chiocca et al., 1990; Dobson et al., 1990). Despite the fact that these virus mutants only efficiently express the other four IE genes but not E or L genes, and an apparent reduction of cytotoxicity in certain cell types

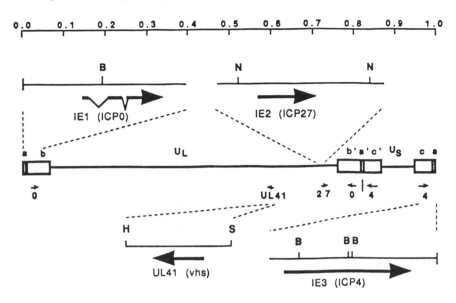

FIGURE 2. HSV gene products affecting gene expression and cytotoxicity. The HSV genome consists of a long and short component. The long component is comprised of the unique long (U_L) sequence bracketed by inverted copies of the "ab" sequences. The short component is comprised of the unique short (U_S) sequence bracketed by inverted copies of the "ca" sequences. The "a" sequences are directly repeated at the genomic termini. The genes for ICP4 (IE3), ICP0 (IE1), ICP27 (IE2) and UL41 (vhs) are shown to scale relative to their map locations on the HSV-1 genome. Note that ICP0 and ICP4 are present in two copies per genome due to their location in the "b" and "c" sequences, respectively. The regions encoding these genes are expanded showing the location of the sequences encoding the indicated mRNAs, and also giving some restriction enzyme cleavage sites as landmarks. The ICP0 mRNA is spliced in two places as shown in the figure. The sites are: Bam HI (B), Hind III (H), Nru I (N), Sal I (S).

relative to wild-type virus (DeLuca et al., 1985), ICP4 mutants result in the death of most of the infected cells (Johnson et al., 1992) in cell culture.

Three types of viral genes or gene products which function or are expressed in ICP4 deficient viruses, may contribute to the cytotoxicity of these mutants. They are: (1) components of the virion itself, (2) the low, but easily detectable levels of many of the early mRNAs or proteins, and (3) the four other IE genes and ICP6. These are considered in turn below (see Fig. 2).

The HSV virion is comprised of an envelope containing approximately 10 different viral proteins, an icosahedral nucleocapsid comprised of approximately 7 different proteins, and a region between the nucleocapsid and the envelope, termed the tegument, which contains possibly a dozen viral proteins (Roizman and Sears, 1990). Ultraviolet-irradiated viruses are not cytotoxic, and have been used to bio-chemically transform cells (Leiden et al., 1980), suggesting that structural compo-nents of the virion do not greatly contribute to cytotoxicity. However, the UV sensitivity of specific virion proteins possessing regulatory activities have not been examined. Therefore, it remains a possibility that specific virion proteins contribute directly to the cytotoxicity of the virus. Two tegument localized regulatory proteins have been extensively studied. They are the products of the UL41 gene (vhs: virion host shutoff) and UL48 (VP16, α-TIF, Vmw65). The vhs function acts along with cellular factors to degrade both viral and cellular mRNA molecules, resulting in a dramatic reduction in host cell protein synthesis even under conditions where viral transcription is inhibited (Kwong and Frenkel, 1987). Mutants in the vhs function have been isolated and do not exhibit the shutoff of cell protein synthesis (Read and Frenkel, 1983). However, inactivating the vhs function even in the background of an ICP4 mutant does not eliminate the cytotoxicity (Johnson et al., 1992). VP16 is another virion protein that may contribute to cytotoxicity. The transcription of the five IE genes of HSV occurs without prior viral protein synthesis, and is stimulated by VP16 (Campbell et al., 1984; Post et al., 1981) which binds, along with Oct 1 and other host cell proteins to TAATGARAT elements located upstream of IE TATA boxes (Cordingly et al., 1983; Mackem and Roizman, 1982). VP16 may contribute to cytotoxicity by promoting high level expression of the IE genes and hence, gene products.

In the absence of ICP4, expression of viral E and L genes is dramatically reduced. However, it is possible to detect 1% to 5% of wild-type levels of early mRNA and proteins in an ICP4 mutant background (DeLuca and Schaffer, 1988). Early genes encode a number of proteins that are directly involved in the replication of the viral nucleic acid (Roizman and Sears, 1990) as well as proteins affecting nucleotide metabolism. It is also possible that low level expression of other viral late genes may occur in an ICP4 deficient mutant and contribute to cytotoxicity. In theory this low level gene expression could be eliminated by inactivating the two other genes encoding the IE proteins ICP27 and ICP0, which are known to promote elevated and regulated levels of viral early and late genes.

The four remaining IE proteins, ICP27, ICP0, ICP22, and ICP47, are all overproduced in an ICP4 mutant background. ICP22 and 47 are dispensable for viral growth and no known function or activity have been described for them. ICP27 and ICP0 have been shown to inhibit neomycin transformation in cotransfection assays, suggestive of their cytotoxic potential (Farkas et al., 1987). In addition their known activities in altering gene expression are not compatible with extended cell survival.

ICP0 is not absolutely required for growth in cell culture, but viruses containing mutations in this gene are partially impaired for gene expression in general, are slow growing (Sacks and Schaffer, 1987), and show some impairment in experimental models of latency (Leib et al., 1989). It has been postulated that ICP0 substitutes for a cellular function (Cai and Schaffer, 1991). In transient assays, ICP0 is a promiscuous activator, and in some circumstances works synergistically with ICP4 (Quinlan and Knipe, 1985). It is highly likely that ICP0 contributes to the elevated levels of IE gene expression seen in an ICP4 deficient virus. Moreover, it is also likely that it contributes to the residual levels of E and L gene expression.

ICP27 is another immediate early regulatory protein that is involved in altering cellular function. Unlike ICP0, it is absolutely required for viral growth (Sacks et al., 1985). Viruses that do not express ICP27 activity are deficient in late gene expression (McCarthy et al., 1989; Sacks et al., 1985). Mechanisms invoked for ICP27 action involve transcriptional (McCarthy et al., 1989; Rice et al., 1989; Rice et al., 1988) and post-transcriptional modes (Sandri-Golden and Mendoza, 1992). In transient assays, it can either help or hinder activation of selected HSV promoters by ICP0 and ICP4 (Rice et al., 1989; Sekulovich et al., 1988). It has also been implicated in altering the phosphorylation state of other proteins in the cell, notably, ICP4 (Su and Knipe, 1989). Given the complex genetics of this protein and the potential to alter phosphorylation states of other proteins, it may be that ICP27 affects gene expression and possibly other processes, at multiple levels.

While HSV is a rapidly replicating and cytotoxic virus in its lytic, or productive, mode it also has the capacity in vivo to establish a latent infection in the sensory ganglia of nerves that project to the primary site of productive infection. In this state the virus is relatively silent from a metabolic and cytotoxic standpoint, with the genome persisting in a potentially functional form for many years. The latency-associated transcript (LAT) region of the genome is the only one that has been found to be abundantly active during latency in peripheral ganglia, but low level expression of specific viral lytic functions cannot be ruled out given the complexity of the HSV genome and the sensitivity of existing detection methods. It remains possible that viral regulatory proteins may affect host cell metabolism during latency. By a process mediated by an unknown mechanism, latent virus may be reactivated in vivo to produce a lytic infection. Given the great difference between viral transcription in the lytic and latent state, it is reasonable to predict that virus encoded regulatory proteins may be involved in determining the occurrence of these two states. Therefore, from the standpoint of efficient gene transfer and genome persistence, viral regulatory mechanisms must be circumvented if HSV is be generally useful as a vector.

From the above discussion, it is clear that HSV has the potential to alter host cell metabolism, and hence survival, by a number of mechanisms. ICP4 mutants also deficient in ICP0 and ICP27 should result in greatly reduced IE and ICP6 gene expression and also eliminate residual E and L gene expression. In addition, elimination of the nonessential vhs function should also reduce cytotoxicity. Efforts are currently underway to construct such viruses in order to produce noncytotoxic vector backbones for general gene transfer purposes.

VIRAL GENE EXPRESSION DURING LATENCY

One of the most important aspects of vector development concerns strategies for driving persistent, inducible or regulated therapeutic gene expression. In some instances constitutive expression of the therapeutic gene product will be sufficient although high or low levels of gene product may be required. In other cases, it may

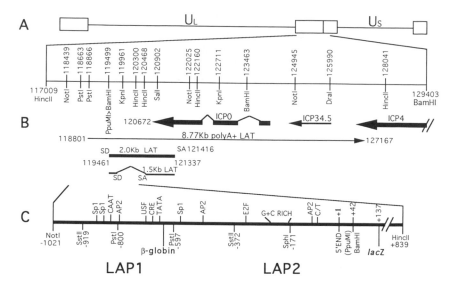

FIGURE 3. Transcription within the HSV-1 LAT region. (A) The genomic location and restriction map of the LAT region with the location of relevant restriction sites numbered according to the nucleotide position from the left-hand end of the prototype genome. (B) Transcription pattern of the LAT region. The 8.77 kb polyadenylated LAT transcript, present during productive infection is depicted. The stable 2 kb LAT transcript, also detected during productive infection, is the major transcript during latency, and the smaller 1.5 kb transcript is a spliced variant found exclusively during latent infection. (C) An expansion of the LAT promoter regions displaying the cis-acting sites within LAP1 and LAP2. LAP1 contains a TATA box, several Sp1 sites, a CRE, a USF-1 site and is located over 600 bp upstream from the 5'end of the stable 2 kb LAT (Batchelor and O'Hare,1990; Batchelor and O'Hare,1992; Devi-Rao et al., 1991; Leib et al.,1991; Zwaagstra et al.,1990; Zwaagstra et al. ,1991). The site at which ß-globin gene was inserted downstream of LAP1 in the LAP1-ß-globin expression vector (Dobson et al.,1989) is depicted. LAP2, located just upstream of the 5'end of the 2 kb stable LAT (Goins et al.,1993), lacks a TATA box consensus yet displays sequence similarity to several eukaryotic RNA polII housekeeping gene promoters such as those for the human NGF (Sehgal et al.,1988) and EGF (Ishii et al.,1985) receptors, proto-oncogenes such as PIM-1 (Meeker et al.,1990), c-myc (Kolluri et al.,1992) and murine C-Ki-ras (Hoffman et al.,1987) and the TATAless Adenovirus IVa2 gene promoter (Tamura and Mikoshiba,1991). A C/T rich element which is present within these promoters is also located within LAP2. The location of the *lacZ* insertion downstream of LAP2 in the RH142 recombinant virus (Ho and Mocarski,1989b) is denoted.

be necessary to induce expression of the gene by administration of a hormone or drug, or depending on the cellular environment, the cell itself may control expression of the foreign gene. Each of these cases requires different tactics of promoter design and the construction of promoter elements which can respond to these different needs. The natural ability of the virus to express the LATs enables the exploitation of a latency active promoter for continuous expression of foreign genes from the latent viral genome in neurons. During latency the viral genome is sequestered in the nucleus of the neuron in a manner that ensures its long term maintenance. This entails the formation of chromatin through the deposition of nucleosomes on the viral DNA (Deshmane and Fraser, 1989) and the methylation of sequences which are not transcriptionally active (Dressler et al., 1987). These processes silence the majority of genes in the viral genome, while allowing gene expression of a limited region localized to the inverted repeats flanking the unique long (U_L) segment of the genome (see Fig. 3).

During latency, a series of stable non-polyadenylated, apparently intranuclear LATs are transcribed off the DNA strand opposite the ICPO regulatory gene; their 3' ends overlap the 3' end of the ICPO transcript. The major species detected during both lytic and latent infection is approximately 2 kb in size depending on the virus strain and animal model used (Stevens et al., 1987; Wagner et al., 1988; Wechsler et al., 1988) and available evidence indicates that the major LAT is a stable intron spliced from a larger 8.77 kb polyadenylated primary transcript (Farrell et al., 1991). Two additional species of 1.45 and 1.5 kb, detected solely during latency, are believed to be derived from the 2 kb species via RNA splicing since they are co-terminal with the 2 kb RNA (Mitchell et al., 1991; Wagner et al., 1988, Wechsler et al., 1988). The 8.77 kb polyadenylated transcript is readily detected during lytic infection, but is present in exceedingly low abundance in latently infected neurons (Devi-Rao et al., 1991; Dobson et al., 1989; Zwaagstra et al., 1990).

The promoter which drives expression of the LATs represents a plausible promoter-regulator for expression of foreign genes from the viral vector backbone. Various studies have been performed to map and characterize the cis-acting regulatory elements (Dobson et al., 1989). The region proximal to the 5' end of the 2 kb LAT RNA species is devoid of a TATA box consensus sequence found upstream of most RNA polymerase class II genes. The nearest TATA homology is present almost 700 bp upstream of this site with the 5' end of the large 8.77 kb transcript mapping 25 bp downstream of this element. Several laboratories have identified LAT promoter regulatory elements within a region encompassing the TATA box and this promoter region has been designated LAP1 or latency-active promoter 1 (Batchelor and O'Hare, 1990; Devi-Rao et al., 1991; Zwaagstra et al., 1990). Additional regulatory elements include several Sp1 sites, a CCAAT box homology, a cyclic AMP response element (CRE), a USF-1 site and a neuronal "enhancer" region (Batchelor and O'Hare, 1992; Leib et al., 1991; Zwaagstra et al., 1991). A viral recombinant in which the β-globin genomic DNA was inserted downstream of the LAP1 TATA box produced β-globin specific mRNA in latently infected PNS neurons (Dobson et al., 1989). In addition, deletion of a 203 bp fragment containing the LAP1 TATA box eliminated LAT expression in latently infected PNS neurons as detected by Northern blot analysis (Devi-Rao et al., 1991; Dobson et al., 1989). Together, these experiments support the existence of a TATA box containing promoter over 700 bp upstream of the 5' end of the 2 kb major LAT and is consistent with the hypothesis that the 2 kb LAT is an intron processed from the larger 8.77 kb transcript.

Other evidence supports the existence of a second promoter region immediately 5' of the stable LATs. Ho and Mocarski (1989b) constructed a viral recombinant containing the β-galactosidase (lacZ) gene inserted 137 bp downstream of the 5' end of the 2 kb LAT which resulted in lacZ expression in latently infected trigeminal ganglion neurons. Moreover, RNAse mapping studies established that the 5' end of the chimeric LAT:lacZ mRNA mapped near the 5' end of the stable 2 kb major LAT, rather than immediately downstream of the LAP1 TATA box. This finding suggests the presence of a promoter more proximal to the major LAT coding sequence. Recently, we have shown that a recombinant containing the 203 bp LAP1 deletion is capable of producing LAT as determined by reverse-transcriptase polymerase chain reaction (rT-PCR) assay of RNA samples isolated from mouse trigeminal ganglia harboring the latent mutant virus genomes despite the fact that LATs were not detected by in situ hybridization (X. Chen, W. Goins, and J. Glorioso, unpublished data). While the LATs are not absent, their expression is, however, substantially reduced. These data suggest that other sequences may also play a role in the production of the stable LATs. Although the 5' region proximal to the 2 kb LAT is devoid of a TATA box element, this region has been shown to possess promoter activity in transient gene expression transfection analyses (Goins et al., 1993). This second promoter region, between LAP1 and the 5' end of the 2 kb LAT, has been designated the latency active promoter 2 or LAP2. In contrast to other HSV lytic promoters, LAP2 is repressed by the viral transactivators ICP4 and ICP0 (Goins et al., 1993). The sequence of LAP2 is extremely GC rich and bears striking similarity to various TATAless cellular housekeeping gene products (see Fig. 3).

LAP2 is capable of driving lacZ gene expression in the trigeminal ganglion of latently infected mice in both an ectopic glycoprotein C (gC) gene locus (Goins et al., 1993) as well as in its natural LAT locus. The size of the lacZ mRNA produced neurons in culture infected by a recombinant containing the LAP2-lacZ gene cassette in the native locus was consistent with initiation from LAP2 rather than LAP1 (X. Chen, W. Goins and J. Glorioso, unpublished data). It may be possible that LAP1 and LAP2 are not independent promoter elements but function as parts of a larger promoter-regulatory complex. The LAT promoters are under study in order to understand their unique ability to drive expression during latency and it is likely that at least certain elements within the LAT region will prove useful in activating expression of otherwise silent but nevertheless strong promoters in other circumstances. In general, the mechanistic questions to be addressed for expression of genes from the latent HSV genome are similar to issues related to expression of any foreign gene introduced into the cell.

EXPRESSION OF FOREIGN GENES FROM THE HSV GENOME

Early studies of HSV-mediated foreign gene expression demonstrated the production of foreign gene products from the context of the viral genome in vitro. Shih et al. (1984) produced hepatitis B surface antigen, Smiley and co-workers (Panning and Smiley, 1989; Smiley et al., 1987) expressed α and β globin genes, and Palella et al. (1988) demonstrated the production of hypoxanthine phosphoribosyltransferase (HPRT) in cell culture systems using HSV promoters to drive the expression of the foreign gene products. In each of these cases, the time course of gene expression followed the kinetics typical of HSV early genes.

Similar viruses were then used to express foreign genes in vivo. Palella et al. (1989) produced human HPRT mRNA in mouse brain following intracranial inoculation of an HSV recombinant carrying the HPRT gene, and Fink et al. (1992) produced functional β-galactosidase in rat hippocampus after introducing the virus by stereotatic inoculation. Following the kinetics of early gene expression, the transgene products could be detected up to 4 days after inoculation, but the animals either died or expression was lost following the establishment of latency in hippocampal neurons. Long-term expression of reporter gene constructs in the peripheral ganglia was achieved by insertion of the foreign gene downstream of the LAP1 or LAP2 promoters, which resulted in expression that could be detected in those PNS neurons 3 weeks (Dobson et al., 1989) to 8 weeks (Ho and Mocarski, 1989b) after peripheral inoculation. Our laboratory has shown that the LAP2 promoter (Goins et al., 1993) can express β-galactosidase during latency in the trigeminal ganglia for at least 300 days post-inoculation (see above).

Later experiments suggested that there might be important differences between long-term gene expression from the viral genome in the central nervous system (brain, brain stem, and spinal cord) and that seen in the peripheral sensory ganglia. Using a construct in which both copies of ICP4 were replaced by the lacZ gene under the control of the Moloney murine leukemia virus LTR, Dobson et al. (1990) showed that while lacZ expression in the trigeminal ganglion remained relatively stable, expression in the hypoglossal nucleus of the brain stem decreased 10-fold over the course of a month, despite the persistence of latent viral genomes in that region of the brain as detected by LAT expression. Similarly, our laboratory has found that replication defective HSV vectors containing the rous sarcoma virus (RSV) LTR driving expression of α-interferon failed to express beyond seven days post-inoculation in rat hippocampus (J. Mester, D. Fink, and J. Glorioso, unpublished data).

Direct inoculation of HSV vectors carrying foreign genes into specific regions of brain have confirmed that time course of expression. Breakefield and co-workers (Anderson et al., 1992; Chiocca et al., 1990), using several different replication impaired vectors with the lacZ gene under the control of a variety of different promoters demonstrated that expression was maximal early after inoculation, but diminished substantially or disappeared entirely by 2 weeks after inoculation. We have observed a similar time course of lacZ expression in hippocampal neurons following direct intracranial inoculation with a variety of impaired replicating or nonreplicating viral vectors, employing either endogenous HSV promoters, or other nonHSV viral promoter elements. Expression peaked at 2 days following inoculation, and disappeared by 7 days (Fink et al., 1992). Initial studies with PCR detection of viral genomes and rT-PCR detection of LATs demonstrated that, despite the absence of *lacZ* expression, viral genomes persist in the injected brain at least 1 year post-inoculation. In other laboratories, a few isolated cells expressing the *lacZ* gene product have been shown at 1 to 4 months after inoculation using the mammalian nerve specific enolose (NSE) promoter in striatum (Anderson et al., 1992) or the LAP1 promoter in brainstem (Wolfe et al., 1992). Together these results show that either the viral genomes are not persisting or that these promoters do not remain sufficiently active in the brain to produce detectable mRNA by in situ hybridization or gene product by enzyme assay.

To further explore whether the HSV genomes persist in a latent state at times when gene expression could not be detected, we performed quantitative PCR and rT-PCR studies using DNA and RNA isolated from rat hippocampus infected with a mutant defective for both the large and small subunit genes for ribonucleotide reductase. The results showed that the number of viral genomes in injected hippocampus decreased 5-fold from 2 days to 7 days post-inoculation, but then remained stable for at least 8 weeks postinoculation (R. Ramakrishnan, M. Levine, D. Fink, and J. Glorioso, unpublished data). The amount of LAT RNA was relatively constant at all three time points examined. These results suggest that a substantial number of viral genomes persist (approximately 5×10^6 genome equivalents per hippocampus) and continue to express LATs during viral latency; the outstanding problem is to establish continuous expression of the foreign gene from the viral genomes that are present.

PROMOTER STRATEGIES

We attempted to express foreign genes from the latent HSV genome taking advantage of one or both of the LAT promoters. As described above, insertion of a reporter gene into the LAT region downstream of either LAP1 or LAP2 provided for long-term gene expression in neurons of the peripheral nervous system. Long-term expression following infection of the CNS, however, was less satisfactory. While the natural LAT RNAs could be detected by in situ hybridization for approximately 10 days post inoculation in the absence of lytic gene mRNA, detection of LAT by this procedure was not possible after this time indicating that the LAT promoters were quite weak in brain. However, the fact that the LATs persisted for long periods of time as detected by rT-PCR, indicated that the LAT promoters were not completely inactive in brain neurons. These findings suggested that a more complete understanding of the functional elements of these promoters might be useful in the construction of strongly latency-active recombinant promoters by insertion of LAT promoter latency specific elements into stronger promoters such as the HCMV immediate early gene promoter thereby maintaining their activity long term. Such a strategy has recently been reported by Inder Verma and colleagues (Dai et al., 1992), who introduced the muscle creatine kinase (MCK) enhancer element into the HCMV promoter, which allowed it to remain active long term in differentiated myoblasts in vivo. The HCMV promoter may be attractive for this purpose since we have shown that this promoter is vigorously active for 2-5 days post inoculation of various brain regions of rats even when carried by viral mutants which are incapable of replication or expression of delayed early and late genes (see Fig. 4). Thus far, it appears that such strong promoters will not be useful without further modification.

Another approach for expression of foreign genes from the latent HSV genome may involve the use of housekeeping gene promoters such as those expressing actin (Galski et al., 1991: Morishita et al., 1991) or HPRT (Johnson and Friedmann, 1990; Rincon-Linas et al., 1991) or polIII promoters such as that of the VA1 RNA of Adenovirus (Mathews and Shenk, 1991). These promoters may be promising since they are normally constitutively active in many cell types including neurons. Whether they will be inactivated in the viral genome during latency is uncertain although experiments are ongoing to test this possibility. The VA1 promoter is capable of robust expression in an HSV background that is blocked at a very early point in the HSV regulatory cascade (Meaney and Glorioso, unpublished data). In addition, VA1 is transcribed from the viral genome in the absence of prior viral protein synthesis, as demonstrated by its efficient expression in anisomycin treated cells (see Fig. 5).

The difficulties in expressing foreign genes during HSV latency have encouraged the development of additional approaches for solving the problem of maintaining persistent gene expression. Several reports have demonstrated that the transcriptional transactivating component of the HSV VP16 gene product can be fused to the yeast GAL4 DNA binding domain in a manner to activate transcription driven from a simple promoter containing multiple copies of the GAL4 binding element (Chasman et al., 1989; Sadowski et al., 1988). Moreover, GAL4 can bind to its cognate site even when bound by nucleosomes and thus the formation of chromatin does not block the transcriptional activity of the recombinant transactivating protein (Taylor et al., 1991; White et al., 1992; Workman et al., 1991). Thus, it is likely that a similar recombinant gene encoding a GAL4-VP16 fusion protein would be capable of transactivating its own promoter provided that it contained GAL4 binding sites upstream of the transcription start site. In this way the gene would be capable of maintaining its own transcription. We are in the process of testing such virus recombinants for auto-induced gene expression during latency. If a second gene were placed upstream of this fusion protein coding sequence, separated by an internal ribosome binding site from picornavirus (Ghattas et al., 1991; Kim et al., 1992), both the therapeutic gene and the transcriptional activator could be transcribed from a single promoter. This system should be capable of persistent gene expression and could be further modified by altering either the GAL4 binding domain or the cis-acting site to regulate the level of expression. This example of an auto-induced promoter or the use of strong promoters carrying sequences which may interfere with nucleosome binding or methylation, particularly those derived form the LAT promoter, offer several attractive strategies which may be useful in overcoming difficulties related to persistent gene expression from the latent HSV genome.

A

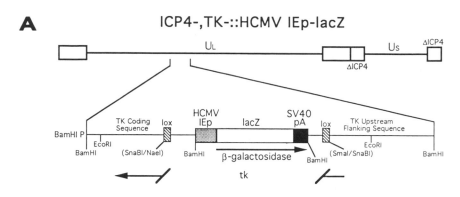

ICP4-,TK-::HCMV IEp-lacZ

B

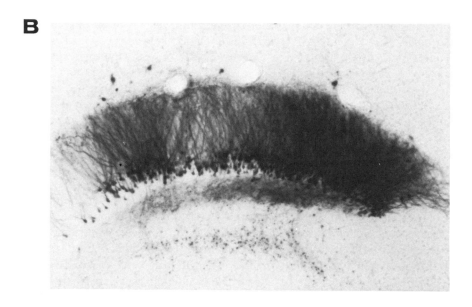

FIGURE 4. In vivo expression of lacZ from the HCMV IE promoter in rat CNS following stereotactic inoculation of a mutant defective in the essential gene ICP4. The HCMV IE promoter-lacZ reporter gene cassette was recombined into the tk locus of the ICP4 defective virus ICP4-,tk::lox [a derivative of d120 (N. DeLuca)] using cre-lox recombination (Gage et al.,1992) to produce the recombinant ICP4-,TK-::HCMV IEp-*lac*Z. Stereotactic inoculation of 5μl containing 5x10^7 pfu of this recombinant into rat hippocampus resulted in intense staining of granule cell neurons of the dentate gyrus at 2 days post inoculation. Although expression of *lac*Z was transient disappearing by day 7, *lac*Z expression could not be detected in either the contralateral hippocampus or other brain regions with projections to the hippocampal region, confirming the inability of this recombinant to spread. In addition, we have been unable to detect any significant pathology resulting from this mutant even in long-term animals.

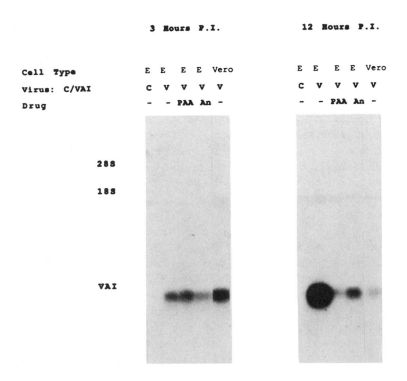

FIGURE 5. Expression of the adenovirus VA1 gene from replication defective HSV-1 vectors. VA1 transcripts were detected in cytoplasmic extracts following infection (MOI 10) with ICP4-, TK-::HCMVlacZ (C) or ICP4-,TK-::VA₁(V). RNAs were collected three and twelve hours following infection, four mg of each sample was separated on a 2% formaldehyde-agarose gel, blotted, and probed with a ^{32}P-labeled VA_1 fragment. RNAs were examined during productive infections of the complementing E5 (E) cell line (DeLuca and Schaffer, 1988) and in non-productive infections of Vero cells. It can be seen that this gene is expressed in both cell types at early and late times following infection. A slight inhibition of VA_1 expression at early times in cells treated with the protein synthesis inhibitor anisomycin (An, 100 mM) suggests that viral immediate early proteins may effect transcription of this gene. The influence of viral DNA replication on VA_1 expression was also examined using the inhibitor of viral DNA synthesis phosphonoacetic acid (PAA, 300 mg/ml). VA_1 signal in productive infection was dramatically reduced in this case, likely reflecting reduced numbers of genome copies per cell. Differences in VA_1 levels twelve hours following infection of cells treated either with PAA or anisomycin further suggest that expressed viral proteins may affect accumulation of this transcript.

CONCLUSIONS

Our experiments thus far suggest that HSV is quite attractive as a gene transfer system for brain. It is a large human virus with considerable capacity for packaging of foreign DNA (>20 kb) even without the removal of accessory and essential viral functions. The foreign DNA packaging capabilities can be increased by deletion of regions of the genome nonessential for virus replication in cell culture. The virus can be grown to very high titers (10^{10} PFU/ml) and can be injected into precise locations in the brain where latency can be established at these specific sites. Latency can be readily established by a replication defective virus and the viral genomes can be maintained for the life of the cell in an episomal nonintegrated state. As detailed above, all indications are that the virus should be rendered nonpathogenic by removal of several key genes from the genome. The resulting defective virus can be replicated only in complementing cell lines. The virus stocks can be made entirely free of replicating virus which would make HSV one of the safest vectors available. The factors regulating foreign gene expression are still under study, however, there are a number of possible strategies for long term and even regulated gene expression during latency. Research related to understanding the functioning of the LAT promoter elements, for example, should reveal a wealth of information on the molecular basis of HSV gene expression during latency. These insights should provide important clues for designing suitable promoters for foreign gene expression within various postmitotic cell types including neurons.

REFERENCES

Akli S, Caillaud C, Vigne E, Stratford-Perricaudet LD, Poenaru L, Perricaudet M, Peschanski MR (1993): Transfer of a foreign gene into the brain using adenovirus vectors. *Nature Genet* 3:224-228

Anderson JK, Garber DA, Meaney CA, Breakefield XO (1992): Gene transfer into mammalian central nervous system using herpesvirus vectors: extended expression of bacterial *lac*Z in neurons using the neuron-specific enolase promoter. *Hum Gene Ther* 3:487-499

Bajocchi G, Feldman SH, Crystal RG, Mastrangeli A (1993): Direct in vivo gene tranfer to ependymal cells in the central nervous system using recombinant adenovirus vectors. *Nature Genet* 3:229-234

Batchelor AH, O'Hare PO (1990): Regulation and cell-type-specific activity of a promoter located upstream of the latency-associated transcripts of herpes simplex virus type 1. *J Virol* 64:3269-3279

Batchelor AH, O'Hare PO (1992): Localization of cis-acting sequence requirements in the promoter of the latency-associated transcripts of herpes simplex virus type 1 required for cell-type-specific activity. *J Virol* 66:3573-3582

Cai W, Schaffer PA (1991): A cellular function can enhance gene expression and plating efficiency of a mutant defective in the gene for ICP0, a transactivating protein of HSV-1. *J Virol* 65:4078-4090

Campbell MEM, Palfreyman JW, Preston, CM (1984) Identification of herpes simplex virus DNA sequences which encode a trans-acting polypeptide responsible for the stimulation of immediate early transcription. *J Mol Biol* 180:1-19

Chasman DJ, Leatherwood J, Carey M, Ptashne M, Kornberg RD (1989): Activation of yeast RNA polymerase II transcription by a herpesvirus VP16 and GAL4 derivative in vitro. *Mol Cell Biol* 9:4746-4749

Chiocca AE, Choi BB, Cai W, DeLuca NA, Schaffer PA, DeFiglia M, Breakefield XO, Martuza RL (1990): Transfer and expression of the *lac*Z gene in rat brain neurons by herpes simplex virus mutants. *New Biol* 2:739-746

Cordingly MG, Campbell MEM, Preston CM (1983): Functional analysis of a herpes simplex virus type 1 promoter: Identification of far-upstream regulatory sequences. *Nucleic Acids Res* 11:2347-2365

Dai Y, Roman M, Naviaux RK, Verma IM (1992): Gene therapy via primary myoblasts: long-term expression of factor IX protein following transplantation in vivo. *Proc Natl Acad Sci USA* 89:10892-10895

Davidson BL, Allen ED, Kozarsky KF, Wilson JM, Roessler BJ (1993): A model system for in vivo gene transfer into the central nervous system using an adenoviral vector. *Nature Genet* 3:219-223

DeLuca NA, McCarthy A, Schaffer PA (1985): Isolation and characterization of deletion mutants of herpes simplex virus type 1 in the gene encoding immediate-early regulatory protein ICP4. *J Virol* 56:558-570

DeLuca NA, Schaffer PA (1985): Activation of immediate-early, early, and late promoters by temperature-sensitive and wild-type forms of herpes simplex virus type 1 protein ICP4. *Mol Cell Biol* 5:558-570

DeLuca NA, Schaffer, PA (1988): Physical and functional domains of the herpes simplex virus transcriptional regulatory protein ICP4. *J Virol* 62:732-743

Deshmane SL, Fraser NW (1989): During latency herpes simplex virus type 1 DNA is associated with nucleosomes in a chromatin structure. *J Virol* 63:943-947

Devi-Rao GB, Goodard SA, Hecht LM, Rochford R, Rice MK, Wagner EK, Feldman LT (1991): Relationship between polyadenylated and nonpolyadenylated herpes simplex virus type 1 latency-associated transcripts. *J Virol* 65:2179-2190

Dixon RAF, Schaffer PA (1980): Fine-structure mapping and functional analysis of temperature-sensitive mutants in the gene encoding the herpes simplex virus type 1 immediate early protein VP175. *J Virol* 36:189-203

Dobson AT, Margolis TP, Sederati F, Stevens JG, Feldman LT (1990): A latent, nonpathogenic HSV-1-derived vector stably expresses β-galactosidase in mouse neurons. *Neuron* 5:353-360

Dobson AT, Sederati F, Devi-Rao G, Flanagan WM, Farrell MJ, Stevens JG, Wagner EK, Feldman LT (1989): Identification of the latency-associated transcript promoter by expression of rabbit β-globin mRNA in mouse sensory nerve ganglia latently infected with a recombinant herpes simplex virus. *J Virol* 63:3844-3851

Dressler GR, Rock DL, Fraser NW (1987): Latent herpes simplex virus type 1 DNA is not extensively methylated in vivo. *J Gen Virol* 68:1761-1765

Everett RD (1984): Transactivation of transcription by herpes virus product: requirements for two HSV-1 immediate-early polypeptides for maximum activity. *EMBO* 3:3135-3141

Farkas DH, Block TM, Hart PM, Huges Jr RG (1987): Sequences of herpex simplx virus type 1 that inhibit formation of stable TK⁺ transformants. *J Virol* 1987:2989-2996

Farrell MJ, Dobson AT, Feldman LT (1991): Herpes simplex virus latency-associated transcript is a stable intron. *Proc Natl Acad Sci USA* 88:790-794

Fink DJ, Sternberg LR, Weber PC, Mata M, Goins WF, Glorioso JC (1992): In vivo expression of β-galactosidase in hippocampal neurons by HSV-mediated gene transfer. *Hum Gene Ther* 3:11-19

Gage PJ, Sauer B, Levine M, Glorioso, JC (1992): A cell-free recombination system for site-specific integration of multigenic shuttle plasmids into the herpes simplex virus type 1 genome. *J Virol* 66:5509-5515

Galski H, Merlino GT, Gottesmann MM, Pastan I (1991): Expression of a human multidrug-resistance cDNA (MDR-1) under the control of a β-actin promoter in transgenic mice. *Biotechnology* 16:103-124

Ghattas IR, Sanes JR, Majors JE (1991): The encephalamyocarditis virus internal ribosome entry site allows efficient coexpression of two genes from a recombinant provirus in cultured cells and in embryos. *Mol Cell Biol* 11:5848-5859

Goins WF, Sternberg LR, Croen KD, Krause PR, Hendricks RL, Fink DJ, Straus SE, Levine M, Glorioso JC (1993): A novel latency active promoter is contained within the herpes simplex virus type 1 U_L flanking repeats. (Submitted for Publication)

Goldberg YP, Rommens JM, Andrew SE, Hutchinson GB, Lin B, Theilmann J, Graham R, Glaves ML, Starr E, McDonald H, Nasir J, Schappert K, Kalchman MA, Clarke LA, Hayden MR (1993): Identification of an Alu retrotransposon event in close proximity to a strong candidate gene for Huntington's disease. *Nature* 362:370-373

Ho DY, Mocarski ES (1989a): β-galactosidase as a marker in the peripheral neural tissues of the herpes simplex virus-infected mouse. *Virology* 167:279-283

Ho DY, Mocarski ES (1989b): Herpes simplex virus latent RNA (LAT) is not required for latent infection in the mouse. *Proc Natl Acad Sci USA* 86:7596-7600

Hoffman EK, Trusko SP, Freeman NA, George DL (1987): Structural and functional characterization of the promoter region of the mouse c-ki-ras gene. *Mol Cell Biol* 7:2592-2596

Holland LE, Anderson KP, Shipman C, Wagner, EK (1980): Viral DNA synthesis is required for the efficient expression of specific herpes simplex virus type 1 mRNA species. *Virology* 101:10-24

Honess RW, Roizman B (1974): Regulation of herpes virus macromolecular synthesis. I. Cascade regulation of the synthesis of three groups of viral proteins. *J Virol* 14:8-19

Ishii S, Xu X-H, Stratton RH (1985): Characterization and sequence of the promoter region of the human epidermal growth factor receptor gene. *Proc Natl Acad Sci USA* 82:4920-4924

Johnson P, Friedmann T (1990): Limited bidirectional activity of two housekeeping gene promoters: human HPRT and PGK. *Gene* 88:207-213

Johnson P, Miyanohara A, Levind F, Cahill T, Friedmann T (1992): Cytotoxicity of a replication defective mutant herpes simplex virus type 1. *J Virol* 66:2952-2965

Kim DG, Kang HM, Jang SK, Shin H-S (1992): Construction of a bifunctional mRNA in the mouse by using the internal ribosome entry site of the encephalomy O carditis virus. *Mol Cell Biol* 12:3636-3643

Kolluri R, Torrey TA, Kinniburgh AJ (1992): A CT promoter element binding protein: definition of a double-strand and a novel-strand DNA binding motif. *Nucl Acids Res* 20:111-116

Kwong AD, Frenkel N (1987): Herpes simplex virus-infected cells contain a function(s) that destablizes both host and viral mRNAs. *Proc Natl Acad Sci USA* 84:1926-1930

LeGal LaSalle G, Robert JJ, Berrard S, Ridoux V, Stratford-Perricaudet LD, Perricaudet M, Mallet J (1993): An adenovirus vector for gene transfer into neurons and glia in the brain. *Science* 259:988-990

Leib DA, Coen DM, Bogard CL, Hicks KA, Yager DR, Knipe DM, Tyler KL, Schaffer PA (1989): Immediate early regulatory mutants define stages in the establishment and reactivation of herpes simplex virus latency. *J Virol* 63:759-768

Leib DA, Nadeau KC, Rundle SA, Schaffer PA (1991): Promoter of the latency-associated transcripts of herpex simplex virus type 1 contains a functional cAMP-response element: role of the latency-associated transcripts and cAMP in reactivation. *Proc Natl Acad Sci USA* 88:48-52

Leiden JM, Frenkel N, Rapp F (1980): Identification of the herpes simplex virus DNA sequences present in six herpex simplex virus thymidine kinase-transformed mouse cell lines. *J Virol* 33:272-285

Mackem S, Roizman B (1982): Structural features of the herpes simplex virus alpha gene 4, 0, and 27 promoter-regulatory sequences which confer alpha regulation on chimeric thymidine kinase genes. *J Virol* 44:939-949

MacDonald ME, Ambrose CM, Duyao MP, Myers RH, Lin C, Srinidhi L, Barnes G, Taylor SA, James M, Groot N, MacFarlane H, Jenkins B, Anderson MA, Wexler NS, Gusella JF, Bates GP, Baxendale S, Hummerich H, Kirby S, North M, Youngman S, Mott R, Zehetner G, Sedlacek Z, Poustka A, Frischauf A-M, Lehrach H, Buckler AJ, Church D, Doucette-Stamm L, O'Donovan MC, Riba-Ramirez L, Shah M, Stanton VP, Strobel SA, Draths KM, Wales JL, Dervan P, Housman DE, Altherr M, Shiang R, Thompson L, Fielder T, Wasmuth JJ, Tagle D, Valdes J, Elmer L, Allard M, Castilla L, Swaroop M, Blanchard K, Collins FS, Snell R, Holloway T, Gillespie K, Datson N, Shaw D and Harper PS (1993): A novel gene containing a trinucleotide repeat that is expanded and unstable on Huntington's disease chromosomes. *Cell* 72:971-983

Mathews MB, Shenk T (1991): Adenovirus virus-associated RNA and translational control. *J Virol* 65:5657-5662

McCarthy AM, McMahan L, Schaffer PA (1989): Herpes simplex virus type 1 ICP27 deletion mutants exhibit altered patterns of transcription and are DNA deficent. *J Virol* 63:18-27

McGeoch DJ, Dolan A, Donald S, Brauer DHK (1986): Complete DNA sequence of the short repeat region in the genome of herpes simplex virus type 1. *Nucleic Acids Res* 14:1727-1744

Meeker TC, Loeb J, Ayres M, Sellers W (1990): The human PIM-1 gene is selectively transcribed in different hemato-lymphoid cell lines in spite of a G+C-rich housekeeping promoter. *Mol Cell Biol* 10:1680-1688

Mitchell WJ, Lirette RP, Fraser NW (1990): Mapping of low abundance latency-associated RNA in trigeminal ganglia of mice latently infected with herpes simplex virus type 1. *J Gen Virol* 71:125-132

Morishita H, Nakamura N, Yamakawa T, Ogino H, Nobuhara M, Namba M (1991) Stable expression of human tissue-type plasminogen activator regulated by β-actin promoter in three human cell lines: HeLA, WI-38 VA13 and KMS-5. *Biochem Biophys Acta* 1090:216-222

O'Hare P, Hayward GS (1985): Three trans-acting regulatory proteins of herpes simplex virus modulate immediate-early gene expression in a pathway involving positive and negative feedback regulation. *J Virol* 56:723-733

Palella TD, Hidaka Y, Silverman LJ, Levine M, Glorioso JC, Kelley WN (1989): Expression of human HPRT mRNA in brains of mice infected with a recombinant herpes simplex virus type 1 vector. *Gene* 80:137-144

Palella TD, Silverman LJ, Schroll CT, Homa FL, Levine M, Kelley WN (1988): Herpes simplex virus-mediated human hypoxanthine-guanine phosphoribosyltransferase gene transfer into neuronal cells. *Mol Cell Biol* 8:457-460

Panning B, Smiley JR (1989): Regulation of cellular genes transduced by herpes simplex virus. *J Virol* 63:1929-1937

Post LE, Mackem S, Roizman B (1981): Regulation of alpha genes of HSV: expression of chimeric genes produced by fusion of thymidine kinase with alpha gene promoters. *Cell* 24:555-565

Preston CM (1979): Control of herpes simplex virus type 1 mRNA synthesis in cells infected with wild-type virus or the temperature-sensitive mutant tsK. *J Virol* 29:275-284

Quinlan M, Knipe D (1985): Stimulation of expression of a herpes simplex virus DNA-binding protein by two viral functions. *Mol Cell Biol* 5:957-963

Read GS, Frenkel N (1983): Herpes simplex virus mutants defective in the virion-associated shutoff of host polypoptide synthesis and abnormal synthesis of a (immediate-early) viral polypeptides. *J Virol* 46:498-512

Rice SA, Knipe DM (1988): Gene-specific transactivation by herpes simplx virus type 1 alpha protein ICP27. *J Virol* 62:3817-3823

Rice SA, Su L, Knipe DM (1989): Herpes simplex virus alpha protein ICP37 possesses separable positive and negative regulatory acivities. *J Virol* 63:3399-3407

Rincon-Limas DE, Krueger DA, Patel PI (1991): Functional characterization of the human hypoxanthine phosphoribosyltransferase gene promoter: evidence for a negative regulatory element. *Mol Cell Biol* 11:4157-4164

Roizman B, Sears A (1990): Herpes simplex viruses and their replication. In: *Virology, Second Edition*. Fields BN, Knipe DM, Chanock RM, Hirsch MS, Melnick JL, Monath TP, Roizman B, eds. New York: Raven Press

Rosen DR, Siddique T, Patterson D, Figlewicz DA, Sapp P, Hentati A, Donaldson D, Goto J, O'Regan JP, Deng H-Z, Rahmani Z, Krizus A, McKenna-Yasek D, Cayabyab A, Gaston SM, Berger R, Tanzi RE, Halperin JJ, Herzfeldt B, Van der Bergh R, Hung W-Y, Bird T, Deng G, Mulder DW, Smyth C, Laing NG, Soriano E, Pericak-Vance MA, Haines J, Rouleau GA, Gusella JS, Horvitz HR, Brown RH (1993): Mutations in Cu/Zn superoxide dismutase gene are associated with familial amyotropic lateral sclerosis. *Nature* 362:59-62

Sacks WR, Schaffer PA (1987): Deletion mutants in the gene encoding the herpes simplex virus type 1 immediate-early protein ICP0 exhibit impaired growth in cell culture. *J Virol* 61:829-839

Sacks WR, Greene CC, Aschman DA, Schaffer PA (1985): Herpes simplex virus type 1 is an essential regulatory protein. *J Virol* 55:796-805

Sadowski I, Ma J, Triezenberg S, Ptashne M (1988): GAL4-VP16 is an unusually potent transcriptional activator. *Nature* 335:563-564

Sandri-Golden RM, Mendoza GE (1992): A herpesvirus regulatory protein appears to act protein ICP27 can act as a *trans*-activator in combination with ICP4 and ICP0. *J Virol* 62:4510-4522

Sehgal A, Patil N, Chao M (1988): A constitutive promoter directs expression of the nerve growth factor receptor gene. Mol Cell Biol 8:3160-3167

Sekulovich RR, Leary K, Sandri-Goldin RM (1988): The herpes simplex virus type 1 α protein ICP27 can act as a *trans*-activator in combination with ICP4 and IVP0. *J Virol* 62:4510-4522

Shih M-F, Arsenakis M, Tiollais P, Roizman B (1984): Expression of hepatitis B virus S gene by herpes simplex virus type 1 vectors carrying α- and β-regulated gene chimeras. *Proc Natl Acad Sci USA* 81:5867-5870

Smiley JR, Smibert C, Everett RD (1987): Expression of a cellular gene cloned in herpes simplex virus: rabbit β-globin is regulated as an early viral gene in infected fibroblasts. *J Virol* 61:2368-2377

Stevens JG, Wagner EK, Devi-Rao GB, Cook ML, Feldman LT (1987): RNA complimentary to α herpes virus a gene mRNA is prominent in latently infected neurons. *Science* 235:1056-1059

Su L, Knipe DK (1989): Herpes simplex virus a protein ICP27 can inhibit or augment viral gene transactivation. *Virology* 170:496-504

Tamura T, Mikoshiba K (1991): Role of a GC-rich motif in transcription regulation of the adenovirus type 2 IVa2 promoter which lacks a typical TATA-box element. *FEBS Lett* 282:87-90

Taylor ICA, Workman JL, Schuetz TJ, Kingston RE (1991): Facilitated binding of

GAL4 and heat shock factor to nucleosomal templates: differential function of DNA-binding domains. *Genes and Dev* 5:1285-1298

Wagner EK, Flanagen WM, Devi-Rao GB, Zhang YF, Hill JM, Anderson KP, Stevens JG (1988): The herpes simplex virus latency-associated transcript is spliced during the latent phase of infection. *J Virol* 61:4577-4585

Watson RJ, Clements JB (1978) Characterization of transcription-deficient temperature sensitive mutants of herpes simplex virus type 1. *Virology* 91:364-379

Wechsler SL, Nesburn AB, Watson R, Slanina SM, Ghiasi H (1988): Fine mapping of the latency-related gene of herpes simplex virus type 1: alternative splicing produces distinct latency-related RNAs containing open reading frames. *J Virol* 62:4051-4058

White J, Brou C, Wu J, Lutz Y, Moncollin V, Chambon P (1992): The acidic transcriptional activator GAL4-VP16 acts on preformed template-committed complexes. *EMBO J* 11:2229-2240

Wildy P, Field HJ, Nash AA (1982): Classical herpes virus latency revisited. In: *Virus Persistence*. Mahy BWJ, Minson AC, Darby GK eds. Cambridge University Press

Wolfe JH, Deshmane SL, Fraser NW (1992): Herpes virus vector gene transfer and expression of β-glucuronidase in the central nervous system of MPS VII mice. *Nature Genetics* 1:379-384

Workman JL, Taylor ICA, Kingston RE (1991): Activation domains of stably bound GAL4 derivatives alleviate repression of promoters by nucleosomes. *Cell* 64:533-544

Zwaagstra JC, Ghiasi H, Nesburn AB, Wechsler SL (1991): Identification of a major regulatory sequence in the latency-associated transcript (LAT) promoter of herpex simplex virus type 1 (HSV-1). *Virology* 182:287-297

Zwaagstra JC, Ghiasi H, Slanina SN, Nesburn AB, Wheatley SC, Lillycrop K, Wood J, Latchman DS, Patel K, Wechsler SL (1990): Activity of herpes simplex virus type 1 latency-associated transcript (LAT) promoter in neuron-derived cells: evidence for neuron specificity and for a large LAT transcript. *J Virol* 64:5019-5028

DIRECT GENE TRANSFER AND CATHETER BASED GENE DELIVERY SYSTEMS: APPLICATIONS TO CARDIOVASCULAR DISEASES AND MALIGNANCY

Gregory E. Plautz, Elizabeth G. Nabel, and Gary J. Nabel

INTRODUCTION

Gene transfer has been utilized as a powerful research tool to analyze the effects of novel gene expression by transduced cells in vitro and in vivo. A goal of gene therapy is to apply this technology to the treatment of human diseases. In addition to its logical role for the correction of inherited diseases caused by a missing or defective gene product, gene therapy also holds promise for treatment of acquired disorders. The critical pathology in many acquired diseases, such as cardiovascular diaease and cancer, is anatomically localized. Recombinant genes can be delivered to specific anatomic sites in vivo via a catheter. Site-specific gene transfer can be utilized to provide therapy for acquired diseases, using recombinant gene products as biologic effectors.

Cardiovascular diseases remain the leading cause of mortality among adults in the industrialized world. Although atherosclerosis is a systemic disorder, critical lesions in most instances are located at specific sites in the circulation. These lesions can be isolated and treated using intravascular catheters; however, current therapies, including percutaneous transluminal angioplasty, are often complicated by restenosis or thrombosis. An approach to therapy of atherosclerosis is the localized introduction of recombinant genes into vascular cells which encode proteins to inhibit cell proliferation or thrombogenesis.

Many types of malignancy are poorly responsive to current therapeutic modalities, including surgery, radiotherapy, and chemotherapy. Biologic therapy has been demonstrated to be effective for several types of malignancy, most notably melanoma. Recombinant gene products with stimulatory effects on the immune system, or direct inhibitory or toxic effects on tumor cells have been administered systemically to patients. Gene transfer into tumor cells or vascular cells supplying the tumor and cellular effectors which can infiltrate tumors may increase the therapeutic efficacy and decrease the systemic toxicity of biologic therapy by delivering high local concentrations of the active protein to the tumor bed. The immune system can also recognize and respond to antigens on tumor cells, and this response can be augmented by the introduction of novel antigens into tumors. Di-

Gene Therapeutics: Methods and Applications of Direct Gene Transfer
Jon A. Wolff, Editor • ©1994 *Birkhäuser Boston*

rect transfer of highly immunogenic genes into tumor cells in vivo can, therefore, stimulate an immune response against tumors.

The application of gene therapy to acquired diseases, such as cardiovascular disease and malignancy, has different requirements than the correction of an inherited gene defect. For acquired diseases, transient rather than lifelong gene expression is acceptable and in many cases desirable. The pathology in many acquired diseases is anatomically localized which allows direct gene transfer in vivo into the affected site. This chapter will describe the development of direct gene transfer in vivo into vascular cells and its application to the study and treatment of vascular diseases. The use of direct gene transfer into melanomas to provide immunotherapy will also be described.

DIRECT GENE TRANSFER IN VIVO: STRATEGIES AND METHODS

A goal of gene therapy for acquired diseases is to achieve expression of genes within somatic cells of subjects which will attenuate or reverse the disease process. A therapeutic effect can result from expression of novel genes, heterotopic gene expression, or overexpression of normally active genes. Two strategies have been used to introduce recombinant genes: cell-mediated gene transfer and direct gene transfer. Cell-mediated gene transfer provides an opportunity to isolate and characterize a defined cell type prior to reintroduction into the host. For some disorders, the critically affected cells can be easily removed from a patient, transduced with the relevant gene, then replaced in the body. Disadvantages of this approach include the difficulty and time required to derive cell lines for many tissues and immunologic incompatibility for outbred animal models. Characteristics of cell lines, such as their ability to proliferate autonomously and to produce or respond to growth factors, may also change during ex vivo culture. Many potential clinical applications of gene transfer would not permit previous preparation of cells in culture. Direct gene transfer overcomes these obstacles and can streamline the process of gene transfer.

Several criteria must be met to optimize direct gene transfer in vivo. An efficient delivery system, including a viral or chemical vehicle, as well as a device to deposit the gene in proximity to the target cells, must be available. The gene must be combined with regulatory and processing signals which permit expression by the target cells. The biologic effect of the gene product on the pathophysiology of the disorder should be characterized, and an animal model for the disease should provide measurable parameters to assess the potential risks and benefits of the treatment. The gene must be delivered directly to the affected cells or provide a systemic effect from transfected tissue. Finally, the procedure of gene transfer and the expression of the introduced gene should not cause adverse effects. Expression should be regulatable when appropriate.

Several alternative gene transfer techniques have been successfully utilized in vivo, including viral vectors, physical methods and chemical methods. Several modified viruses have served as vectors for in vivo gene transfer, including retroviruses (Price et al., 1987; Nabel et al., 1990; and Culver et al., 1992), herpes viruses (Palella et al., 1989; Chiocca et al., 1990; and Breakefield and DeLuca, 1991), adenoviruses (Rosenfeld et al., 1991; Rosenfeld et al., 1992; and Jaffe et al., 1992), and adeno-associated viruses (Samulski et al., 1991). Direct injection of DNA has allowed expression of recombinant genes in skeletal or cardiac myocytes(Wolff et al., 1990; Lin et al., 1990; and Acsadi et al., 1991). DNA has also been complexed with polylysine coupled to asialoorosomucoid for receptor mediated uptake by the asialoglycoprotein receptor (Wu and Wu, 1987). An additional approach employing DNA complexed with cationic liposomes has been used to transfer recombinant genes directly into vascular cells and tumor cells in vivo (Nabel et al., 1990, Brigham et al., 1989, Holt et al., 1990, and Plautz et al., 1993).

Retroviral vectors and DNA liposome complexes have been utilized to introduce recombinant genes into vascular cells and into tumors. Each provides different features which may influence their utility for gene transfer in vivo. Retroviral vectors are largely derived from the Moloney murine leukemia virus from which coding sequences for gag, pol, and env genes have been replaced with recombinant genes. These vectors, when transfected into packaging cell lines (Miller, 1990 and Danos and Mulligan, 1988), can produce helper virus free viral particles. Retroviral vectors have several features which are advantageous for gene transfer. Retroviral vectors containing amphotropic or xenotropic envelope proteins can infect many cell types from most species, serving to integrate the recombinant gene into the recipient cell chromosomal DNA. There are, however, several limitations to the use of retroviral vectors for in vivo gene transfer. For instance, there are constraints on the size of introduced genes (7-13 kb), and transcription from the viral LTR may be inefficient in certain cell types. Retroviral vectors also require replication of target cells to become integrated into chromosomal DNA and subsequently expressed. For some applications, minimal proliferation of terminally differentiated target cells might limit the efficiency of retroviral mediated gene transfer. Although current retroviral packaging cell lines are usually free of replication competent helper virus, the formation of such a virus prior to instillation or through recombination with endogenous retroviruses in vivo is possible. Viral proteins are also immunogenic, and sensitization of the host might limit the efficacy of repeated treatments.

Liposomes complexed to plasmid DNA provide another method of direct gene transfer in vivo. The cationic liposome, Lipofectin® (Bethesda Research Laboratories, Gaithersburg, MD), is a mixture of DOTMA (N-[2,3-dioleyloxy)propyl]-N,N,N-trimethylammonium chloride) and DOPE (dioleoyl phosphatidylethanolamine) (Felgner et al., 1987), and has been used to introduce recombinant genes into vascular cells in peripheral (Nabel et al., 1990) and coronary (Lim et al., 1991) arteries in vivo. Another cationic liposome preparation, comprised of DC-cholesterol (3b[N-(N'N'-dimethylaminoethane)-carbamoyl] cholesterol) and DOPE (Gao and Huang, 1991), has also provided efficient gene transfer into vascular cells and into malignant tumors (Plautz et al., 1993) in vivo. These cationic liposomes can be prepared in large batches by sonication to provide particles with a diameter of approximately 250 nm, and they maintain activity in aqueous solution for several months. An electrostatic interaction, which is highly dependent on the molar ratio between the DNA and liposomes (Stewart et al., 1992), forms a complex which can interact with the plasma membrane of target cells. The mechanisms by which the DNA is released into the cell and directs transcription are not well understood (Felgner and Ringold, 1989). Unlike other liposomes which are primarily cleared by the reticuloendothelial system (Liu et al., 1992), cationic liposomes are often inactivated by serum (Felgner et al., 1989) and transduce cells most effectively at the site of delivery.

Liposomes have several features which can facilitate direct gene transfer. Because viral sequences are not necessary, there are few constraints on the enhancer/promoter elements or size of the vectors. DNA-liposome complexes form rapidly in aqueous solution without extensive preparation, and therefore, it is possible to rapidly analyze a series of vectors for activity in vitro or in vivo. In contrast to retroviral-mediated gene transfer, replication of the target cell is not necessary, allowing recombinant gene expression in terminally differentiated somatic cells. The DC-cholesterol preparation is not toxic to cells over a wide range of concentrations in vitro, and is metabolized in vivo (Gao and Huang, 1991). The DC-cholesterol liposome preparation has been demonstrated as safe in vivo after extensive toxicity testing (Stewart et al., 1992 and Nabel et al., 1992a). Retroviral vectors and DNA-liposome complexes have been applied to demonstrate direct gene transfer into vascular cells and tumors in vivo, and to develop novel therapeutic approaches for vascular diseases and malignancy.

DIRECT GENE TRANSFER INTO VASCULAR CELLS

Cardiovascular diseases are desirable candidates for novel approaches to treatment, such as gene transfer, because many people are afflicted each year and current therapies are often insufficient. The critical lesions in many patients with atherosclerosis involve the coronary circulation. Coronary angioplasty by balloon dilatation has been used successfully since the late 1970s (Gruntzig et al., 1977), and recently additional methods such as use of atherectomy devices (Safian et al., 1990 and Ellis et al., 1991), laser photo-ablation (Bresnahan et al., 1991), and intraluminal stenting (Sigwart et al., 1987) have been employed. Each of these methods causes endovascular trauma, however, and these procedures are complicated by angiographic evidence of restenosis in up to 50% of patients (Nobuyoshi et al., 1988, Roberts et al.., 1990, Fourrier et al., 1989, Rothbaum et al., 1991 and Spears et al., 1993). There have been many clinical trials examining the prevention of restenosis by calcium antagonists (Corcos et al., 1985), β-adrenergic blockers (Johansson et al., 1990), corticosteroids (Pepine et al., 1990), anticoagulants (Ellis et al., 1989), and antiplatelet agents (Schwartz et al., 1988), all with disappointing results. The mechanisms which contribute to restenosis are complex and include growth factors, cytokines and angiogenic factors. Direct gene transfer into vascular cells in vivo provides a model to examine the physiologic response to recombinant gene expression, such as growth factor genes. Such studies may be useful to investigate the pathophysiology of vascular disease, and to provide the basis for novel therapeutic interventions for restenosis or atherosclerosis.

Multiple cell types are located within arteries; however, two important targets for gene transfer are endothelial cells and vascular smooth muscle cells. Endothelial cells form a monolayer on the luminal surface of blood vessels. They regulate hemostasis (Esmon, 1987 and Rodgers, 1988), and by regulated expression of cell surface adhesion proteins, they modulate adherence and trafficking of cells involved in the inflammatory response (Osborn et al., 1989, Bevilacqua et al., 1989 and Elices et al., 1990). Vascular smooth muscle cell tone and proliferation are also regulated by the endothelium (Furchgott and Zawadzki, 1980; Berk et al., 1986; and Palmer et al., 1987). Thus, endothelial cells can deliver therapeutic gene products with anticoagulant, anti-inflammatory, vasodilatory, or antiproliferative effects.

Vascular smooth muscle cells comprise the media of arteries and exert the contractile force that provides arterial tone. Smooth muscle cells proliferate in the intima in response to vessel injury and contribute to the development of restenosis and atherosclerosis. Because of their central role in stenotic vascular lesions, smooth muscle cells are important targets for gene transfer. In addition, whereas the endothelium exists as a monolayer of approximately 10^5 cells per square centimeter, smooth muscle cells are multilayered in arteries, providing a larger reservoir for synthesis of recombinant gene products.

Cell-mediated gene transfer and direct gene transfer have both been used to introduce recombinant genes into the vasculature. Initially, using cell-mediated gene transfer, primary cultures of vascular cells were transduced in vitro and reimplantated onto localized denuded segments of vessels through a double balloon catheter. This method has provided expression of recombinant genes in vivo by endothelial cells (Nabel et al., 1989) and smooth muscle cells (Plautz et al., 1991 and Lynch et al., 1992). The location of recombinant gene expression in the artery wall in cell-mediated gene transfer experiments depended on the type of cell introduced. Microscopic analysis of artery sections demonstrated that reimplanted endothelial cells were found primarily in the intimal layer (Nabel et al., 1989), whereas transduced vascular smooth muscle cells were present in the media and in areas of intimal proliferation (Plautz et al., 1991 and Lynch et al., 1992). Approaches to seeding endothelial cells which express recombinant genes onto implantable biomedical devices also show promise (Wilson et al., 1989; Dichek et al., 1989; and Dichek et al., 1991).

Direct gene transfer provides a powerful tool to modify endogenous vascular cells in order to examine the effects of recombinant gene expression in vivo. To develop a method by which vascular cells could be transduced with recombinant genes in vivo, retroviral vectors or DNA-liposome complexes were instilled into localized arterial segments (Nabel et al., 1990). Using a porcine model, a segment of the iliofemoral artery was isolated from the systemic circulation using a double balloon catheter. A central protected space between the two balloons was flushed to remove residual serum, which can neutralize both retroviral vectors and lipo-somes (Felgner et al., 1989). A concentrated suspension of amphotropic Moloney murine leukemia viral vector expressing the β-galactosidase gene (infectious titer 1-8 x 10^5) was instilled in the arterial segment for thirty minutes prior to removal of the catheter. Following gene transfer, recombinant gene expression was present in endothelial cells, vascular smooth muscle cells, and adventitial cells in trans-duced arteries. Expression of β-galactosidase decreased with time but was clearly present up to 21 weeks following retroviral gene transfer. Recombinant gene ex-pression was confined to the localized site of instillation and was not detected in the downstream arterial segment or in other tissues by PCR analysis. In these experiments, helper virus was not detected in the viral stocks prior to instillation, and helper virus was not isolated from serum or lymphocytes of experimental ani-mals receiving the retroviral vector.

DNA liposome complexes also provided localized efficient direct gene trans-fer in vivo. The Lipofectin® (DOTMA/DOPE) reagent (Felgner et al., 1987) was incubated with the β-galactosidase containing plasmid BAG (Price et al., 1987) in minimal essential media. This mixture was instilled through the central port of the double balloon catheter for thirty minutes prior to reestablishment of blood flow. Transduced arteries demonstrated extensive β-galactosidase staining, limited to the site between the two balloons. Microscopic analysis of the transduced arteries demonstrated β-galactosidase expression, in endothelial cells and vascular smooth muscle cells, confirmed by immunohistochemical staining. Independent studies using Lipofectin® complexed with either the β-galactosidase plasmid or the firefly luciferase genes have confirmed the ability to transduce peripheral arteries and have extended this technique to coronary arteries in a canine model (Lim et al., 1991).

APPLICATIONS OF DIRECT GENE TRANSFER INTO VASCULAR CELLS

Direct gene transfer is being used to investigate the pathogenesis of vascular disor-ders. A significant advantage of localized direct gene transfer for animal models of vascular disease is that the biological effects of introduced genes can be ana-lyzed in intact animals using the contralateral vessel as a control. Immune-medi-ated vasculitis is a poorly understood disorder and effective therapy is lacking. To develop an animal model for immune-mediated vasculitis, a human major histo-compatibility complex (MHC) gene, HLA-B7, was introduced into the iliofemoral artery of pigs using retroviral vectors or DNA liposome complexes (Nabel et al., 1992b). Using either delivery system, expression of the HLA-B7 protein was demonstrated within vascular cells by immunohistochemistry. Ex-pression of the foreign histocompatibility antigen stimulated an intense inflamma-tory response in the recipient animal. Mononuclear cells were observed in the adventitia and media 17 to 21 days following gene transfer. At 75 days, chronic inflammation was noted in the transduced arteries. Further studies determined that porcine T lymphocytes specifically recognized the foreign antigen and produced the inflammatory response. Control arteries transduced with the β-galactosidase gene did not develop inflammatory histologic changes or an immune response. The histologic and immunologic responses induced by HLA-B7 were similar for both retroviral and liposome mediated gene transfer, confirming that each method can provide appropriate and biologically active gene expression. Foreign histocompatibility antigens are also presented on vascular cells in the setting of organ transplantation. Rejection of organ grafts usually involves severe vasculitis and is a limitation of organ transplantation. Cell-mediated immune vasculitis induced by focal expression of a foreign histocompatibility gene provides a novel animal model to study this disorder and to test therapeutic interventions.

The physiological response to recombinant growth factor gene expression in normal and injured arteries is currently under study. The endothelial cell growth factor, fibroblast growth factor-1 (FGF-1) induces endothelial cell proliferation in vitro (Burgess and Maciag, 1989) and is angiogenic in vivo (Ausprunk and Folkman, 1977). FGF-1 lacks a classical signal sequence for secretion which has made study of its effects as an extracellular protein difficult. A chimeric gene, comprised of the signal sequence from the FGF-4 gene fused to the coding sequence of FGF-1, complexed with Lipofectin®, was transfected into porcine arteries (Nabel et al., 1992c). The transfection was performed with low instillation pressure (150 mmHg) to minimize trauma to the vessel. Presence of the introduced DNA was confirmed 21 days after transfection by PCR and protein expression by immunohistochemistry. The secreted FGF-1 gene induced intimal proliferation, and in several vessels capillary formation was observed in the neointima. Such angiogenesis has been observed in atherosclerotic plaques (Barger et al., 1984); however, mechanisms to explain this observation have previously been lacking.

Platelet-derived growth factor (PDGF) B chain has also been implicated in the generation of atherosclerosis. This growth factor does not have mitogenic effects on endothelial cells, due to the absence of the PDGF receptor, in contrast to its mitogenic effects on vascular smooth muscle cells (Heldin et al., 1981). A plasmid expression vector encoding the human PDGF B gene was introduced into porcine arteries using Lipofectin® at low instillation pressures (Nabel et al., 1993). The presence of introduced DNA was confirmed by PCR analysis of recombinant PDGF B mRNA. Immunohistochemistry revealed human PDGF BB protein expression in the intima and media whereas control arteries transduced with β-galactosidase lacked staining. Quantitative morphometry of intimal and medial thickness demonstrated a sevenfold increase in the intimal to medial ratio compared to β-galactosidase transduced vessels. Unlike the FGF-1 transduced arteries, the intimal thickening was not associated with neocapillary formation. These studies provide a method to examine the effects of recombinant growth factor gene expression on vascular physiology in normal and injured arteries. Such studies also provide a model to investigate inhibition of intimal proliferation using growth factor or receptor antagonists.

DIRECT GENE TRANSFER INTO TUMORS TO PROVIDE IMMUNOTHERAPY

Cancer treatment with surgery, radiotherapy, and chemotherapy is often unsuccessful. Immunotherapy has shown promise as an adjuvant approach for treating malignancy. Tumors display unique antigens which can be recognized by humoral and cellular components of the immune system (Hellstrom and Hellstrom, 1991 and van der Bruggen et al., 1991). Cellular effectors with nonspecific antitumor activity, such as natural killer (NK) cells (Herberman, 1986) and lymphokine activated killer (LAK) cells (Lotze et al., 1981 and Grimm et al., 1982), participate in tumor cell destruction. Tumor-specific cytolytic T cells mediate MHC restricted lysis and can be isolated from peripheral blood (Knuth et al., 1989 and Anichini et al., 1989) and the tumor (Anichini et al., 1989; Yron et al., 1980; Rosenberg et al., 1986; and Spiess et al., 1987). Strategies to augment existing host immune response against tumors through systemic administration of cytokines, such as IL-2 (Lotze et al., 1985 and Lotze et al., 1986), interferon-α (Quesada et al., 1984; Foon et al., 1984; and Bunn et al., 1986), or IFN-γ (Ernstoff et al., 1987; Creagan et al., 1987; and Perez et al., 1988), have shown efficacy in animal tumor models and human trials. Intralesional instillation of nonspecific immune potentiators, such as BCG, can also induce systemic protection against several types of tumors (Morton et al., 1970 and Herr et al., 1987). Recently, a series of studies using cell-mediated gene transfer have demonstrated that expression of IL-2 (Fearon et al., 1990 and Gansbacher et al., 1990a), IL-4 (Tepper et al., 1989), TNF-α (Asher et al., 1991), and IFN-γ (Gansbacher et al., 1990b and Restifo et al., 1992) by tumor cells can stimulate a vigorous immune response which leads to rejection of the inoculum of modified tumor cells. In many cases, this immune response provides protection against rechallenge with nontransduced tumor cells. The potential clinical applicability of cell-mediated gene transfer approaches might be limited, however, by the time, cost, and in some cases, inability to establish cell lines from human tumors. Direct gene transfer, which obviates some of these problems, has now been used to introduce a gene encoding an allogenic class I major histocompatibility complex (MHC) protein into tumors in vivo (Nabel et al., 1992d).

Class I MHC glycoproteins are displayed on the surface of nearly all somatic cells where they present peptide fragments of endogenously synthesized proteins (Jardetzky et al., 1991). The combination of the peptide fragment and class I MHC protein are recognized by specific T cell receptors on CD8+ T cells (Townsend and Bodmer, 1989). Transplanted allogeneic tissue is highly immunogenic due to a high precursor frequency of lymphocytes capable of recognizing allogeneic MHC molecules (Skinner and Marbrook, 1976 and Lindahl and Wilson, 1977). To stimulate a strong immune response within a tumor, a murine class I MHC gene was introduced directly into the parenchyma of tumors in vivo (Plautz et al., 1993). Preparations containing retroviral vectors or DC-cholesterol liposome plasmid complexes were delivered to subcutaneous tumor nodules by intratumoral injection. Expression of a allogeneic class I MHC gene by tumor cells induced a specific CD8+ cytolytic T cell response. More importantly, animals treated with the allogenic MHC gene, but not a control gene, developed a CD8+ cytolytic T-cell response against antigens present on nontransduced tumor cells. In animals presensitized to this foreign antigen, direct gene transfer into growing established tumors could attenuate tumor growth and in some cases lead to complete tumor regression. These studies demonstrate the ability to transduce an allogeneic MHC gene into tumors in vivo, and the protective effect that the response to this gene can provide.

The acute and long-term toxicity of DNA-liposome complexes has been studied extensively in animal models. DC-cholesterol liposomes (Gao and Huang, 1991) were injected into mice intravenously or intratumorally, and the anatomic location of plasmid was determined by PCR analysis of tissues two to three weeks later. Plasmid could be detected in mice receiving intravenous DNA-liposome complexes from heart and lung tissue in most cases and occasionally in kidney, whereas intratumoral injection resulted in isolation of plasmid occasionally in heart, lung, and spleen. Organs from these mice did not demonstrate any histopathology, and electrocardiography during the liposome injection and at followup was normal. Serum enzyme studies of liver, heart and kidney function were also normal acutely and at followup (Stewart et al.., 1992). The potential for inadvertent introduction of recombinant genes into germline tissue is a concern for gene therapy. To address this question, forty-two rabbits and pigs were injected intravenously or intraarterially with DNA-liposome complexes. Transfected DNA was not isolated from gonadal tissue using PCR, despite its presence in the transduced artery segments and occasionally in other tissues, as previously observed (Nabel et al., 1992a). Analysis of a panel of serum enzymes did not reveal any abnormalities up to 120 days after gene transfer with DNA-liposome complexes. An important question regarding the potential for autoimmune phenomena induced by transfer of a foreign Class I MHC gene was also addressed in mice which received intravenous, subcutaneous, or intraperitoneal injection of either an allogeneic MHC gene or a β-galactosidase gene complexed to DC-cholesterol. Mice receiving the allogeneic MHC gene all generated a specific CTL response to this gene; however, there was no histopathologic evidence of organ toxicity (Nabel et al., 1992a). These studies demonstrate that uptake and expression of recombinant genes, including a foreign MHC gene, are not associated with generalized autoimmunity, toxicity, or gonadal localization. The method of DNA-liposome mediated gene transfer therefore appeared suitable for human gene therapy.

A phase I/II clinical trial (Nabel et al., 1992d) based on the strategy of direct transfer of an allogeneic MHC gene into tumors in vivo to provide immunotherapy was approved by the Recombinant DNA Advisory Committee in January 1992. This clinical trial has commenced and patients with metastatic melanoma and subcutaneous tumor nodules have undergone treatment. The treatment protocol consists of intratumor injection of a preparation of the human class I MHC gene, HLA-B7, complexed with DC-cholesterol liposomes. Four study groups received escalating doses of the DNA liposome complex (Table 1).

TABLE 1. Protocol for Clinical Protocol: Direct Gene Transfer for Immunotherapy of Malignancy

Group	Number of Injections Per Treatment	Volume of Injection (ml)	Times of Repeated Treatment	Total Number of Treatments
I	1	≤ 0.2	2 wk.	3
II	3	≤ 0.2	2 wk.	3
III	5	≤ 0.2	2 wk.	3
IV	5	≤ 0.2	2 wk.	4

Gene transfer and expression are examined by analysis of recombinant DNA, RNA and protein in tumor biopsies obtained two weeks after each treatment. The immunologic response of peripheral blood lymphocytes to HLA-B7 (expressed on syngeneic EBV immortalized B cells) and tumor cells will also be analyzed. The objectives of this ongoing clinical trial are to: 1) establish a safe and effective dose to introduce a recombinant gene, HLA-B7, into tumors by DNA liposome transfection; 2) to confirm expression of this class I MHC gene by tumor cells following direct gene transfer in vivo; and 3) to analyze the immune response against this antigen and other tumor antigens.

Direct gene transfer into tumors is a new approach to tumor immunotherapy. Introduction of cytokine genes with direct antitumor or immunostimulatory effects, alone or in combination with MHC genes, may augment the immune response within a tumor. Delivery of recombinant genes to tumors may also be conducted by an intravascular catheter. These modifications to existing tumor immunotherapy gene therapy protocols offer promise for future clinical trials.

CONCLUSIONS

Direct transfer of recombinant genes in vivo has been demonstrated for vascular cells and tumor cells using retroviral vectors and DNA-liposome complexes. Expression of transduced genes is limited to specific anatomic sites through localized delivery of the vectors. Expression of recombinant genes by transduced cells produces biologic responses which provide a system to study the pathophysiology of diseases. Direct gene transfer for tumor immunotherapy has been established in animal models. A clinical trial using this approach in patients with metastatic melanoma is in progress. Direct gene transfer is a promising approach to gene therapy for many acquired and inherited disorders.

REFERENCES

Acsadi G, Jiao SS, Jani A, Duke D, Williams P, Chong W, Wolff JA(1991): Direct gene transfer and expression into rat heart in vivo. *New Biol* 3:71-81

Anichini A, Mazzocchi A, Fossati G, Paramiani G (1989): Cytotoxic T lymphocyte clones from peripheral blood and from tumor site detect intratumor heterogeneity of melanoma cells. Analysis of specificity and mechanisms of interaction. *J Immunol* 142:3692-3701

Asher AL, Mule JJ, Kasid A, Restifo NP, Salo JC, Reichert CM, Jaffe G, Fendly B, Kriegler M, Rosenberg SA (1991): Murine tumor cells transduced with the gene from tumor necrosis-a: evidence for paracrine immune effects of tumor necrosis factor against tumors. *J Immunol* 146:3227-3234

Ausprunk DH, Folkman J (1977): Migration and proliferation of endothelial cells in preformed and newly formed blood vessels during tumor angiogenesis. *Microvasc Res* 14:53-65

Barger AC, Beeuwkes R, Lainey LL, Silverman RJ (1984): Hypothesis: Vasa vasorum and neovascularization of human coronary arteries. A possible role in the pathophysiology of atherosclerosis. *N Engl J Med* 310:175-177

Berk BC, Alexander RW, Brock TA, Gimbrone Jr MA, Webb RC (1986): Vasoconstriction: a new activity for platelet-derived growth factor. *Science* 232:87-90

Bevilacqua MP, Stengelin S, Gimbrone MA, Seed B (1989): Endothelial leukocyte adhesion molecule1: an inducible receptor for neutrophils related to complement regulatory proteins and lectins. *Science* 243:1160-1165

Breakefield XO, DeLuca NA (1991): Herpes simplex virus for gene delivery to neurons. *New Biol* 3:203-218

Bresnahan JF, Litvack F, Margolis J, Rothbaum D, Kent K, Untereker W, Cummins F (1991): Excimer laser coronary angioplasty initial results of a multicenter investigation in 958 patients. *J Am Coll Cardiol* 17:30A

Brigham KL, Meyrick B, Christman B, Magnuson M, King G, Berry LC (1989): In vivo transfection of murine lungs with a functioning prokaryotic gene using a liposome vehicle. *Am J Med Sci* 298:278-281

Bunn PA, Ihde DC, Foon K (1986): The role of recombinant interferon-alpha-2a in the therapy of cutaneous T-cell lymphomas. *Cancer* 57:1689-1695

Burgess WH, Maciag. T (1989): The heparin-binding (fibroblast) growth factor family of proteins. *Annu Rev Biochem* 58:575-606

Chiocca EA, Choi BB, Cai WZ, DeLuca NA, Schaffer PA, DiFiglia M, Breakefield XO, Martuza RL (1990): Transfer and expression of the lacZ gene in rat brain neurons mediated by herpes simplex virus mutants. *New Biol* 2:739-746

Corcos T, David PR, Val PG, Renkin J, Dangoisse V, Rapold HG (1985): Failure of diltiazem to prevent restenosis after percutaneous transluminal coronary angioplasty. *Am Heart J* 109:926-931

Creagan ET, Ahmann DL, Long HJ, Frytak S, Sherwin SA, Chang MN (1987): Phase II study of recombinant interferon-gamma in patients with disseminated malignant melanoma. *Cancer Treat Rep* 71:843-844

Culver KW, Ram Z, Wallbridge S, Ishii H, Oldfield EH, Blaese RM (1992): In vivo gene transfer with retroviral vector-producer cells for treatment of experimental brain tumors. *Science* 256:1550-1552

Danos O, Mulligan RC (1988): Safe and efficient generation of recombinant retroviruses with amphotropic and ecotropic host ranges. *Proc Natl Acad Sci USA* 85:6460-6464

Dichek DA, Nussbaum O, Degen SJ, Anderson WF (1991): Enhancement of the fibrinolytic activity of sheep endothelial cells by retroviral vector-mediated gene transfer. *Blood* 77:533-541

Dichek DA, Neville RF, Zwiebel JA, Freeman SM, Leon MB, Anderson WF (1989): Seeding of intravascular stents with genetically engineered endothelial cells. *Circulation* 80:1347-1353

Elices MJ, Osborn L, Takada Y, Crouse C, Luhowskyj S, Hemler ME, Lobb RR (1990): VCAM-1 on activated endothelium interacts with the leukocyte inegrin VLA-4 at a site distinct from the VLA-4/fibronectin binding site. *Cell* 60:577-584

Ellis SG, Roubin GS, Wilentz J, Douglas Jr JS, King SB (1989): Effect of 18 to 24-hour heparin administration for prevention of restenosis after uncomplicated coronary angioplasty. *Am Heart J* 117:777-782

Ellis SG, de Cesare NB, Pinkerton CA, Whitlow P, King SB, Ghazzel ZM, Kerelakes DJ, Popma JJ, Menke KK, Topol EJ (1991): Relation of stenosis morphology and clinical presentation to the procedural results of directional coronary atherectomy. *Circulation* 84:644-653

Ernstoff MS, Trautman T, Davis CA, Reich SD, Witman P, Balser J, Rudnick S, Kirkwood JM (1987): A randomized phase I/II study of continuous versus intermittent intravenous interferon gamma in patients with metastatic melanoma. *J Clin Oncol* 5:1804-1810

Esmon CT (1987): The regulation of natural anticoagulant pathways. *Science* 235:1348-1352

Fearon ER, Pardoll DM, Itaya T, Golumbek P, Levitsky HI, Simons JW, Karasuyama H, Vogelstein B, Frost P (1990): Interleukin-2 production by tumor cells bypasses T helper function in the generation of an antitumor response. *Cell* 60:397-403

Felgner PL, Ringold GM (1989): Cationic liposome-mediated transfection. *Nature* 337:387-388

Felgner PL, Holm M, Chan H (1989): Cationic liposome mediated transfection. *Proc West Pharmacol Soc* 32:115-121

Felgner PL, Gadek TR, Holm M, Roman R, Chan HW, Wenz M, Northrop JP, Ringold GM, Danielsen M (1987): Lipofection: a highly efficient, lipid-mediated DNA-transfection procedure. *Proc Natl Acad Sci USA* 84:7413-7417

Foon KA, Sherwin SA, Abrams PG, Longo DL, Fer MF, Stevenson HC, Ochs JJ, Bottino GC, Schoenberger CS, Zeffren J (1984): Treatment of advanced non-Hodkin's lymphoma with recombinant leukocyte A interferon. *N Engl J Med* 311:1148-1152

Fourrier JL, Bertrand ME, q Auth DC, Lablanche JM, Gommeauz A, Bertrand JM (1989): Percutaneous coronary rotational angioplasty in humans: preliminary report. *J Am Coll Cardiol* 14:1278-1282

Furchgott RF, Zawadzki JV (1980): The obligatory role of endothelial cells in the relaxation of arterial smooth muscle by acetylcholine. *Nature* 288:373-376

Gansbacher B, Zier K, Daniels B, Cronin K, Banner R, Gilboa E (1990a): Interleukin 2 gene transfer into tumor cells abrogates tumorigenicity and induces protective immunity. *J Exp Med* 172:1217-1224

Gansbacher B, Bannerji R, Daniels B, Zier K, Cronin K, Gilboa E (1990b): Retroviral vector-mediated g-interferon gene transfer into tumor cells generates potent and long lasting antitumor immunity. *Cancer Res* 50:7820-7825

Gao X, Huang L (1991): A novel cationic liposome reagent for efficient transfection of mammalian cells. *Biochem Biophys Res Commun* 179:280-285

Grimm EA, Mazumder A, Zhang HZ, Rosenberg SA (1982): Lymphokine-activated killer cell phenomenon: Lysis of natural killer-resistant fresh solid tumor cells by interleukin-2-activated autologous human peripheral blood lymphocytes. *J Exp Med* 155:1823-1841

Gruntzig AR, Senning A, Siegenthaler WE (1977): Nonoperative dilatation of coronary-artery stenosis: percutaneous transluminal coronary angioplasty. *N Engl J Med* 301:61-68

Heldin CH, Westermark B, Wasteson A (1981): Specific receptors for platelet-derived growth factor on cells derived from connective tissue and glia. *Proc Natl Acad Sci USA* 78:3664-3668

Hellstrom KE, Hellstrom I (1991): Principles of Tumor Immunity: Tumor Antigens. In *Biologic Therapy of Cancer*. VT DeVita Jr., S Hellman, SA Rosenberg, editors. J.B. Lippincott Co., Philadelphia. 35-52

Herberman RB (1986): Natural killer cells. *Annu Rev Med* 37:347-352

Herr HW, Laudone VP, Whitmore Jr WF (1987): An overview of intravesical therapy for superficial bladder tumors. *J Urol* 138:1363-1368

Holt CI, Garlick N, Cornel E (1990): Lipofection of cDNAs in the mbryonic vertebrate central nervous system. *Neuron* 4:203-214

Jaffe HA, Danel C, Longenecker G, Metzger M, Setoguchi Y, Rosenfeld MA, Gant TW, Thorgeirsson SS, Stratford-Perricaudet LD, Perricaudet M, Pavirani A, Lecocq JP, Crystal RG (1992): Adenovirus-mediated in vivo gene transfer and expression in normal rat liver. *Nature genetics* 1:372-378

Jardetzky TS, Lane WS, Robinson RA, Madden DR, Wiley DC (1991): Identification of self peptides bound to purified HLA-B27. *Nature* 353:326-329

Johansson SR, Lamm C, Bondjers G, Emanuelsson H, Hjalmarson A (1990): Role of beta-adrenergic blockers after percutaneous transluminal coronary angioplasty. *Am Heart J* 66:915-920

Knuth A, Wolfel T, Klehmann E, Boon T, Meyer zum Buschenfelde KH (1989): Cytolytic T-cell clones against an autologous human melanoma: Specificity study and definition of three antigens by immunoselection. *Proc Natl Acad Sci USA* 86:2804-2808

Lim CS, Chapman GD, Gammon RS, Muhlestein JB, Bauman RP, Stack RS, Swain JL (1991): Direct in vivo gene transfer into the coronary and peripheral vasculatures of the intact dog. *Circulation* 83:2007-2011

Lin H, Parmacek MS, Morle G, Bolling S, Leiden JM (1990): Expression of recombinant genes in myocardium in vivo after direct injection of DNA. *Circulation* 82:2217-2221

Lindahl KF, Wilson DB (1977): Histocompatibility antigen-activated cytotoxic T lymphocytes I. Estimates of the absolute frequency of killer cells generated in vitro. *J Exp Med* 145:500-522

Liu D, Mori A, Huang L (1992): Role of liposome size and RES blockade in controlling biodistribution and tumor uptake of GM1-containing liposomes. *Biochim Biophys Acta* 1104:95-101

Lotze MT, Grimm EA, Mazumder A, Strausser JL, Rosenberg SA (1981): Lysis of fresh and cultured autologous tumor by human lymphocytes cultured in T-cell growth factor. *Cancer Res* 41:4420-4425

Lotze MT, Matory YL, Rayner AA, Ettinghausen SE, Vetto JT, Seipp CA, Rosenberg SA (1986): Clinical effects and toxicity of interleukin-2 in patients with cancer. *Cancer* 58:2764-2772

Lotze MT, Matory YL, Ettinghausen SE, Rayner AA, Sharrow SO, Seipp CA, Custer MC, Rosenberg SA (1985): In vivo administration of purified human interleukin-2. II. Half-life, immunologic effects, and expansion of peripheral lymphoid cells in vivo with IL-2. *J Immunol* 135:2865-2875

Lynch CM, Clowes MM, Osborne WR, Clowes AW, Miller AD (1992): Long-term expression of human adenosine deaminase in vascular smooth muscle cells of rats: a model for gene therapy. *Proc Natl Acad Sci USA* 89:1138-1142

Miller AD (1990): Retrovirus packaging cells. *Hum Gene Ther* 1:5-14

Morton DL, Eilber FR, Malmgren RA, Wood WC (1970): Immunological factors which influence response of immunotherapy in malignant melanoma. *Surgery* 68:158-164

Nabel EG, Gordon D, Xang ZY, Xu L, San H, Plautz GE, Gao X, Huang L, Nabel GJ (1992a): Gene transfer in vivo with DNA-liposome complexes: lack of autoimmunity and gonadal localization. *Hum Gene Ther* 3:649-656

Nabel EG, Plautz G, Nabel GJ (1990): Site-specific gene expression in vivo by direct gene transfer into the arterial wall. *Science* 249:1285-1288

Nabel EG, Plautz G, Nabel GJ (1992b): Transduction of a foreign histocompatibility gene into the arterial wall induces vasculitis. *Proc Natl Acad Sci USA* 89:5157-5161

Nabel EG, Plautz G, Boyce FM, Stanley JC, Nabel GJ (1989): Recombinant gene expression in vivo within endothelial cells of the arterial wall. *Science* 244:1342-1344

Nabel EG, Liptay S, Yang Z, Gordon D, Haudenschild C, Nabel GJ (1993): Recombinant platelet-derived growth factor b gene expression in porcine arteries induces intimal hyperplasia in vivo. *J Clin Invest* 91:1822-1829

Nabel EG, Yang Z, Plautz G, Forough R, Zhan X, Haudenschild CC, Maciag T, Nabel GJ (1992c): Recombinant fibroblast growth factor-1 gene expression in porcine arteries induced intimal hyperplasia and angiogenesis in vivo. *Nature* 362:844-846

Nabel GJ, Chang A, Nabel EG, Plautz G, Fox BA, Huang L, Shu S (1992d): Clinical protocol. Immunotherapy of malignancy by in vivo gene transfer into tumors. *Hum Gene Ther* 3:399-410

Nobuyoshi M, Kimura T, Nosaka H, Mioka S, Ueno K, Yokoi H, Hamasaki N, Horiuchi H, Ohishi H (1988): Restenosis after successful percutaneous transluminal coronary angioplasty: serial angiographic follow-up of 229 patients. *J Am Coll Cardiol* 12:616-623

Osborn L, Hession C, Tizard R, Vassallo C, Luhowskyj S (1989): Direct expression of cloning of vascular cell adhesion molecule 1, a cytokine-induced endothelial protein that binds to lymphocytes. *Cell* 59:1203-12011

Palella TD, Hidaka Y, Silverman LJ, Levine M, Glorioso J, Kelly WN (1989): Expression of human HPRT mRNA in brains of mice infected with a recombinant herpes simplex virus-1 vector. *Gene* 80:137-144

Palmer RM, Ferrige AG, Moncada S (1987): Nitric oxide release accounts for the biological activity of endothelium-derived relaxing factor. *Nature* 327:524-526

Pepine CJ, Hirshfeld JW, MacDonald RG, Henderson MA, Bass TA, Goldberg S, Savage MP, Vetrovec G, Cowley M, Taussig AS (1990): A controlled trial of corticosteroids to prevent restenosis after coronary angioplasty. *Circulation* 81:1753-1761

Perez R, Lipton A, Harvey HA, Simmonds MA, Romano PJ, Imboden SL, Giudice G, Downing MR, Alton NK (1988): A phase I trial of recombinant human gamma interferon (IKFN-g4A) in patients with advanced malignancy. *J Biol Response Modif* 7:309-317

Plautz GE, Yang ZY, Gao X, Haung L, Nabel GJ (1993): Immunotherapy of malignancy by in vivo gene transfer into tumors. *Proc Natl Acad Sci USA* 90:4645-4649

Plautz G, Nabel EG, Nabel GJ (1991): Introduction of vascular smooth muscle cells expressing recombinant genes in vivo. *Circulation* 83:578-583

Price J, Turner D, Cepko C (1987): Lineage analysis in the vertebrate nervous system by retrovirus-mediated gene transfer. *Proc Natl Acad Sci USA* 84:156-160

Quesada JR, Reuben J, Manning JT, Hersh EM, Gutterman JU (1984): Alpha interferon for induction of remission in hairy-cell leukemia. *N Engl J Med* 310:15-18

Restifo NP, Spiess PJ, Karp SE, Mule JJ, Rosenberg SA (1992): A nonimmunogenic sarcoma transduced with the cDNA for interferon γ elicits CD8+T cells against the wild-type tumor: correlation with antigen presentation capability. *J Exp Med* 175:1423-1431

Roberts W, Potkin B, Solus D, Reddy S (1990): Mode of death, frequency of healed and acute myocardial infarction, number of major epicardial coronary arteries severely narrowed by atherosclerotic plaque and heart weight in fatal atherosclerotic coronary artery disease: analysis of 889 patients studied at necropsy. *J Am Coll Cardiol* 15:196-203

Rodgers GM (1988): Hemostatic properties of normal and perturbed vascular cells. *FASEB J* 2:116-123

Rosenberg SA, Spiess P, Lafreniere R (1986): A new approach to the adoptive immunotherapy of cancer with tumor infiltrating lymphocytes. *Science* 233:1318-1321

Rosenfeld MA, Yoshimura K, Trapnell BC, Yoneyama K, Rosenthal ER, Dalemans W, Fukayama M, Bargon J, Stier LE, Stratford-Perricaudet L, et al. (1992): In vivo transfer of the human cystic fibrosis transmembrane conductance regulator gene to the airway epithelium. *Cell* 68:143-155

Rosenfeld MA, Siegfried W, Yoshimura K, Yoneyama K, Fukayama M, Stier LE, Paakko PK, Gilardi P, Stratford-Perricaudet LD, Perricaudet M, et al. (1991): Adenovirus-mediated transfer of a recombinant alpha 1-antitrypsin gene to the lung epithelium in vivo. *Science* 252:431-434

Rothbaum D, Linnemeier T, Landin R, Morgan S (1991): Eximer laser coronary angioplasty: angiographic restenosis rate at 6 month follow-up. *J Am Coll Cardiol* 17:205A

Safian RD, Gelbfish JS, Erny RE, Schnitt SJ, Schmidt DA, Baim DS (1990): Coronary atherectomy. Clinical, angiographic, and histologic findings and observations regarding potential mechanisms. *Circulation* 82:69-79

Samulski RJ, Zhu X, Xiao X, Brook JD, Housman DE, Epstein N, Hunter LA (1991): Targeted integration of adeno-associated virus (AAV) into human chromosome 19 [published erratum appears in EMBO J 1992 Mar;11(3):1228]. *EMBO J* 10:3941-3950

Schwartz L, Bourassa MG, Lesperance J, Aldridge HE, Kazim F, Salvatori VA, Henderson M, Bonan R, David PR (1988): Aspirin and dipyridamole in the prevention of restenosis after percutaneous transluminal coronary angioplasty. *N Engl J Med* 318:1714-1719

Sigwart U, Puel J, Mirkovitch V, Joffre F, Kappenberger L (1987): Intravascular stents to prevent occlusion and restenosis after transluminal angioplasty. *N Engl J Med* 316:701-706

Skinner MA, Marbrook J (1976): An estimation of the frequency of precursor cells which generate cytotoxic lymphocytes. *J Exp Med* 143:1562-1567

Spears JR, Reyes VP, Wynne J, Fromm BS, Sinofsky EL,,rus S, Sinclair IN, Hopkins BE, Schwartz L, Aldridge HE (1993): Percutaneous coronary laser balloon angioplasty: initial results of a multicenter experience. *J Am Coll Cardiol* 16:293-303

Spiess PJ, Yang JC, Rosenberg SA (1987): In vivo antitumor activity of tumor-infiltrating lymphocytes expanded in recombinant interleukin-2. *J Natl Cancer Inst* 79:1067-1075

Stewart MJ, Plautz GE, Del Buono L, Yang ZY, Xu L, Gao X, Huang L, Nabel EG, Nabel GJ (1992): Gene transfer in vivo with DNA-liposome complexes: safety and acute toxicity in mice. *Hum Gene Ther* 3:267-275

Tepper RI, Pattengale PK, Leder P (1989): Murine interleukin-4 displays potent anti-tumor activity in vivo. *Cell* 57:503-512

Townsend A, Bodmer H (1989): Antigen recognition by Class I-restricted T lymphocytes. *Ann Rev Immunol* 7:601-624

van der Bruggen P, Traversari C, Chomez P, Lurquin C, De Plaen E, Van den

Eynde B, Kuth A, Boon T (1991): A gene encoding an antigen recognized by cytolytic T lymphocytes on a human melanoma. *Science* 254:1643-1647

Wilson JM, Birinyi LK, Salomon RN, Libby P, Callow AD, Mulligan RC (1989): Implantation of vascular grafts lined with genetically modified endothelial cells. *Science* 244:1344-1346

Wolff JA, Malone RW, Williams P, Chong W, Acsadi G, Jani A, Felgner P (1990): Direct gene transfer into mouse muscle in vivo. *Science* 247:1465-1468

Wu GY, Wu CH (1987): Receptor-mediated in vitro gene transformation by a soluble DNA carrier system. *J Biol Chem* 262:4429-4432

Yron I, Wood TA, Spiess PJ, Rosenberg SA (1980): In vitro growth of murine T cells. V. The isolation and growth of lymphoid cells infiltrating syngeneic solid tumors. *J Immunol* 125:238-245

GENE THERAPY FOR ARTHRITIS

Christopher H. Evans and Paul D. Robbins

INTRODUCTION: WHY GENE THERAPY FOR ARTHRITIS?

Arthritis is the most frequently reported chronic condition among American females, and the second most frequently reported overall (Praemer et al., 1992; Yelin,
1992). Although arthritis rarely kills, chronic rheumatoid arthritis (RA) is associated with lower life expectancy (Pincus and Callahan, 1992) and a dramatically
impaired quality of life. Over 30 million Americans suffer from this disease, a
number which will increase as the greying of society continues. Approximately
50% of those over the age of 65 years have arthritis; according to the National
Center for Health Statistics (1987), arthritis is more common than hypertension,
hearing impairment and heart conditions among this age group.

Despite an extensive rheumatologic armamentarium and a number of surgical
options, arthritis remains incurable. Consequently, joint replacement surgery becomes the final recourse for many patients. By 1988, out of a total of 1.3 million
Americans having prosthetic joints, 778,000 artificial joints had been implanted as
a result of arthritis (Praemer et al., 1992).

Statistics such as these serve to illustrate the pressing and widespread need for
improved treatments of arthritis. The failure of traditional ways of dealing with
this disease encourages the pursuit of novel, experimental modalities. With the
exception of familial osteoarthritis (OA) (Ala-kokko et al., 1990), arthritis is probably not a genetic disease. Nevertheless, we have proposed gene therapy as a new
approach to treating this disease (Bandara et al., 1992a). In this context, we envisage the use of gene transfer techniques as delivery systems for anti-arthritic proteins. Our present emphasis is on the delivery of genes to synovium. The properties
of this interesting tissue have been reviewed recently by Simkin (1992) and Hung
and Evans (1994).

Drug delivery is one of the major weaknesses of existing anti-arthritic therapeutics. Whether the therapeutic agent is administered orally or by s.c., i.p., i.m.,
or i.v. injection, its delivery to the joint relies upon the vascular perfusion of the
synovium (Hung and Evans, 1994). Drugs carried within the synovial capillaries
diffuse passively via the synovium into the joint cavity and thence the articular
cartilage, an avascular tissue. The absence of any pumping mechanism or other
means of selectively transporting solutes from the synovial capillaries into the

Gene Therapeutics: Methods and Applications of Direct Gene Transfer
Jon A. Wolff, Editor • ©1994 *Birkhäuser Boston*

joint limits the efficiency of this process. Furthermore, as the vascularity of synovium falls markedly in chronic RA (Stevens et al., 1991), drug delivery becomes even less efficient in the very joints where it is most needed. These problems are compounded by the rapid clearance of materials from the joint space. Thus, although direct intra-articular injection obviates the above limitations to drug delivery, its usefulness is severely reduced by the short intraarticular half-life of most materials. (Fig. 1A).

These inefficiencies presently require the repeated, systemic administration of large concentrations of anti-arthritic drugs in order to achieve stable, therapeutic levels within the joint. Exposure of non-target tissues in this way exacerbates the tendency, for which anti-arthritic drugs are already notorious, to produce unpleasant side effects. Delivery problems also limit the chemical range of useful drugs to small, diffusible molecules. This excludes most proteins from serious consideration, an omission which becomes all the more glaring as recent research identifies increasing numbers of proteins with potential anti-arthritic properties (see section III).

Finally, we draw attention to the chronicity of arthritis; it is a disease that can last for decades, if not a lifetime. The ideal treatment should have a matching chronicity of effect. If a drug cannot be administered orally, present delivery strategies require frequent injection. In terms of unpleasantness, repeated injection becomes undesirable in the order i.a.>i.v.>i.p.>i.m.>s.c. Although diabetics adapt to daily self-injection of insulin, one clinical trial in which arthritic patients were required to self-administer the drug by s.c. injection (Lebsack et al., 1991) suffered a high drop-out rate. Patient compliance can even be problematic when an orally active agent is available.

To address these issues, we have proposed inserting into the synovial lining of arthritic joints, genes which code for therapeutic proteins (Fig. 1B). Such a system would solve the targeting problem, as the joint itself would now be the site of synthesis of the drug. Side effects should be greatly reduced, as the highest concentration of the gene product would be within the joint. In addition, the stable insertion and expression of these genes would ensure a long-lasting effect; indeed, it may prove possible to maintain and express the therapeutic genes for the lifetime of the patient, in which case the treatment becomes effectively a cure. Under these circumstances, regulated, rather than constitutive, expression of the therapeutic genes would permit its downregulation during periods of remission.

As an additional advantage, this type of gene therapy can exploit the tremendous potential that many proteins have as anti-arthritic agents. Not only are proteins difficult to deliver to joints, but those with the most promising therapeutic.properties are.outrageously expensive. Because a gene can be transcribed and translated many millions of times into the protein for which it codes, and because genes are metabolically more stable than most proteins, the cost of a therapeutic gene is intrinsically far less than the cost of its corresponding protein. These arguments in support of a gene therapy treatment for arthritis are summarized in Table 1.

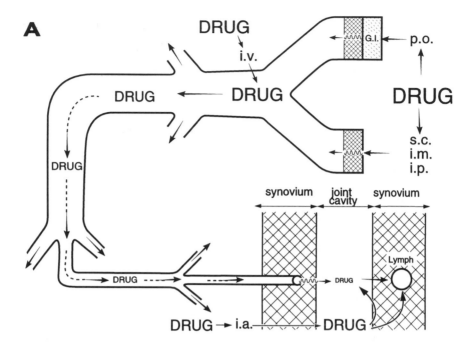

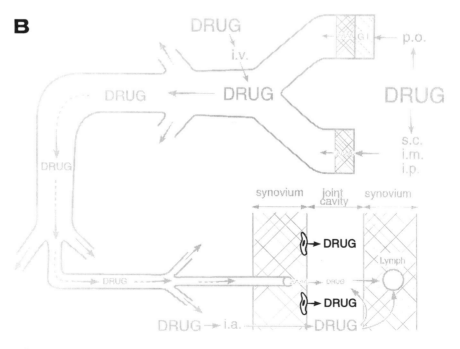

FIGURE 1. See figure legend, opposite page.

TRANSFERRING GENES TO JOINTS

Two approaches for transfer of therapeutic genes to the synovial lining of the joint have been proposed for local gene therapy of connective tissue diseases (Bandara et al., 1992a; Bandara et al., 1993; Evans et al., 1992). These two methods involve an in vivo or direct approach and an ex vivo or indirect approach to gene delivery within the joint. The ex vivo approaches involves the removal of cells from the synovium and their subsequent propagation in culture. The therapeutic gene is then delivered by viral or non-viral means and the genetically altered cells are subsequently reintroduced into the synovium by intraarticular injection (Evans et al., 1992). The in vivo approach involves the direct transfer of genes to the synovial lining by injection of the appropriate vector directly into the joint cavity where it can come in contact with the synovial lining. The in vivo method is technically simple, but it may be difficult to regulate the efficiency of transduction and the level of gene expression. The ex vivo method is more technically complex, but it is potentially easier to regulate the level of transduction as well as the level of expression. A number of viral and nonviral vectors are particularly suited for either the ex vivo and/or the in vivo methods. A brief description of the vectors that can be used to deliver therapeutic genes to synovial cells will be presented and their advantages and disadvantages for gene therapy for connective tissue diseases discussed (see Table 2).

Retroviral vectors

The best characterized viral vector for gene transfer is the retroviral vector derived from Moloney Murine Leukemia Virus (MoMLV), approved for gene therapy for ADA-deficiencies and immunotherapy for AIDS and cancer (for reviews see, Mulligan, 1991; Miller, 1992). The MoMLV retroviral particle contains two copies of a RNA genome encapsulated into a virus capsid. Upon infection of the target cell, mediated by an interaction between the viral envelope protein and a specific receptor protein, the RNA is uncoated and reverse transcribed in the cytoplasm by

FIGURE 1. How drugs get into joints. (A) Following oral administration, the drug encounters the acidic conditions of the stomach and the diffuses via the wall of the G.I. into the blood. Drugs delivered by s.c., i.m., or i.p. injection avoid the G.I., and enter the blood by diffusing through surrounding tissue. Direct i.v. injection avoids both the G.I. and tissue barriers to the blood stream. On its way to the synovial capillaries the drug is diluted and substantial amounts are diverted into the systemic circulation. Drugs diffuse from the synovial capillaries into the joint from which they are rapidly cleared. Intraarticular injection avoids delivery problems, but the injected drug is still rapidly removed from the joint space. Repeated i.a. injection is not a reasonable clinical option. (B) To circumvent the problems indicated in (A) above, we have proposed using gene transfer technology to insert genes which code for therapeutic proteins directly into the synovial lining cells. In this way, the synovium becomes the site of sustained synthesis of the drug.

a virally encoded reverse transcriptase. The resulting double-stranded DNA is then transported to the nucleus where it integrates stably into the host genome. The stably integrated genome is transcribed and the viral-specific proteins are then used to package the RNA into virions that are released by budding. MoMLV normally encodes three proteins termed gag, pol, and env that are required in trans for viral replication. However, if the three proteins are provided in trans, only the long terminal repeats (LTR), and a packaging sequence (psi) are required in cis for viral replication. Therefore, genes of interest can be inserted into the virus in place of gag pol and env so that the therapeutic gene is expressed from the viral long terminal repeat (LTR). Alternatively, a heterologous promoter can be inserted so that an internal promoter drives expression of the therapeutic gene. Infectious recombinant viruses can be produced by the introduction of the recombinant provirus into a packaging cell line that expresses, in trans, the retroviral proteins required for encapsulation of the RNA into virions.

We have used retroviral vectors extensively for gene delivery to synovial cells. A simplified retroviral vector termed MFG (P.D.R., B. Guild, and R. C. Mulligan, unpublished; Ohashi et al., 1992; Ferry et al., 1992; Bandara et al., 1993) that expresses the cDNA of interest from the LTR was used to express the IL-1 receptor antagonist protein (IL-1ra or IRAP; Arend, 1991), a protein that is potentially therapeutic for arthritis (Schwab et al., 1991). The vector has been constructed so that the ATG of the therapeutic gene is fused to the ATG of the viral envelope gene, resulting in a chimeric RNA that resembles the normal spliced message of the envelope gene (MFG-IRAP; Fig. 2). A high titer amphotropic CRIP producer was generated with MFG-IRAP and used to infect primary synovial cells in culture. A similar virus expressing the LacZ marker gene (MFG-LacZ; Fig. 2) was also used to determine the efficiency of synovial cell infection. Approximately 20% of the

---

TABLE 1. How gene therapy overcomes problems with traditional methods of drug delivery.

TRADITIONAL METHODS	GENE THERAPY
Targeting difficult	Once gene in place, no targeting problems
Side effects high	Side effects minimized
Short lasting effect; frequent administration	Long lasting effect, infrequent administration (potentially only once)
Not easily adapted to deliver proteins as drugs	Proteins are the active gene products

primary synovial cells could be infected with the MFG-LacZ amphotropic virus having a NIH 3T3 cell titer of 10^6. Moreover, MFG-IRAP infected synovial cells produced 100-300 ng of IRAP per 10^6 cells per 24 hours. Analysis of synovial fluid of rabbits transplanted with autologous synovial cells infected with the MFG-IRAP virus has detected expression of IRAP for at least one month. These results are described in greater detail in section IV.

Our results demonstrate that rabbit synovial cells can be readily infected in culture with retroviral vectors and high levels of the therapeutic proteins can be obtained in vitro and in vivo. The disadvantage of retroviral vectors is that they can only be used to infect dividing cells and thus may not be applicable to the in vivo approach to synovial cell gene transfer. However, it is possible that in the arthritic joint synovial cells, which normally would be nondividing (Coulton et al., 1980), may be dividing at a rate that will permit efficient retroviral infection. Experiments to determine whether retroviral infection can be obtained by co-injecting cytokines which provoke synovial cell division are currently being performed.

TABLE 2. Viral and Nonviral Systems for Gene Transfer to Synovium.

VIRUS VECTORS	NONVIRUS METHODS
Retrovirus[A]	Calcium Phosphate[C]
Adenovirus[A]	Electroporation[C]
Adeno-associated Virus[A]	DEAE-Dextran[C]
Herpes Simplex Virus[A]	Polybrene[D]
SV40[B]	Liposomes [C,E]
Polyoma Virus[B]	Protoplast Fusion[D]
Papilloma Virus[B]	Microinjection[D]
Picornavirus[B]	Polysine/DNA conjugates[D] Naked DNA[E]

[A] Demonstrated to infect rabbit synovial cells in culture.
[B] Not tested for ability to infect synovial cells.
[C] Demonstrated to transfect type B synovial cells in culture.
[D] Not tested for ability to transfect synovial cells.
[E] Demonstrated to transfect type A cells in vivo.

    Given that multiple joints are affected in certain connective tissue diseases, it may be necessary to express a therapeutic product systemically. One target tissue used for systemic delivery is the bone marrow, where either the stem cell or more differentiated cell types such as T-cells can be transduced. Retroviruses have been successfully utilized for the introduction of therapeutic genes into mouse stem cells that are then used to reconstitute an irradiated mouse recipient (Ohashi et al., 1992). We have efficiently infected mouse stem cells with the MFG-IRAP virus and generated long-term reconstituted mice with the infected cells. The mice are constitutively producing high levels of IL-1 receptor antagonist in their serum at thirteen months post-transplant without deleterious affects to their immune system. The IRAP-expressing mice are currently being tested in a mouse model for arthritis to determine if they are resistant to the onset and progression of the disease (See following section). If the results prove promising, it will be worth examining more clinically acceptable routes of systemic delivery. Candidates include transduction of cells in peripheral blood, such as the CD34[+] population, myoblasts, and direct i.m. injection of plasmid DNA (Wolff et al., 1990; Wolff, 1994).

DNA vectors

A number of DNA viruses have been modified so that they can be used as vectors to deliver therapeutic genes to cells, as summarized in Table 2. These viruses included SV40, polyoma, bovine and human papilloma viruses, adenovirus, adeno-associated virus, herpes simplex viruses, and vaccinia viruses (See Table 2). Although only adenovirus has been approved for human gene therapy experiments, it is possible that other DNA viruses will be utilized in the future in clinical trials. Adenovirus is advantageous in that it has a wide host range and is able to infect nondividing cells. It has been modified so that genes can be inserted into the E1A region of the virus where they are efficiently expressed after viral infection (Rosenfeld et al., 1992). An adenovirus containing the LacZ gene driven by a CMV promoter has been used to infect efficiently rabbit synovial cells in culture (our unpublished data) and thus could be applied for gene transfer in the ex vivo approach. In addition, we have recently shown that adenovirus vectors are able to infect synovial cells in vivo. However, the expression from adenovirus vectors is transient and a low level of viral proteins are also expressed in the infected cells. In an inflamed joint, the presence of viral antigens may be incompatible with treatment of the disease state.

    Adeno-associated virus (AAV) has been recently modified for use as a vector for gene transfer (Walsh et al., 1992). AAV is a single-stranded DNA virus that requires adenovirus as a helper to replicate in co-infected cells. Similar to retroviruses, the AAV-encoded rep and cap proteins that are needed for replication and packaging can be supplied in trans; only the terminal repeats of the virus are needed in cis for propagation of AAV. Various genes have been inserted into AAV under the regulation of heterologous promoters and infectious virus generated by co-transfection with a plasmid expressing cap and rep, and infection with an aden-

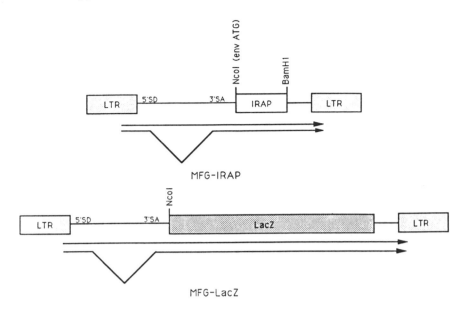

FIGURE 2. Structure of the MFG-IRAP and MFG-LacZ vectors used for infection of rabbit synovial cells. The MFG retroviral vector contains gag sequences up to a NarI site at position 1035 in MoMLV, the 3' env splice acceptor, a 5' NcoI cloning site at the env ATG, and a 3' BamHI cloning site. The therapeutic gene is inserted to that the ATG of the encoded proteins fused to the ATG of the env protein at the NcoI site. Thus the therapeutic protein is expressed from a LTR-driven, spliced message that is similar in structure to the normal env message found in MoMLV infected cells. The cDNAs for human IL-1 receptor antagonist (IRAP) and ß-galactosidase were inserted into MFG so that their initiation codons are fused to the env ATG at the NcoI site.

ovirus helper. Wild type AAV has been shown to integrate preferentially at a specific site on human chromosome 19, although recombinant AAV does not show the same specificity (Samulski et al., 1991). AAV also is thought to infect nondividing cells, making it suitable for gene transfer to synovial cells using the in vivo approach. We have generated a recombinant AAV virus able to express a neo[r] marker gene and the gene for viral IL-10, an immunosuppressive cytokine encoded by Epstein-Barr Virus. Primary synovial cells and the HIG-82 line of lapine synoviocytes cells (Georgescu et al., 1988) can be infected with this virus in culture and G418-resistant cells selected that express high levels of active vIL-10. However, the inability to generate a high titer virus stock has so far precluded analysis of the ability of AAV to infect synovial cells in vivo.

Herpes Simplex viruses (HSV) are large DNA viruses that can infect, and are found in, neuronal cells in humans. These viruses currently are being modified so that they can be used as vectors to transfer genetic material for human gene therapy applications (Glorioso 1994, Chapter 15). The advantages of HSV vectors are that they can carry large DNA fragments (>50 kb), have a very high titer (>10^{10}) and can infect a variety of dividing and nondividing cell types. A virus carrying a deletion in the immediate early gene ICP4 (d120; DeLuca et al., 1985) and a LacZ marker gene was used to infect rabbit synovial cells in culture. The synovial cells could be infected with the virus and express the LacZ marker, but the continued presence of the defective virus was still toxic to rabbit synoviocytes. Further inactivation of the virus, including mutations in other immediate early proteins such as ICP27 and ICP0, is required before HSV can be utilized for gene transfer to synovial cells. The ability to generate high titers make a non-toxic, defective HSV a potential vector for gene delivery to synovium in vivo.

Other DNA viruses have also been used as vectors for gene delivery including papilloma viruses, SV40, polyoma, and vaccinia. Of these viruses, the ones potentially suitable for gene delivery to synovial cells using the indirect, ex vivo approach are the papilloma viruses. These viruses establish themselves as stable, episomal elements in infected cells and continue to replicate and express genes for the life span of the cell. Although the papilloma viruses have been shown to be transforming in culture, the virally encoded proteins responsible for viral replication, E1 and E2, that are distinct from the transforming proteins, and the cis-acting origin of replication have been identified (Yang et al. 1991). It should be possible in the near future to generate modified viruses or DNA vectors that can replicate episomally using the E1 and E2 proteins of bovine papilloma virus and/or human papilloma virus (HPV) in combination with its origin of replication. Given that HPV normally replicates in human skin fibroblasts, it is likely that HPV would be able to replicate efficiently and stably in human synovial fibroblasts.

Non viral vectors

A variety of chemical methods for introducing DNA into cells are available and are summarized in Table 2. These include calcium phosphate precipitation (Chang 1984), DEAE Dextran, electroporation, lipofection, protoplast fusion, and ligand/ DNA conjugates. In addition, direct microinjection of DNA directly into the cells is an efficient way to introduce DNA (Capecchi, 1980). The majority of these techniques are designed for introducing DNA into cells in culture and therefore are suitable for the ex vivo method for gene delivery to synovial cells. Of these different methods, the most efficient for introduction of DNA into synovial cells, as determined by our laboratory, has been lipofection utilizing a DC cholesterol form of cationic liposomes (Gao and Huang, 1991). Using the appropriate ratio of a CMV-LacZ marker DNA to liposome, approximately 20% of cultured synovial cells can be transfected. However, the expression is transient so LacZ expression is lost if the cells are maintained in culture.

The transfer of genes to cells in vivo using liposome-mediated delivery has been demonstrated in several systems (Singhal and Huang, 1994). In particular, the DC chol liposomes efficiently transfer DNA to melanoma cells, resulting in expression of a HLA B7 gene in the transfected cells (Nabel et al, 1993). We have used the DC chol liposome to deliver LacZ and IL-1β expression vectors to synovial cells in vivo by injection of the complex intraarticularly. Interestingly, the type A synovial macrophage is predominately LacZ positive in these in vivo liposome experiments compared to the type B fibroblast that was so efficiently transfected in culture. However, the ability to transfect type A synovial cells efficiently in vivo still allowed for expression of biologically active IL-1β in the joint, resulting in a stimulation in cellular infiltrate and cartilage breakdown in the transfected rabbit knee (our unpublished data). Thus liposomes may be applicable to both the in vivo and ex vivo approaches to synovial cell gene transfer.

One difficulty with the non-viral methods of gene transfer such as the use of cationic liposomes is that only a percentage of the transferred DNA actually makes it to the nucleus and is expressed; moreover the expression is transient. Approaches to circumvent this problem involve the use of stronger promoters, or modified expression systems, inclusion of chemicals to facilitate release of the DNA from the lysosome, or approaches to increase the frequency of stable integration. To increase expression, methodologies designed to allow for expression of the therapeutic gene in the cytoplasm are currently being designed. The bacteriophage T7 polymerase has been demonstrated to be transcriptionally active in mammalian cells in the cytoplasm. The use of T7 polymerase-dependent promoter in conjunction with a plasmid expressing T7 polymerase also from a T7 promoter, should allow for sustained expression in the cytoplasm. Preliminary experiments have shown that expression from the T7-driven system does indeed result in high sustained levels of IRAP expression in liposome transfected synovial cells in culture (our unpublished data).

As an alternate approach to obtaining high and stable levels of expression after transfection, plus-strand picornaviruses are currently being modified so that they can be used to express a therapeutic gene as well as continue to express the viral proteins required for replication of the RNA in the cytoplasm. In this manner, it may be possible to maintain indefinitely a self-replicating RNA encoding a therapeutic gene. In addition, the utilization of the integration systems of certain viruses, such as that from AAV, may be utilized in the transfection system to increase the percentage of the transfected DNA that is stably integrated into the host genome. These methods may allow for high levels and longer-term expression of therapeutic genes after liposome-mediated transfection in the synovial cells.

In addition to the use of chemical means to introduce DNA, conjugates between DNA, polylysine and specific antibodies or DNA conjugated to specific receptor binding proteins such as asialoglycoproteins can be formed (Wu 1994; Singhal and Huang 1994). In this manner, the DNA can be targeted to cells that express a cell-specific surface protein recognized by the antibody or protein. In addition, complexes containing poly-lysine, DNA and inactivated adenovirus can be used (Wagner et al., 1992; Curiel 1994). It has been demonstrated that the presence of the adenovirus facilitates the uptake and uncoating of the DNA in the lysosome after internalization. These methodologies may be readily applied to gene transfer to the synovial lining by intraarticular injection of the complexes. Surprisingly, we have also demonstrated that naked DNA itself can be taken up and expressed by what appears to be type A synovial cells in vivo. Intraarticular injection of a LacZ expression vector DNA results in blue-staining type A synovial macrophage cells. Moreover, injection of an IL-1β expression vector DNA alone into the joint results in IL-1β expression and an increase in the level of cellular infiltrate. However, the level of expression and cellular infiltrate detected after injection with naked DNA was far less than that observed for the DNA-liposome complexes (our unpublished data). The observation that the synovial macrophages can be transfected by naked DNA in vivo is similar to what has been observed for myoblasts in vivo (Wolff et al., 1990).

WHICH GENES ARE ANTI-ARTHRITIC?

Two main pathologies afflict the joint during arthritis. One is inflammation, which occurs as a synovitis and a voluminous, cellular, effusion. The other is breakdown of the articular cartilage. These can occur in the same joint, as in RA, or independently from each other. In OA, for example, extensive destruction of the cartilages is associated with little or no inflammation. Patients with lupus, on the other hand, suffer inflammation of the joints without cartilage loss. Nearly all the pharmacologic effect has traditionally addressed the problem of inflammation, with scant attention to protecting the cartilage (chondroprotection). The flaw in this approach is reflected in its results. Despite reasonably satisfactory pharmacologic control of joint inflammation, the underlying disease process in arthritis has not been arrested. Indeed, over 90% of the reduction in RA morbidity during the last two decades has come from better surgical techniques (Paulus, 1992).

Inhibiting cartilage degradation and inflammation promises to arrest the disease process but, unless administered early, it will not repair the damage inflicted upon the joint prior to treatment. As articular cartilage has very limited reparative ability, the identification of proteins which promote cartilage regeneration is an urgent complimentary task. As discussed later, they may be the key ingredient in any gene treatment for OA.

Cytokines and cytokine inhibitors

Recent research has identified a number of cytokines as potential mediators of articular inflammation. These include interleukin-1 (IL-1), tumor necrosis factor α (TNF-α), interleukin-8 (IL-8), and transforming growth factor-β (TGF-β) (Arend and Dayer, 1990). The importance of IL-1 and TNF-α is increased by their additional ability to stimulate cartilage breakdown and inhibit cartilage repair (Saklatvala, 1986). No known other cytokines share this property, although additional ones may be identified by future research (Bandara et al., 1992b). Thus antagonists of IL-1 and TNF-α hold particular promise as anti-arthritic agents. Agents which block the biological activity of IL-1 include soluble forms of the IL-1 receptors (Dower et al., 1989) and the interleukin-1 receptor antagonist protein

(Arend, 1991). Soluble receptors presently hold the greatest promise as antagonists of TNF-α (Novick et al., 1989). Because TNF-α induces IL-1, it has been suggested that TNF-α should be the primary target of therapeutic attack.

An alternative approach to blocking directly these cytokines, is to do so indirectly using proteins with countervailing properties. For example, IL-4 and IL-10 appear to counteract the inflammatory properties of IL-1. Part of their anti-inflammatory activity may involve concomitant down regulation of IL-1 synthesis and induction of IRAP (Vannier et al., 1992).

Antagonists of articular cartilage degradation

Degradation of articular cartilage is thought to involve the extracellular digestion of the matrix by proteinases (Evans, 1991) and, perhaps, oxygen-derived free radicals such as superoxide, hydroxyl radical or nitric oxide (Stefanovic-Racic et al., 1993) and its derivatives. Antagonists of these mediators include proteinase inhibitors such as the various inhibitors of metalloproteinases (TIMPs, LIMP and IMPs), plasminogen activator inhibitors PAI-1, PAI-2, PAI-3 (Cawston et al., 1981; Apodaca et al., 1990; Hart and Fritzler, 1989) and inhibitors of cysteine proteinases. Free radical damage may be prevented by genes coding for enzymes such as superoxide dismutase, or for other proteins which serve as anti-oxidants. Cartilage repair may be stimulated by insulin-like growth factor-1 (IGF-1; Luyten et al., 1988), basic fibroblast growth factor (bFGF; Cuevas et al, 1988) and TGF-β (Morales and Roberts, 1988). Thus, depending on the type of arthritis and its severity, genes coding for one or more antiinflammatory, chondroprotective or chondroreparative protein may need to be administered. These potentially therapeutic proteins for arthritis are summarized in Table 3.

Anti-adhesion molecules

Increasing evidence implicates various types of cell surface adhesion molecule in the arthritic process. Such molecules include CD18 (Jasin et al., 1992), ICAM-1 (Iigo et al., 1991) and CD44 (Galea-Lauri et al., 1993). Genes coding for soluble forms of these molecules, or other blocking proteins, could be of future therapeutic use. These potentially therapeutic proteins for arthritis are summarized in Table 3.

EXPERIMENTAL PROGRESS

Introduction

Nearly all the present experimental data have come from studies with rabbits. Small enough to house cheaply and conveniently, yet large enough for experimental surgery, this animal has long been a favorite of orthopaedic researchers. In terms of gene transfer, the rabbits' knees are large enough both to provide sufficient synovium for the ex vivo approach, and to permit intraarticular injection of the genetically modified cells or of vectors used in the in vivo approach. As we look ahead to human trials, we can bear in mind that the rabbits' knee joint is approximately the same size as the human proximal interphalangeal joint, one of the most common sites of RA.

In order to establish some ground rules, our investigations until now have been limited to the normal knee joint. However, we will soon extend these studies to include the arthritic joint, where some of these rules may change. The only deviation from the rabbit has been to use mice for means of systemic gene delivery. This move takes advantage of the syngeneic animals that are readily available for mice, but unavailable for rabbits.

The ex vivo approach

As described in a previous section ("Transferring Genes to Joints"), this approach involves the in vitro genetic manipulation of synoviocytes prior to their transplantation to the recipient joint. There are two major classes of synoviocyte (reviewed in Hung and Evans, 1994). The type A cell closely resembles a macrophage and does not grow under standard cell culture conditions. The type B cell is fibroblastic and grows readily in vitro. However, the small size of the synovium imposes severe limits on the numbers of synoviocytes available for use. Thus we have made free use of an established line of lapine synovial fibroblasts, known as HIG-82 (Georgescu et al., 1988).

Both primary cultures of lapine synovial fibroblasts and HIG-82 cells are readily infected by amphitropic retroviruses derived from MoMLV. Two such viruses have been used to transduce synoviocytes in vitro prior to transplantation to the rabbit's knee joint. One, a BAG virus, has LacZ and neo^r genes under the regulation of the viral long terminal repeat and the SV40 early promoter, respectively. The second retrovirus, MFG, carries a cDNA coding for human IRAP (Section IIa and III) under the control of the viral LTR. Sequential infection with these two viruses produces cultures of lac Z$^+$, neo^r, IRAP$^+$ cells as indicated in Figure 3.

In a first series of experiments, such cultures were allografted to recipient knees. In the absence of any literature on the subject, we predicted that intraarticular injection of the donor cells should lead to colonization of the host synovium (Bandara et al., 1992a; Evans et al., 1992). This prediction has been confirmed in several ways. Studies with BrdU-labelled synoviocytes have identified the donor cells within the recipient synovium one week after transplant. Furthermore, colonies of LacZ$^+$, neo^r, IRAP$^+$ cells can be grown from synovia receiving transplanted, transduced (Figure 3) synoviocytes (Bandara et al., 1993). However, the longevity of the transplant is unknown.

IRAP is a secreted protein which, unlike β-galactosidase and neomycin phosphotransferase, can be detected in joint lavages. When allografted primary or HIG-82 IRAP$^+$ cells are introduced into the recipient rabbit's knee, there is an initial vigorous intraarticular production of IRAP protein. However, in vivo pro-

TABLE 3. Candidate Gene Products for Treating Arthritis.

PROTEIN	RATIONALE
IRAP/IL-1ra	Antagonize IL-1 Antiinflammatory and Chondroprotective
IL-1 soluble receptors	Antagonize IL-1 Antiinflammatory and Chondroprotective
TNF-α soluble receptors	Antagonize TNF-α Antiinflammatory and Chondroprotective
IL-4	Antiinflammatory Induces IRAP/IL-1ra
IL-10	Antiinflammatory Induces IRAP/IL-1ra
γ-IFN	Inhibits MMP induction in chondrocytes
TGF-β	Antagonizes responses of chondrocytes and synoviocytes to IL-1 Promotes cartilage matrix synthesis. Immunosuppressive but causes intraarticular inflammation
TIMPs, LIMP, IMPs	Inhibit matrix metalloproteinases
Superoxide dismutase, etc.	Antagonize oxygen-derived free radicals
Soluble ICAM-1, CD44 etc.	Block cell-cell, cell-matrix interactions
IGF-1	Promotes cartilage matrix synthesis Antagonizes catabolic effect of IL-1
bFGF	Promotes cartilage matrix synthesis

This list is illustrative, not exhaustive.

duction of IRAP is temporary and by 14 days post-transplantation neither the primary synoviocytes nor the HIG-82 cells are producing detectable levels of IRAP (Bandara et al., 1993).

Possible causes of this extinction include loss or down-regulation of the gene and loss of the transplanted cells. Both are possible. Others have noted that the expression of genes driven by viral promoters in fibroblasts in vivo is temporary. Alternatively, the cells could be lost through migration or death. The latter could involve immune recognition of the allografted cells, or their human gene product, by the host animal. We have preliminary evidence (unpublished) that immune recognition indeed occurs, a finding which contradicts the widely held belief that the joint is an immunologically privileged site. Rabbits' knees are big enough to permit the autografting of synoviocytes from one knee to the other. When immune rejection of the cells is eliminated in this way, expression of IRAP is prolonged. So far, we have succeeded in maintaining intraarticular IRAP production for 5 weeks (Fig. 4).

Although allografted cells produce IRAP intraarticularly for only 10-12 days, this provides ample opportunity to test the biological efficacy of the system. Intraarticular injection of IL-1β into the rabbit's knee elicits a well characterized series of biological responses which begin with the influx of PMNs within a few hours, and which spontaneously reverse within a few days (McDonnell et al., 1992). Using this as an assay, it has been possible to demonstrate quite clearly that transfer of the IRAP gene to the knee protects it from the deleterious effects of an intraarticular injection of human, recombinant IL-1β (Hung et al., 1993). This proof of principal encourages further development of the approach.

The in vivo approach

Synovial cell transplantation looks promising as a means of delivering genes to joints, but it is cumbersome and unsuited to mass treatment of the millions of individuals with arthritis. The in vivo approach offers to streamline gene delivery by eliminating ex vivo genetic manipulation and subsequent transplantation of the cells.

We have confirmed that retroviruses do not transduce the synovial lining cells of the normal rabbit knee following i.a. injection (our unpublished data). This presumably reflects the low mitotic rate of the cells. However, in the inflamed synovium there may be sufficient cell division to support in situ transduction in this way. As alternative transducers of the synovial lining of normal, rabbit knee joints, we are evaluating adenovirus, herpes simplex virus, adeno-associated virus and other viral vectors as well as liposomes for their ability to transfer DNA to nondividing cells (see earlier section, "Transferring Genes to Joints").

A cationic liposome "DC-chol" (Gao and Huang, 1991) has proved very effective in transferring a CMV-LacZ plasmid to cultures of synovial fibroblasts, with approximately 20% of the cells turning blue. Evaluation of in vivo efficacy has been hampered by the tendency of lapine synovium to stain positively for the

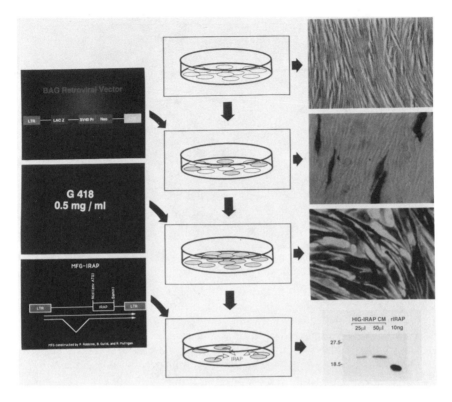

FIGURE 3. Preparation of transduced synoviocytes for ex vivo gene transfer to joints. Synovial cells are removed from the joint and placed into cell cultures (top center). No cells spontaneously express β-galactosidase (top right). Follow infection with BAG-lac Z-neo, a few percent of the cells stain positively for β-galactosidase (2nd panel, right). Addition of G418 to the culture medium (left, middle) leads to cultures where nearly all cells are lac Z⁺ (3rd panel, right). A second infection with MFG-IRAP (left, bottom) produces neoʳ, lac Z⁺, IRAP⁺ cultures (center, bottom). Western blot of conditioned medium (bottom panel, right) confirms the presence of human IRAP. This runs slower than the recombinant human IRAP used as a standard, because of glycosylation.

presence of β-galactosidase in the absence of the LacZ gene. Liposomes generate especially problematic background staining. To demonstrate unequivocally the presence of LacZ⁺ synoviocytes following in vivo transduction, it is necessary to digest the synovium with collagenase and to put the synoviocytes into cell culture. After the cells have attached and spread, they can be stained for the presence of β-galactosidase without background. Use of this tedious procedure has confirmed that cationic liposomes indeed transfer DNA to synoviocytes in vivo. Staining of the cells ex vivo in the manner described above, identifies the type A synoviocytes as the transduced cells. This is an interesting and potentially useful difference from the ex vivo method which transfers DNA to type B synoviocytes. In performing

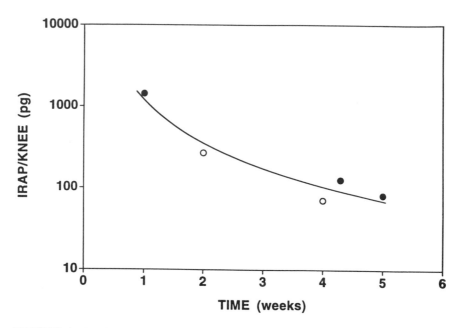

FIGURE 4. In vivo expression of IRAP as a function of time following transplant of autografted, IRAP⁺ synoviocytes. ELISA assay of joint lavages demonstrates the in vivo production of IRAP for at least 5 weeks. Reprinted with permission from Bandara et al., 1993.

the control experiments for these studies, we also noted that naked DNA had a certain ability to transduce synoviocytes in vivo. The use of liposomes to transfer the IRAP gene in this way is under investigation.

Systemic delivery

Rheumatoid arthritis is a polyarticular disease. Thus the individual transduction of each joint in the manner discussed so far is not ideally suited to this form of arthritis. Although section I discussed the side effects associated with systemic exposure to antiarthritic drugs, one potentially anti-arthritic protein, IRAP, is of such surprisingly low toxicity, that we have recently considered a more general delivery technique for this protein (Evans and Robbins, 1994a, b). Thus, as indicated in Figure 5, we are supplementing local delivery with the systemic delivery of suitable genes. Systemic delivery could involve the transduction of a variety of cells including fibroblasts, blood cells, myoblasts, and bone marrow cells.

We have recently achieved the stable introduction of a cDNA coding for IRAP into the bone marrow stem cells of mice. At the time of writing this chapter, we have a group of mice which, for the past 13 months, have been living with high constitutive levels of endogenous human IRAP production. Retroviral-mediated transduction of an IRAP cDNA into their bone marrow stem cells has led to serum

IRAP levels over 200 ng/ml. Surprisingly, these animals have gained weight normally, have not fallen victim to the animal room pathogens, do not appear to suffer from problems associated with immune recognition of human IRAP, and look set to complete their natural life span. It is not possible to measure their intraarticular IRAP levels but it is known that IRAP introduced i.v. in experimental animals antagonizes IL-1 in the joint (Henderson et al., 1991). Furthermore, the type A synoviocyte is derived from stem cells in the bone marrow (Revell, 1989). We are presently confirming the biological activity of the IRAP produced by these mice, as a prelude to testing their resistance to experimental arthritis.

Delivery to chondrocytes

Recent research has identified families in which OA is genetically transmitted (Ala-Kokko et al., 1990). In affected individuals, the genes coding for type II collagen are defective. Future research may well detect defects in additional genes which code for key components of the extracellular matrix. As this matrix is synthesized by chondrocytes, these are the cells which need to be genetically repaired. Transferring genes to chondrocytes will be much more complicated than transferring them to synovium, as chondrocytes are sparsely distributed throughout an abundant, highly anionic extracellular matrix which excludes molecules greater than 60,000 in molecular weight. Under these conditions we favor an ex vivo approach in which the existing cartilage is removed and the joint resurfaced with allo- or autografted chondrocytes or mesenchymal stem cells (Caplan, 1991).

BEYOND ARTHRITIS

Other disorders of bones and joints

Arthritis is not the only pathological condition of joints amenable to gene treatment. In particular, the healing and repair of ligaments (Evans et al., 1993) and cartilage defects may respond to suitable gene products.

The anterior cruciate ligament (ACL) of the knee provides a particularly enticing target. Rupture of the ACL is the most common sporting injury, being particularly prevalent in skiers and football players. It never repairs or regenerates spontaneously. Orthopaedic treatment of the ACL-deficient knee ranges from conservative physical therapy to aggressive use of artificial ligaments. The latter have been something of a clinical disaster, due to rupture of the prosthesis and an adverse synovial reaction to its wear particles (Olson et al., 1989; Klein and Jensen, 1992; Greis et al., 1992). However, there is reason to believe that, given the correct cytokine environment, the ACL could be induced to regenerate. A search for the appropriate cytokines is underway (Evans et al., 1993). Alternatively, cytokines might improve the cellular colonization and ligamentization of the ACL allografts presently implanted into many patients. Gene treatment of ligament healing is simplified by the probability that in the ACL-deficient joint, unlike the arthritic joint,

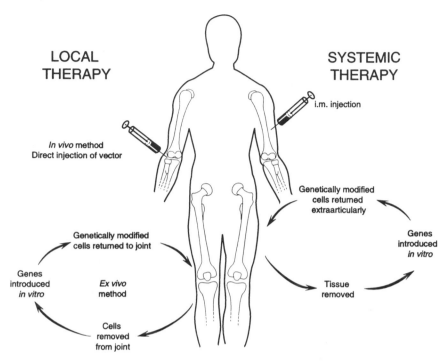

FIGURE 5. Gene delivery for arthritis. Local delivery to the joint by in vivo and ex vivo methods are indicated on the left. Systemic delivery is indicated on the right.

the transgene need only be expressed for the limited time that it takes for healing to occur. In these circumstances, the transient expression of genes that are carried episomally may be an advantage.

As articular cartilage does not repair well, defects in the cartilage as a result of injury or OA are difficult to treat. Present approaches include the transplant of osteochondral plugs and drilling into the subchondral bone to stimulate filling of the defect. Although each method has its advocates, neither is generally accepted, as the both the transplanted cartilage and the new cartilage which fills the drill holes tends to degenerate with time. Transplanted cartilage may fail to assimilate into the surrounding host cartilage, or may suffer immunological rejection. The new cartilage stimulated by drilling fails because it is fibrocartilage rather than hyaline cartilage.

Genes could improve the outcome of both approaches by, for example, coding for cytokines which stimulate the formation of new, hyaline cartilage. Alternatively, they could be used in conjunction with transplanted chondrocytes or mesenchymal stem cells. In this context, the appropriate genes are introduced into the chondrocytes or stem cells prior to their introduction into the defect. Suitable genes may code for cytokines which promote the growth and differentiation of cells, as well as cytokines which stimulate matrix synthesis. Alternatively, the transgenes could code for the proteins which constitute the extracellular matrix of cartilage, such as type II collagen, aggrecan core protein and so on. Placing such genes under the control of a heterologous promoter would permit their independent regulation.

Our ability to express genes in bone marrow (see subsection "Systemic Delivery") suggests that various types of bone disease, such as osteoporosis, osteogenesis imperfecta and fracture non-unions, also may be susceptible to the type of genetic therapies we are discussing.

Joint biology and animal models

The ability to express specific genes in joints has additional uses. In particular it should enable the biology of the diarthrodial joint to be studied in ways that were not previously possible. For example, the articular roles of selected cytokines can be evaluated individually in a biologically authentic manner. Presently, the responses of joints to such molecules are studied intrusively, by injecting the cytokine intraarticularly or by the use of an infusion pump. The sustained intraarticular production of protein that follows delivery of the appropriate gene should permit more accurate analysis of the biological function of the gene product. A number of cytokines vie for early analysis in this way; the list includes IL-1, TNF-α, IL-6 and IL-8. This approach should also generate useful models of joint disease with which to evaluate anti-arthritic drugs.

ACKNOWLEDGMENTS

The authors' work in this area has been supported by a University Exploratory Research Program grant from Procter and Gamble, and grant number RO1 DK46640 from NIDDK. Mrs. Lou Duerring kindly typed the manuscript.

REFERENCES

Ala-kokko L, Baldwin GT, Moskowitz RW, Prockop DJ (1990): Single base mutation in the type II procollagen gene (COL 2A1) as a cause of primary osteoarthritis associated with a mild chondrodysplasia. *Proc Natl Acad Sci USA* 87:6565-6568

Apodaca G, Rutka JT, Bouhara K, Berens ME, Gribbin JR, Rosenblum ML, McKerrow JH, Banda MJ (1990): Expression of metalloproteinases and metalloproteinase inhibitors by fetal astrocytes and glioma cells. *Cancer Res* 50:2322-2329

Arend WP (1991): Interleukin-1 receptor antagonist. A new member of the interleukin-1 family. *J Clin Invest* 88:1445-1451

Arend WP, Dayer JM (1990): Cytokines and cytokine inhibitors or antagonists in rheumatoid arthritis. *Arthritis Rheum* 33:305-315

Bandara G, Robbins PD, Georgescu HI, Mueller GM, Glorioso JC, Evans CH (1992a): Gene transfer to synoviocytes: Prospects for gene treatment of arthritis. *DNA Cell Biol* 11:227-231

Bandara G, Lin CW, Georgescu HI, Evans CH (1992b): The synovial activation of chondrocytes: evidence for complex cytokine interactions involving a possible novel factor. *Biochim Biophys Acta* 1134:309-318

Bandara G, Mueller GM, Galea-Lauri J, Tindal MH, Georgescu HI, Suchanek MK, Hung GL, Glorioso JC, Robbins PD, Evans CH (1993): Intraarticular expression of biologically active interleukin-1 receptor antagonist protein by ex vivo gene transfer. *Proc Natl Acad Sci USA* (In Press)

Capecchi MR (1980): High efficiency transformation by direct microinjection of DNA into cultured mammalian cells. *Cell* 22:479-485

Caplan A (1991): Mesenchymal stem cells. *J Orthop Res* 9:641-650

Cawston TE, Galloway WA, Mercer E, Murphy G, Reynolds JJ (1981): Purification of rabbit bone inhibitor of collagenase. *Biochem J* 195:159-165

Chang PL, (1994): Calcium Phosphate-Mediated DNA Transfection. In: *Gene Therapeutics* (Jon A. Wolff, ed.). Boston: Birkhäuser Boston

Coulton LA, Henderson B, Bityensky L, Chayer L (1980): DNA synthesis in human rheumatoid and non-rheumatoid synovial lining. *Ann Rheum Dis* 39:241-247

Curiel DT (1994): Receptor-Mediated Gene Delivery Employing Adenovirus-Polylysine-DNA Complexes. In: *Gene Therapeutics* (Jon A. Wolff, ed.). Boston: Birkhäuser Boston

Cuevas P, Burgos J, Baird A (1988): Basic fibroblast growth factor (FGF) promotes cartilage repair in vivo. *Biochem Biophys Res Commun* 156:611-618

DeLuca N, McCarthy AM, Schaffer PA (1985): Isolation and characterization of deletion mutants of herpes simplex virus type 1 in the gene encoding immediate-early regulatory protein ICP4. *J Virol* 56:558-570

Dower SK, Wignall JM, Schooley K, McMahan CJ, Jackson JL, Prickett KS, Lupton S, Cosman D, Sims JE (1989): Retention of ligand binding activity by the extracellular domain of the IL-1 receptor. *J Immunol* 142:4314-4320

Dowty ME, Wolff JA (1994): Possible Mechanisms of DNA Uptake in Skeletal Muscle. In: *Gene Therapeutics* (Jon A. Wolff, ed.). Boston: Birkhäuser Boston

Evans CH (1991): The role of proteinases in cartilage destruction. In: *Drugs in inflammation* (eds. MJ Parnham, MA Bray, WB Van den Berg) pp. 135-152, Birkhäuser Verlag, Basel

Evans CH, Bandara G, Mueller GM, Robbins PD, Glorioso JC, Georgescu HI (1992): Synovial cell transplants for gene transfer to joints. *Transplantation Proc* 24:2966

Evans CH, Bandara G, Robbins PD, Mueller GM, Georgescu HI, Glorioso JC (1993): Gene therapy for ligament healing. In: *The anterior cruciate ligament: current and future concepts* (S Arnoczky, SL-Y Woo, CB Frank, DW Jackson, eds). pp 419-422 Raven Press, New York (In Press)

Evans CH, Robbins PD (1994a): The interleukin-1 receptor antagonist and its delivery by gene transfer. *Receptor* (In Press)

Evans C, Robbins PD (1994b): Prospects for treating arthritis by gene therapy. *J Rheumatol* (In Press)

Furs S, Wu GY, (1994): Receptor-Mediated Targeted Gene Delivery Using Asialoglycoprotein-Polylysine Conjugates. In: *Gene Therapeutics* (Jon A. Wolff, ed.). Boston: Birkhäuser Boston

Ferry N, Duplessis O, Hopussin D, Danos O, Heard J-M (1991): Retroviral-mediated gene transfer into hepatocytes in vivo. *Proc Natl Acad Sci USA* 88:8377-8381

Galea-Lauri J, Wilkinson JM, Evans CH (1993): Characterization of monoclonal antibodies against CD44: Evidence of a role for CD44 modulating synovial metabolism. *Mol Immunol* 30:1383-1392

Gao X, Huang L (1991): A novel cationic liposome reagent for efficient transfection of mammalian cells. *Biochem Biophys Res Commun* 179:280-285

Georgescu HI, Mendelow D, Evans CH (1988): HIG-82: An established cell line from rabbit periarticular soft tissue which retains the "activatable" phenotype. *In Vitro* 24:1015-1022

Glorioso JC, DeLuca NA, Goins WF, Fink DJ (1994): Development of Herpes Simplex Virus Vectors for Gene Transfer to the Central Nervous System. In: *Gene Therapeutics* (Jon A. Wolff, ed.). Boston: Birkhäuser Boston

Greis PE, Georgescu HI, Fu FH, Evans CH (1992): Use of an anticollagenase antibody to study synovial cell interactions with particulate material. In: *Particulate debris from medical implants: Mechanisms of formation and biological consequences.* (ed. KR St. John) pp 200-205, ASTM, Philadelphia, PA

Hart DA, Fritzler MJ (1989): Regulation of plasminogen activators and their inhibitors in rheumatic diseases. *J Rheumatol* 16:1184-1191

Henderson B, Thompson RC, Hardingham T, Lewthwaite J (1991): Inhibition of interleukin-1-induced synovitis and articular cartilage proteoglycan loss in the rabbit knee by recombinant human interleukin-1 receptor antagonist. *Cytokine* 3:246-249

Hung GL, Evans CH (1994): Synovium In: *Knee Surgery* (eds. FH Fu, CD Harner, KG Vince) (In Press)

Hung GL, Galea-Lauri J, Mueller GM, Georgescu HI, Larkin LA, Tindal M, Robbins PD, Evans CH (1993): Suppression of intracellular responses to interleukin-1 by transfer of the interleukin-1 receptor antagonist gene to sinovirus. *Gene Therapy* (In Press)

Iigo Y, Takashi T, Tamatani T, Miyasaka M, Higashida T, Yagita H, Okumura K, Tsukada W (1991): ICAM-1-dependent pathway is critically involved in the pathogenesis of a adjuvant arthritis in rats. *J Immunol* 147:4167-4171

Jasin HE, Lightfoot E, Davis LS, Rothlein R, Faanes RB, Lipsky PE (1992): Amelioration of antigen-induced arthritis in rabbits treated with monoclonal antibodies to leukocyte adhesion molecules. *Arthritis Rheum* 35:541-549

Klein W, Jensen KU (1992): Synovitis and artificial ligaments. *J Arthroscop* 8:116-124

Lebsack ME, Paul CC, Bluedow DC, Burch FX, Sack MA, Chase W, Catalano

MA (1991): Subcutaneous IL-1 receptor antagonist in patients with rheumatoid arthritis. *Arthritis Rheum* 34:S45

Luyten FP, Hascall VC, Nissley SP, Morales TI, Reddi AH (1988): Insulin-like growth factors maintain steady state metabolism of proteoglycans in bovine articular cartilage explants. *Arch Biochem Biophys* 267:416-425

McDonnell J, Hoessner LA, Lark MW, Harper C, Dey T, Lobner J, Eiesmann G, Kazazis D, Singer II, Moore VL (1992): Recombinant human interleukin-1β-induced increase in levels of proteoglycans, stromelysin and leukocytes in rabbit synovial fluid. *Arthritis Rheum* 35:799-805

Miller AD (1992): Human gene therapy comes of age. *Nature* 357:455-460

Morales TI, Roberts AB (1988): Transforming growth factor-β regulates the metabolism of proteoglycans in bovine cartilage organ cultures. *J Biol Chem* 263:12828-12831

Mulligan RC (1991): *Gene Transfer and Gene Therapy Principles, Prospects, and Perspectives* (eds. J Lindstern, U Petterson). Raven Press, Ltd

Nabel EG, Gordon D, Yang Z-Y, Xu L, San H, Plautz GE, Wu B-Y, Gao X, Huang L, Nabel GJ (1992): Gene transfer in vivo with DNA-liposome complexes: Lack of autoimmunity and gonadal localization. *Human Gene Therapy* 3:649-656

National Center for Health Statistics (1987): Vital and Health Statistics Series 10:164

Novick D, Engelmann H, Wallach D, Rubenstein M (1989): Soluble cytokine receptors are present in normal urine. *J Exp Med* 170:1409-1414

Ohashi T, Boggs S, Robbins P, Bahnson A, Patrene K, Wei FS, Wei JF, Li J, Lucht L, Fei Y, Clark S, Kimak M, Huiling H, Mowery-Tushton P, Barranger JA (1992): Efficient transfer and sustained high expression of the human glucocerebrosidase gene in mice and their functional macrophages following transplantation of bone marrow transduced by a retroviral vector. *Proc Nat Acad Sci USA* 89:11332-11336

Olson EJ, Kang JD, Fu FH, Georgescu HI, Mason GC, Evans CH (1988): The biochemical and histological effects of artificial ligament wear particles: in vitro and in vivo studies. *Am J Sports Med* 16:558-570

Paulus HE (1992): New perspectives on the management of rheumatoid arthritis. *Clinical Courier* 10:1-12

Pincus T, Callahan LF (1992): Early motality in RA preducted by poor clinical status. *Bull Rheum Dis* 41:1-4

Praemer A, Furner S, Rice DP (1992): Musculoskeletal conditions in the United States. American Academy of Orthopaedic Surgeons, Park Ridge, IL

Revell PA (1989): Synovial lining cells. *Rheumatol Int* 9:49-51

Rosenfeld MA, Yoshimura K, Trapnell BC, Yoneyama K, Rosenthal ER, Dalemans W, Fukayama M, Bargon J, Stier LE, Strattford-Perricaudet L, Perricaudet M, Guggino WB, Pavirani A, Lecocq JP, Crystal RG (1992): In vivo transfer of the human cystic fibrosis transmembrane conductance regulator gene to the airway epithelium. *Cell* 68:143-155

Saklatvala J (1986): Tumour necrosis factor α stimulates resorption and inhibits synthesis of proteoglycan in cartilage. *Nature* 322:547-549

Samulski RJ, Zhu X, Xiao X, Brook JD, Housman DE, Epstein N, Hunter LA (1991): Targeted integration of adeno-associated virus (AAV) into human chromosome 19. *EMBO J* 10:3941-3950

Schwab JH, Anderle SK, Brown RR, Dalldorf FG, Thompson RC (1991): Pro- and anti-inflammatory roles of interleukin-1 in recurrence of bacterial cell-wall induced arthritis in rats. *Infect Immunol* 59:4436-4442

Simkin P (1992): Physiology of normal and abnormal synovium. *Semin Arth Rheum* 21:179-183

Singhal A, Huang L (1994): Gene Transfer in Mammalian Cells Using Liposomes as Carriers. In: *Gene Therapeutics* (Jon A.Wolff, ed.). Boston: Birkhäuser Boston

Skaleric U, Allen JB, Smith PD, Mergenhagen SE, Wahl SM (1991): Inhibitors of reactive oxygen intermediates suppress bacterial cell wall-induced arthritis. *J Immunol* 147:2559-2564

Stefanovic-Racic M, Stadler J, Evans CH (1993): Nitric oxide and arthritis. *Arthritis Rheum* 36:1036-1044

Stevens CR, Blake DR, Merry P, Revell PA, Levick JR (1991): A comparative study by morphometry of the microvasculature in normal and rheumatoid synovium. *Arthritis Rheum* 34:1508-1513

Vannier E, Miller EC, Dinarello CA (1992): Coordinated antiinflammatory effects of interleukin-4: interleukin-4 suppresses interleukin-1 production but up-regulates gene expression and synthesis of interleukin-1 receptor antagonist. *Proc Natl Acad Sci USA* 89:4076-4080

Wagner E, Zatloukal K, Cotten M, Kirlappos H, Mechtrler K, Curiel DT, Birnstiel ML (1992): Coupling of adenovirus to transferring-polylysine/DNA complexes greatly enhances receptor-mediated gene delivery and expression of transfected genes. *Proc Natl Acad Sci USA* 89:6099-6103

Walsh CE, Liu JM, Xiao X, Young NS, Nienhuis AW, Samulski RJ (1992): Regulated high level expression of a human γ-globulin gene introduced into erythroid cells by an adeno-associated virus vector. *Proc Natl Acad Sci USA* 89:7257-7261

Wolff JA, Malone RW, Williams P, Chong W, Ascadi G, Jani A, Felgner PL (1990): Direct gene transfer into mouse muscle in vivo. *Science* 247:1465-1468

Yang L, Li R, Mohr IJ, Clark R, Botchan MR (1991): Activation of BPV-1 replication in vitro by the transcription factor E2. *Nature* 353:628-632

Yelin E (1992): Arthritis. The cumulative impact of a common chronic condition. *Arthritis Rheum* 35:489-497

GENE THERAPY: THE ADVENT OF ADENOVIRUS

Leslie D. Stratford-Perricaudet and Michel Perricaudet

Adenovirus has been developed as an alternative gene transfer vehicle which has emerged as a potent vector with a promising future. Infection of cells with replication-incompetent adenoviruses allows the production of foreign proteins encoded by the engineered viruses without otherwise affecting the host cell. Of utmost relevance to gene therapy, postmitotic cells seem particularly adapted to gene transfer by adenovirus, since the viral genome is not integrated into the cell's chromosome and presumably persists the life of the cell. Administration of recombinant adenoviruses directly in vivo opens the way to new therapeutic strategies. The first successful somatic gene therapy of a hepatic enzyme deficiency in an animal model was achieved using an adenovirus (Stratford-Perricaudet et al., 1990). Since this initial demonstration of the feasibility of correcting a genetic defect with adenovirus, many potential applications have been imagined. The field has aroused much enthousiasm as reflected at the December 1992 RAC meeting where approval was given to carry out clinical trials using three different recombinant adenoviruses capable of expressing the human CFTR, one of which was constructed in our laboratory (Rosenfeld et al., 1992).

HUMAN ADENOVIRUSES

Human adenoviruses were first discovered in 1953 after a witch hunt was initiated to isolate the causative agent of the common cold (Rowe et al., 1953). Rowe and colleagues, using cultures of human adenoids, isolated a filterable agent capable of inducing cytopathic changes. The previously unidentified viruses were subsequently found to be responsible for only a fraction of acute viral respiratory diseases, and were not the elusive etiologic agents of the common cold. To date, 47 distinct human serotypes have been identified (Ad1 to Ad47) and classified into six subgroups (A to F). Adenoviruses generally infect the differentiated epithelial cells of ocular tissue and of the respiratory and GI tracts. The various serotypes differ markedly in tissue specificity and virulence. The two prototypes of subgroup C, Ad2 and Ad5, have been the most extensively characterized biochemically and genetically, and are commonly at the origin of mild respiratory infections (Straus, 1984; Horwitz, 1990).

Gene Therapeutics: Methods and Applications of Direct Gene Transfer
Jon A. Wolff, Editor • ©1994 *Birkhäuser Boston*

BIOLOGY OF HUMAN ADENOVIRUS

Adenoviruses consist of a complex, nonenveloped icosahedral outer protein capsid harboring a DNA protein core. The linear, duplex 36 kb genome is characterized by a short ITR (inverted terminal repeat) found at each extremity and a small terminal protein covalently linked to the 5' end of each strand, both features being involved in replication (Flint, 1982; Flint and Broker, 1982 and refs. therein). Four major steps are involved in a productive infection, each successive step dependent on the previous one. After adsorption of the virus to its receptor, the viral DNA must be unpackaged and reach the nucleus to be transcribed. A complete cycle of the genetic program in a permissive cell in culture lasts 30 hours and results from an orderly transcription of the viral DNA once it has reached the host cell nucleus. Two phases of transcription (immediate early and early) can then take place, followed by the onset of viral genome replication concomitantly to the late phase of gene expression (Williams, 1986).

The early mRNAs are processed from larger transcripts and are generated from five separate regions making up less than half of the viral genome. The *immediate early gene E1A,* as its name suggests, is the very first transcriptional unit to be expressed. The E1A gene products, in fact, condition the outcome of the infection, since they set the stage for an efficient usurpation of the infected cell. Cellular transcription factors already present become modified such that the promoters of the *delayed* early genes of adenovirus (E1B, E2, E3, E4) are enhanced. The expression of E1B contributes to the preparation of the cell for production of progeny virus. From transcription unit E2, proteins involved in viral DNA replication are synthesized. Expression of the E3 region allows adenovirus-infected cells to evade the host's immune surveillance mechanism in vivo. The attribution of functions to the legion of proteins encoded by the E4 transcriptional unit has been more difficult, but it appears that these polypeptides have a role in late viral gene expression and in virion assembly.

After the onset of viral DNA replication at about 6 to 8 hours following the initial infection, expression from the major late transcriptional unit commences. During this late phase of the productive cycle, host cell protein synthesis is shut off. A giant nuclear RNA extending from map units (mu) 17 to 98 is generated from the major late promoter (MLP). Five families of late mRNAs coding for structural proteins are processed from the large precursor; each message possesses a common tripartite leader sequence which favors their translation. As with the early genes, splicing has an important role in protein expression. The complexity of the intertwining reading frames allows for a methodological appropriation of the infected cell.

All subgroups of adenovirus can transform rodent cells in culture, yet only subgroups A and B can induce tumors in newborn hamsters. The genes essential for transformation are located in the E1 region which is consistently found in transformed cells. Despite this, there is no evidence for any adenovirus-associated neoplasms in humans.

DEVELOPMENT OF ADENOVIRUS AS A CLONING VEHICLE

During the late seventies a major interest in biology rested in the development of viral vectors for the introduction of genetic material into cells growing in culture (for review, see Berkner, 1988). Adenovirus was an interesting candidate due to its large genome which would theoretically allow the transfer of extensive fragments of foreign DNA. With the generation of a cell line (293) expressing the E1 region of Ad5 (Graham et al., 1977), it became possible without the use of a helper virus to construct recombinant adenoviruses lacking this important region. Deletion of a part of region E3 increased the cloning capacity further, but this time without affecting the viability of the virus in culture. The 105 map unit upper packaging limit in the adenovirus capsid, combined with the E1 and E3 deletions, allows for the insertion of about 8 kb of heterologous DNA. As mentioned above, the E1 transcriptional unit is essential for multiplication of the virus. Its deletion leads to a block in the viral genetic program and prevents the other viral genes from being expressed. In turn, viral infection no longer leads to cell death. The 293 cells provide complementing E1 proteins, thus allowing the propagation of mutant viruses.

The cloning of foreign DNA sequences in adenovirus can be carried out following different strategies (Gluzman, 1982; Berkner and Sharp, 1983; Ghosh-Choudhury et al., 1986). The resultant vectors are either defective or not for replication, depending on the deletion in the viral genome. The purpose of this review is to trace the development of replication-incompetent adenovirus as a gene transfer vehicle in vivo and to summarize the potentials emanating from the versatility of the vector.

GENERATION OF HELPER-INDEPENDENT RECOMBINANT ADENOVIRUSES

Insertion of genes in the E1 region of the adenoviral genome may be obtained by either in vitro ligation or in vivo homologous recombination (Figure 1). Either strategy is carried out by manipulation of bacterial plasmids containing viral DNA sequences and the fragment to be cloned. The plasmid harbors the very left-hand end PvuII fragment of Ad5 (mu 0-1.26) which includes the ITR, the origin of replication and packaging signals, as well as the E1A enhancer elements. Immediately 3' to these Ad sequences is the gene to be inserted. For ligation to the Ad genome a Cla I-compatible restriction site is inserted downstream the foreign gene. On the other hand, promotion of homologous recombination with the wild type adenovirus genome requires the gene be followed by a second region from adenovirus extending from the Bgl II site at 9.4 mu to the Hind III site at 17 mu. Transfection of 293 cells with the ligation product, or cotransfection of the plasmid and viral DNA generates E1-defective recombinant adenoviruses. More precisely, the ligation scheme at the Cla I site results in E1A-deleted recombinants, while the second strategy generates recombinants with the foreign sequences replacing both E1A and E1B (Figure 2).

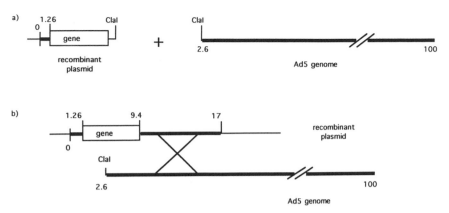

FIGURE 1. Design of Ad5-based recombinant adenoviruses. a) The foreign gene is cloned in a plasmid downstream the left end of Ad (0-1.26 mu). The gene is followed by a ClaI site to allow ligation to ClaI-restricted Ad5 genomic DNA at 2.6 mu. The resultant virus is E1A defective. b) The foreign gene is inserted in a plasmid between the left end of Ad (0-1.26 mu) and 9.4-17 mu of Ad to permit homologous recombination. Cotransfection of the recombinant plasmid and genomic Ad DNA into 293 cells generates an E1-defective recombinant virus. With either scheme the E3 region may be deleted to increase the cloning capacity. Wild type Ad genome: ████████; plasmid: ————; foreign gene: ▭ ; 1 mu = 360 bp.

ADENOVIRUS AS AN EXPRESSION VECTOR IN CELL CULTURE

Infection of cells in culture with various recombinant adenoviruses demonstrates that even when the viral life cycle is blocked at its initial stages due to deletion of the E1 region, generous amounts of the foreign protein are synthesized. The gene products are found to undergo post-translational modifications leading to correct glycosylation and phosphorylation, as appropriate. Requirements for proteolytic cleavage, assembly, and secretion are met, with the resulting recombinant product being identical to the original protein (Ballay et al., 1985; Stratford-Perricaudet et al., 1990; Gilardi et al., 1990; Eloit et al., 1990; Levrero et al., 1991; Ragot et al., 1991). Adenoviral expression control elements such as the E1A promoter and, perhaps more surprisingly, the MLP can be used to drive the expression of the transgene borne by the defective virus. In the context of wild type adenovirus genome, the major late transcription unit is active subsequent to replication. Expression from the ectopic MLP in a replication-defective genome is most likely due to its proximity to the E1A enhancer. The comparison of two recombinant adenoviruses harboring the same foreign gene but differing with respect to their ability to synthesize the E1A proteins, has shown that efficient expression from an ectopic MLP can occur in cells of different species and tissue origins regardless of the expression of the immediate early gene (Levrero et al., 1991). This notion is important because gene transfer followed by cell death has limited applications.

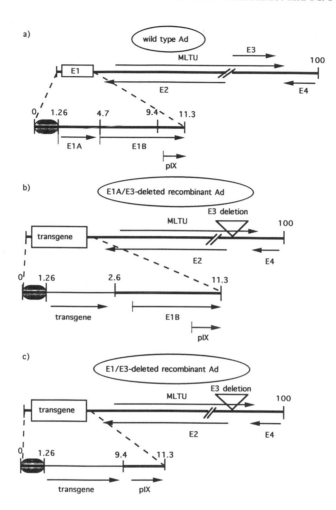

FIGURE 2. Simplified schematic representation of wild type Ad and E1A⁻/E3⁻, E1⁻/E3⁻ recombinant adenovirus genomes. Transcription units are indicated as E1, E2, E3, E4, and MLTU for early regions 1, 2, 3, and 4, and major late transcription unit, respectively. The left end has been enlarged in each case to show transcripts. Map units of the wild type Ad genomic fragments present in each virus are indicated. Recombinants may be up to 105 mu in length. The genomes are not drawn to scale, but merely show relative positions of the various regions. a) Wild type Ad. Detail of the first 11 mu are given to indicate the different regions for comparison with the two types of recombinants in b and c. b) E1A/E3-deleted recombinant adenovirus. The left end is expanded to show the insertion of the foreign gene in the E1 region. The E1B and pIX transcripts are intact, whereas the E1A transcripts are replaced by the transgene. The E3 region may be deleted. c) E1/E3-deleted recombinant adenovirus. An enlargement of the left end is provided where the transgene replaces both E1A and E1B. The E3 region may be deleted. Wild type Ad genome: ▬▬▬▬ ; mu 0 - 1.25 of Ad5: ▬▬▬. This sequence harbors the ITR, encapsidation signals, origin of replication, and the E1A enhancers. 1 mu = 360 bp.

Inasmuch as deletion of the E1 region has no incidence on foreign gene expression, but on the other hand prevents viral induction of cell destruction, E1-defective recombinant adenoviruses become interesting vectors for gene delivery in vivo.

ADENOVIRUS AS A GENE TRANSFER VEHICLE IN VIVO

1. Ad vectors for antigen expression in man and animals

a) anti-HBV vaccine

In an attempt to control epidemics of adenovirus-induced acute respiratory infections in military recruits, an unattenuated bivalent vaccine against serotypes 4 and 7 was developed and found to be highly effective (Chanock et al., 1966; Top et al., 1971a, b). Millions of US military recruits have since been vaccinated using the enteric-coated capsules, and have not manifested any undesirable side effects. The use of live, nondefective adenovirus as a vaccine provides a most important precedent endorsing the administration of adenovirus-based vectors in man. Consequently, we attempted to adapt the replication-defective adenovirus to immunize against other agents. As a model system to evaluate the potential of this vector in vaccination, we developed a vaccine against hepatitis B (HBV) by cloning the hepatitis B surface antigen (HBsAg) gene in place of the E1A gene of Ad5. Anti-HBs antibodies were elicited in rabbits inoculated by the intravenous route with the AdS (M-B) where the expression of the HBsAg-encoding gene is driven by the adenoviral E1A promoter (Ballay et al., 1985). The elicitation of specific anti-HBsAg antibodies reflects an in vivo expression of the cloned gene carried by the vector. Similar results were obtained using the recombinant Ad.MLP.S2 which harbors the same gene but expressed from the adenoviral MLP (Levrero et al., 1988). Clearly, replication-defective adenoviruses may be used to transfer and express genes in living animals (Levrero et al., 1991).

To evaluate efficacy of the novel vaccine, chimpanzees, which are the only animal susceptible to infection by HBV, were inoculated with three intravenous doses of 10^9 plaque-forming units (pfu) of Ad.MLP.S2. Importantly, the immune response elicited by the defective recombinant adenovirus was sufficient to fully protect one of the two vaccinated chimpanzees after an HBV challenge. The second animal experienced a modified HBV-induced disease, demonstrating a partial protection in this case (Levrero et al., 1988). Interestingly, identical results were obtained with a nondefective recombinant adenovirus (Lubeck et al., 1989). Further studies are required to establish the vaccination value of this engineered virus. It may be necessary to increase the doses of vaccinating agent; or possibly necessary to use younger animals; or even use a different mode of administration.

b) anti-EBV vaccine

Because of the strong association of the Epstein-Barr virus (EBV) with Burkitt's lymphoma and nasopharyngeal carcinoma, EBV vaccination may help reduce the incidence of these malignancies. An adenovirus-based EBV vaccine has been developed in our laboratory. Again, the expression of the vaccinating glycoprotein was placed under the control of the adenovirus MLP, and was inserted in the E1 region of the vector. Vaccination of rabbits with the recombinant Ad-gp340 led to high titers of anti-gp340/220 antibodies which persisted for 40 weeks (Ragot et al., 1991). Importantly, the sera from immunized animals were capable of neutralizing EBV in vitro. The ability of Ad-gp340 to protect cottontop tamarins from EBV-induced lymphoma was tested following a series of three intramuscular administrations of Ad-gp340 (5 X 10^9 to 2 X 10^{10} pfu). Although the anti-gp340 antibodies elicited in the vaccinated tamarins were not EBV-neutralizing in vitro, a remarkable protection of the tamarins from EBV-induced tumors was observed, resulting undoubtedly from an efficacious cellular immune response (Ragot et al., 1993a). These results are quite encouraging and support the development of defective adenovirus-based vaccines against other infectious agents for use in man.

c) anti-PRV vaccine

Adenovirus-based vaccines may also have a place in veterinary preventive medicine. In this regard, an attempt at developing a vaccine against the Pseudorabies virus (PRV), which poses severe economic burdens on the swine industry, has been undertaken. Because the gp50 glycoprotein from PRV induces neutralizing antibodies with a protective effect in mice, it is considered a good candidate for a subunit vaccine. A recombinant vaccinia virus expressing this glycoprotein has offered protection to mice challenged with moderate doses of PRV (Marchioli et al., 1987). The use of adenovirus in this system was evaluated by vaccinating mice via different routes with Ad-gp50 which expresses the PRV glycoprotein using the Ad MLP. Analysis of sera 2 weeks post-vaccination revealed strong antibody responses against PRV gp50, whatever the inoculation route. Challenge with lethal doses (at least 30 LD 50) of the neurovirulent PRV strain Kojnok resulted in protection of a proportion of the vaccinated mice despite high antibody titers in all animals, while all control mice died within 3 to 5 days (Eloit et al., 1990). The same modalities of challenge after vaccination with the vaccinia vector remain to be applied to allow a direct comparison of the two vectors.

In the development of viral vectors as carriers of genes encoding vaccinating polypeptides, adenovirus has emerged as a new candidate. The elicitation of an immune response specific of the cloned, foreign gene product in animals injected with various adenoviral gene vectors demonstrates that expression of the gene is independent of transcription of the adenoviral genes, and furthermore, is not hampered by the replication-deficiency. Importantly, the concept of viral-mediated gene transfer may be extended to therapeutic genes so that applications may go beyond the prevention of infectious disease. Applied early in life, gene therapy can in theory prevent the development of numerous genetic diseases, and may possibly reverse diseased states already manifest. In practice, the challenge is to safely transfer enough of the right gene to the right tissue. We have explored the idea of using replication-defective adenovirus vectors to deliver genes in view of gene therapy.

2. Gene therapy: Targets amenable to Ad-mediated transfer in vivo

a) lung, liver, and muscle

It is expected that intravenous administration of a vector leads to its dissemination throughout the animal. Receptors for adenovirus have been reported on a variety of cell types in addition to the pulmonary epithelium, making gene transfer theoretically possible to many organs. We focused on determining which tissues can effectively be infected by recombinant adenoviruses after a direct in vivo administration. To address this question, a virus expressing a nuclearly-targeted ß-galactosidase under constitutive control was constructed (Stratford-Perricaudet et al., 1992a). The in situ histochemical analysis of different tissues after a systemic delivery of the marker-containing virus (Ad.RSVßgal) revealed that the virus can be conducted throughout the mouse, and that the transgene can be expressed in many tissues in addition to the lung, such as the liver and intestine, and even cardiac and skeletal muscles (Stratford-Perricaudet et al., 1992a). The use of high viral titers makes possible efficient infections. Long-term experiments indicate that stability of gene transfer appears to be a function of cell turnover rate. The data reveal that adenovirus is particularly adapted to long-term gene delivery to quiescent cells such as myocytes since ß-galactosidase-positive nuclei were still present in large numbers even over a year after a single IV injection of the viral vector. These findings are analogous to those obtained when plasmid DNA is injected directly into muscle (Wolff et al., 1990). The post-mitotic state seems to offer favorable conditions for stability of the transferred DNA. The adenoviral genome persists as an extrachromosomal entity, and the Rous sarcoma virus LTR used to drive the marker gene remains active.

b) nervous system

The capacity of adenovirus to infect quiescent cells bringing a heterologous gene with it has hinted at the awesome potentials carried by this unexploited virus. It has attracted much attention and hope to effect gene transfer to those organs which until now seemed far from reach. Another tissue of this kind relevant to gene therapy is the nervous system. To assess the behavior of replication-incompetent adenovirus in the CNS, Ad.RSVßgal was stereotactically inoculated into specific cerebral structures of the adult rat (Le Gal La Salle et al., 1993; Akli et al., 1993). Marker gene expression was detected in injected hippocampus, substantia nigra, striatum, and nucleus of the twelfth nerve. A marked blue reaction product was seen in a large number of neural cells including neurons, microglia, astrocytes, and ependymal cells. The feasibility of stable adenovirus-mediated gene transfer to the nervous system was demonstrated since X-gal staining was still present 60 days after injection. Successful marker gene transfer and expression in neurons without cytopathic effects suggests that specific studies aimed at understanding gene expression in the brain may now be undertaken. The future may also hold effective therapeutic interventions for neurological diseases based on the use of adenovirus.

MODEL SYSTEMS FOR GENE DELIVERY USING ADENOVIRUS VEC-
TORS IN VIVO

The wide spectrum of tissues which can undergo efficient gene transfer using adenovirus potentially makes this vector applicable to the treatment of numerous
diseases through gene augmentation (Stratford-Perricaudet and Perricaudet, 1991).
The high titers to which adenovirus grows allows the direct in vivo delivery of the
vector, offering a facile administration without the constraints related to the manipulation of cells ex vivo.

Correction of a hepatic enzyme deficiency in the mouse

Having established the feasibility of gene transfer to various tissues with adenovirus, we turned to an animal model of a human hepatic disorder to evaluate the
reality of correcting a genetic defect with this type of vector. Ornithine
transcarbamylase deficiency is one of the most common hereditary
hyperammonemias in humans leading to death of 75% of affected neonatal males
(Brusilow and Horwich, 1989). A restricted diet and pharmaceutical therapy to
reduce the nitrogen load are not always sufficient to avoid mental retardation or
even death. Liver transplantation is the only real therapy. Ornithine transcarbamylase
(OTC) catalyzes the synthesis of citrulline from ornithine and carbamyl phosphate
in the mammalian urea cycle. OTC, a mitochondrial enzyme, is encoded by an X-
linked gene expressed in the liver and small intestine. Aberrant splicing of the
OTC mRNA in the Spf-ash mutant mouse allows synthesis of only about 5% of
the wild type level of OTC (Hodges and Rosenberg, 1989). The mutant mice are
regarded as a model for OTC deficiency in man due to the similar clinical profiles.
In addition to the classic symptoms which include hyperammonemia,
hypocitrullinemia, and orotic aciduria, Spf-ash mice are hypotrophic and exhibit
sparse fur until weaning. Germinal gene therapy of the Spf-ash mouse established
the rationale for somatic gene augmentation to effect a reversal of diseased state
(Cavard et al., 1988).

An E1A/E3-deficient adenovirus engineered to express the rat OTC cDNA
under the control of the MLP and found to efficiently express OTC in primary rat
hepatocytes, was administered to neonatal Spf-ash mice (Chassé et al., 1988). After a single injection, hepatic OTC activity was monitored at different times in a
number of mice. Values were found to vary anywhere from that of untreated mutant animals to that of normal control (C57BL6) mice, with intermediate values
being the most common. Clearly, adenovirus is able to transfer a gene of therapeutic interest directly to a live animal and thereby ameliorate the diseased condition
(Chassé et al., 1989). A pronounced orotic aciduria is one of the hallmarks of OTC
deficiency. Urine samples collected at intervals during the life of two animals were
assayed for orotic acid. The results provide indirect evidence for a long-term biochemical correction. Even 13 months post-injection the level of orotic acid was
still markedly reduced. Sacrifice of animals at 15 months for an evaluation of

hepatic ornithine transcarbamylase activity conclusively demonstrated that injected animals can express the therapeutic gene at significantly high levels in the liver for extended periods of time (Stratford-Perricaudet et al., 1990). In agreement with this is the finding of specific mRNA in the liver 15 months after therapy. An interesting observation relates to the characteristic sparse fur of Spf-ash animals. Those mice expressing the most important levels of hepatic OTC activity had a normalized fur phenotype before weaning. These results document the first adenovirus-mediated somatic gene therapy leading to an elimination of the phenotypic traits associated with the mutation.

Gene transfer: potential applications to the lung

The lung has several characteristics which make it customized to adenovirus-assisted gene transfer. It is richly populated in terminally differentiated cells which, in fact, represent the natural host for adenovirus and constitute a barrier to retroviral integration. The complex arrangement of the impressive cellular surface makes a direct in vivo approach more realistic than an ex vivo one where cells would be reimplanted after manipulation. Administration of a modified adenovirus to the airways may allow efficient targeting of appropriate cells such that pulmonary disease may be treated or prevented.

Cystic fibrosis emerges as the obvious lung disorder to attempt to treat since the gene responsible for this dreadful disease has now been cloned. In 1988 however, when the first promising results were obtained showing that adenovirus may be used to correct a genetic deficiency in the mouse, the CFTR gene was not yet available, so an alternative cDNA was chosen to address the notion of pulmonary gene therapy. α1-Antitrypsin deficiency leads to emphysema by age 30 to 40 due to the accumulation of neutrophil elastase. Without α1-antitrypsin to inhibit the potent proteolytic enzyme chronically deposited in the lung by resident neutrophils, irreparable lung damage ensues. We constructed an E1A/E3-deleted adenovirus (Ad-α1AT) capable of expressing the human α1-antitrypsin (hα1AT) gene controlled by the Ad MLP to investigate the possibility of using this modified respiratory virus to deliver the gene directly to the lung in vivo. Preliminary studies demonstrated that infection of different cell types in culture led to synthesis and secretion of hα1AT protein (Gilardi et al., 1990). After a single administration of 3×10^7 pfu of Ad-α1AT to the airway of cotton rats, although hα1AT capable of combining with neutrophil elastase could be detected, the actual levels found in the epithelial lining fluid were estimated as being 50-fold below threshold human protective levels (Rosenfeld et al., 1991). It may be possible to attain higher levels by modifying the chimeric gene construct or by simply increasing the administered dose. Nevertheless, the absence of an animal model for α1AT deficiency makes it difficult to evaluate the potential therapeutic benefit of gene delivery to the lung.

A large leap was made towards a treatment for the most common lethal genetic disease in Caucasians when the gene responsible for cystic fibrosis (CF) was identified in 1989 (Boat et al., 1989; Rommens et al., 1989; Riordan et al., 1989). Data showing that gene transfer to mutated cells grown in culture complements the defective chloride secretion spawned justified excitement (Drumm et al., 1990; Rich et al., 1990). The remaining hurdle, however, is undoubtedly the most difficult to surmount. It is not obvious how the normal gene encoding the cystic fibrosis conductance regulator (CFTR) is to be transferred to the patient. Cystic fibrosis is a multifacet disease with manifestations in several organs including the lung, liver, pancreas, and intestine. A working hypothesis for gene therapy in cystic fibrosis is to target the airway, since the pulmonary complications are the life-limiting factor. The exact mechanisms by which the mutations in the CFTR gene lead to the clinical manifestations remain to be clarified, but the absence of cAMP-induced chloride channels is believed to disrupt electrolyte transport. In CF airway epithelial cells, the abnormal mucocilliary clearance is probably a direct consequence of the defective Cl⁻ secretion. Progressive airway destruction occurs resulting from chronic infection and inflammation.

The treatment of cystic fibrosis is a challenge with different requirements from those imposed by $\alpha 1AT$ deficiency. $\alpha 1AT$ is normally synthesized in the liver and transported to the lung. This has led to the development of expensive protein therapy whereby human plasma $\alpha 1AT$ is administered intravenously. Because the CFTR gene product is a subcellular component, an extrapulmonary targeting of the CFTR gene would be inadequate. The success with the Ad-$\alpha 1AT$ to deliver a gene to the lung epithelium of cotton rats made it urgent to substitute CFTR for the h$\alpha 1AT$ gene in the vector. We constructed an E1/E3-deleted recombinant making use of a CFTR cDNA isolated by Transgene, SA (Strasbourg, France). It was shown that a functional CFTR gene product capable of complementing the CF defect is made after infection with Ad-CFTR of cultured epithelial cells (CFPAC-1) derived from CF patients (Rosenfeld et al., 1992). As with Ad-$\alpha 1AT$, expression of the gene carried by the vector could be detected in lung epithelium of experimental animals after intratracheal instillation. Although these results are very suggestive of a strategy to treat the pulmonary manifestations of cystic fibrosis, many key questions remain about the feasibility of gene therapy of CF.

Localization studies have shown that all epithelial cell types making up the non-CF human airway express CFTR at least to some extent, making each one a target potentially important for transfer of the CFTR-encoding gene. It is not clear however, which population contributes the most to disease when the gene is defective. In this regard, experiments using the Ad.RSVßgal recombinant adenovirus as an indicator of gene transfer, have shown that administration of the virus to cotton rats leads to gene delivery to all major categories of the airway epithelium, including ciliated, basal, secretory, and undifferentiated columnar cells (Mastrangeli et al., 1993). In studies carried out in rhesus monkeys however, only exceptionally were basal cells the site of in vivo gene transfer (Bout et al., 1993). Perhaps inaccessibility of submucosal glands explains the absence of gene transfer to these glands in the monkey. What this implies for man remains to be determined in light of the finding that CFTR mRNA and protein in non-CF human bronchus have been detected predominantly in these glands (Engelhardt et al., 1992). It has been hypothesized that the Cl⁻ ions may flow from cell to cell via gap junctions and be secreted across the apical membrane of CFTR-containing cells. Cell-cell coupling may just make gene therapy for CF possible by compensating for gene transfer efficiencies below 100%. Experiments in vitro have suggested that the gene transfer efficiency achieved by bronchoscopic administration of adenovirus to rhesus monkeys would provide the minimal requirement for an efficacious delivery (Bout et al., 1993; Johnson et al., 1992).

Gene transfer: potential applications to muscle

The formidable efficiency of gene delivery to cardiac and skeletal muscle which has been demonstrated with Ad.RSVßgal makes adenovirus an attractive vector for gene therapy for diseases involving these tissues which represent such a large proportion of body mass (Stratford-Perricaudet et al., 1992b). An effective treatment for Duchenne muscular dystrophy (DMD) for example, cannot be one limited to skeletal muscle, and will require addressing cardiomyopathy. In DMD, an X-linked disease, the absence or abnormality of dystrophin leads to a progressive degeneration of skeletal muscle and to cardiac failure with a later onset. As an initial step towards gene therapy of DMD we have evaluated the use of adenovirus to transfer a minigene encoding a truncated form of the human muscle cytoskeletal protein, dystrophin. The 6.3 kb cDNA issued from a Becker muscular dystrophy (BMD) patient and provided by K. Davies (John Radcliffe Hospital, UK) was cloned downstream the RSV LTR into an E1/E3-deleted adenovirus vector (Ragot et al., 1993b). The current adenoviral vectors are inadequate for insertion of either the enormous 2.3×10^6 bp gene or the 11 kb complete cDNA sequence. The BMD individual from which the 6.3 kb minigene was isolated exhibited very mild clinical features, indicating that this truncated form of dystrophin is significantly active and may be sufficient to complement deficient myocytes. Immunoblots performed with myoblast extracts prepared 60 hours after infection in vitro with Ad-RSVmDys demonstrated the capacity of the virus to produce the expected 200 kd truncated dystrophin. To study expression of the transgene in muscle in vivo, the recombinant adenovirus was injected intramuscularly into mdx mice which have a nonsense mutation in the dystrophin gene. Becker dystrophin was localized to the cell membrane of 5 to 50% of myofibers in the injected muscles by immunohistochemical detection using an anti-dystrophin antibody. Importantly, the expression of the transferred dystrophin gene after 13 weeks was still detectable both at the mRNA level using reverse transcriptase-polymerase chain reaction and at the protein level by immunofluorescence (Ragot et al., 1993b).

While these experiments demonstrate that adenovirus may be used to efficiently transfer a minidystrophin gene construct to the mdx mouse by intramuscular injection, it remains to be established whether this Becker protein could provide an adequate phenotypic correction of the defect in man. Normal dystrophin is a very large molecule issued from an extensively spliced mRNA. It would seem less hazardous to develop a novel adenoviral vector capable of carrying a larger insert. Furthermore, natural variants of the protein operating in different muscle tissues may make it necessary to target a different cDNA construct to the heart. Use of a dystrophin gene construct whose expression is controlled by an appropriate muscle specific promoter can restrict protein production using a systemic administration all the while (Quantin et al., 1992). The mdx mouse is not an adequate model to evaluate therapy because an unidentified alternative component assures normal muscle function; future investigations will be directed towards the CXMD golden retriever whose dystrophin deficiency leads to clinical symptoms resembling man's.

DISCUSSION

The past few years have seen the development of new delivery systems aimed at countering the most fundamental villain responsible for disease. Indeed, the medicine of the next century may offer gene augmentation as the standard arsenal to combat maladies. Due to their efficiency, those vectors which have retained the most attention are viral-based. To date, retroviruses have been the most extensively engineered and studied, and have been found to be particularly suited for ex vivo gene transfer of hematopoietic cells. Their essential drawback, however, resides in their dependence on host cell division to integrate and to allow expression of the exogenous gene. This seriously limits their applicability. Other vectors need investigation inasmuch as a number of hereditary and acquired diseases will require gene transfer to quiescent or slowly dividing cells. Adenovirus appears to have filled the gap with its inherent ability to infect these cells (Stratford-Perricaudet et al., 1992a). Table 1 recapitulates the properties of adenovirus rendering it an interesting vector system for gene transfer in vivo, and Table 2 provides examples of applications.

The treatment of disease with gene transfer in general will necessitate particular attention to its immunological consequences. Disorders may be grossly separated into two categories: those which result from a total deficiency of a protein and those where the protein is insufficiently synthesized or is unfunctional. The introduction of a normal gene will in one case arouse the patient's immune system, and in the other will go unnoticed. This will undoubtedly influence the duration of the therapeutic effect achieved by gene transfer whatever the means of delivery. The principle of vaccination illustrates this notion. The presence of a foreign body ellicits a specific immune response for the safeguard of the individual. Experiments have shown that nu/nu mice are more tolerant of grafts and cells modified to produce a foreign protein. This indicates that gene therapy will be most successful in patients of the second category. It is interesting to note that long-term OTC gene transfer with adenovirus was demonstrated in the Spf-ash mouse which has a residual level of ornithine transcarbamylase expression.

For the treatment of individuals with total deficiencies it might prove useful to capitalize on mechanisms already incorporated into adenovirus' genetic pro-

TABLE 1. Properties of Ad allowing its adaptation as a vector for in vivo administration.

- Large host range
- Virus can infect dividing and quiescent cells
- E1 mutants are replication-defective
- Availability of E1-complementing cell line 293
- Cloning capacity of helper-independent vector is 8 kb
- High titer stocks
- Wild type Ad has been largely administered as a vaccine

gram which help adenovirus-infected cells to evade immune destruction (Wold and Gooding, 1991). For example, the E3 region encodes a transmembrane glycoprotein (gp19K) which is localized in the endoplasmic reticulum and binds to class I antigens (Ag) of the MHC. This binding blocks the transport of class I Ag to the surface of the infected cell and prevents class I-restricted cytolysis by CTL (Pääbo et al., 1987 and refs. within; Wold and Gooding, 1989). It would be of interest to compare longevity of in vivo expression of a transgene carried by two Ad vectors differing only in their capacity to express gp19K. Studies have shown that affinity of gp19K for class I Ag varies with different MHC genotypes (Severinsson et al., 1986). This suggests that use of vectors encoding gp19K may not be equally ben-

TABLE 2. Examples of recombinant E1-defective Ad vectors for gene delivery in vivo

Foreign Gene	Promoter	Reference
Secreted Proteins:		
HBsAg	Ad E1A	Ballay et al., 1985
HBsAg	Ad MLP	Levrero et al., 1991
human α1AT	Ad MLP	Gilardi et al., 1990
Intracellular Proteins:		
rat OTC	Ad MLP	Stratford-Perricaudet et al., 1990
lacZ	RSV LTR	Stratford-Perricaudet et al., 1992
lacZ	skeletal α-actin	Quantin et al., 1992
Membranous Proteins:		
PRV gp50	Ad MLP	Eloit et al., 1990
human CFTR	Ad MLP	Rosenfeld et al., 1992
EBV gp340/220	Ad MLP	Ragot et al., 1993a
human dystrophin	RSV LTR	Ragot et al., 1993b

eficial for all individuals. Administration of E1A-deleted viruses may also contribute to a stable gene transfer since this region is responsible for sensitizing Ad-infected cells to lysis by TNFα, NK cells, and activated macrophages (Cook et al., 1987). Different built-in components of the vector could help overcome immune problems without the use of immunocompromisors.

A second potential immunological problem resides in the host's immune response directed towards the vector itself. If repetitive administrations of the recombinant vector are required to assure a durable treatment, the risk of developing immunity to the gene vehicle is probable. Consistent with this is the production of anti-Ad antibodies upon administration of E1/E3-deleted recombinants in animals (Ragot et al., 1993a). Use of a battery of heterotypic recombinants based on antigenically distinct serotypes may be a means around this.

It is obvious that thorough evaluation of the behavior of replication-defective recombinant adenoviruses in humans will require clinical trials. Studies of human adenoviruses in animals cannot provide answers to all questions regarding safety issues. Furthermore, fundamental biological differences between species will make assessment of therapeutic benefit difficult even when animal models of human disease are available.

The biologic property of Ad to dispense with host cell proliferation to express the exogenous gene makes it advantageous for in vivo transfer of genes (Perricaudet and Stratford-Perricaudet, 1993). Demonstration of long-term expression in tissues such as liver, muscle, and brain underscores the multitude of potential applications (Stratford-Perricaudet et al., 1990, 1992a; Ragot et al., 1993b; Le Gal La Salle et al., 1993; Akli et al., 1993). The success of these experiments provides a firm foundation for human gene transfer studies toward the goal of gene therapy. The recent development of replication-incompetent adenoviruses has paved the way for human trials which will hopefully lead to the treatment and prevention of disease.

ACKNOWLEDGMENTS

The studies reported in this review are the fruit of several years supported by the Centre National de Recherches Scientifiques (CNRS), Institut National de la Santé et de la Recherche Médicale (INSERM), Ministère de la Recherche et de la Technologie (MRT), Association Française contre les Myopathies (AFM), Association Françaises pour la Lutte contre la Mucoviscidose (AFLM), Agence Nationale de Recherches sur le SIDA (ANRS) and Association de Recherches sur le Cancer (ARC) to which we are most grateful. Close collaborations with P. Briand (ICGM, Paris), R. Crystal (NIH), A. Kahn (ICGM, Paris), J-C. Kaplan (ICGM, Paris), G. LeGal LaSalle (CNRS, Gif sur Yvette), J. Mallet (CNRS, Gif sur Yvette), J-L. Mandel (CNRS/INSERM, Strasbourg), A. Morgan (University of Bristol), M. Peschanski (INSERM, Creteil), Transgene, SA (Strasbourg), and D. Valerio (TNO, The Netherlands) made these advances possible. This manuscript is dedicated to our daughter, Caroline who is a perfect product of gene transfer in vivo.

REFERENCES

Akli S, Caillaud C, Vigne E, Stratford-Perricaudet LD, Poenaru L, Perricaudet M, Kahn A, Peschanski M (1993): Transfer of foreign genes into the brain using adenovirus vectors. *Nature Genetics* 3:224-228

Ballay A, Levrero M, Buendia MA, Tiollais P, Perricaudet M (1985): In vitro and in vivo synthesis of the hepatitis B virus surface antigen and of the receptor for polymerized human serum albumin from recombinant human adenoviruses. *EMBO J* 4:3861-3865

Berkner KL (1988): Development of adenovirus vectors for the expression of heterologous genes. *BioTech* 6:616-630

Berkner KL, Sharp PA (1983): Generation of adenovirus by transfection of plasmids. *Nucl Acids Res* 11:6003-6020

Boat TF, Welsh MJ, Beaudet AL (1989): Cystic fibrosis. In: *The Metabolic Basis of Inherited Disease*, Scriver CR, Beaudet AL, Sly WS, Valle D, eds. NY: McGraw-Hill

Bout A, Perricaudet M, Baskin G, Imler JL, Scholte BJ, Pavirani A, Valerio D (1993): Lung gene therapy: in vivo adenovirus-mediated gene transfer to rhesus monkey airway epithelium. *Hum Gene Ther* (In Press)

Brusilow S, Horwich AL (1989): Urea cycle disorders. In: *The Metabolic Basis of Inherited Disease*, Scriver CR, Beaudet AL, Sly WS, Valle D, eds. NY: McGraw-Hill

Cavard C, Grimber G, Dubois N, Chassé J-F, Bennoum M, Minet-Thuriaux M, Kamoun P, et Briand P (1988): Correction of mouse ornithine transcarbamylase deficiency by gene transfer into the germ line. *Nucl Acids Res* 16:2099-2110

Chanock RM, Ludwig L, Heubner RJ, Cate TR, Chu L-W (1966): Immunization by selective infection with type 4 adenovirus grown in human diploid tissue culture. I. Safety and lack of oncogenicity and tests for potency in volunteers. *JAMA* 195:445-452

Chassé J-F, Perricaudet M, Minet-Thurriaux M, Briand P, Levrero M (1988): Human recombinant adenovirus to correct a mouse enzyme deficiency. *J Cell Biochem* sup.12B UCLA Symposium on Molecular and Cellular Biology p. 197

Chassé J-F, Levrero M, Kamoun P, Briand P, Perricaudet M (1989): L'adénovirus: vecteur de thérapie génique. *Médecine/ Sciences* 5:331-337

Cook JL, May DL, Lewis Jr AM, Walker TA (1987): Adenovirus, E1A gene induction of susceptibility to lysis by natural killer cells and activated macrophages in infected rodent cells. *J Virol* 61:3510-3520

Drumm ML, Pope HA, Cliff WH, Rommens JM, Marvin SA, Tsui L-C, Collins FS, Frizzell RA, Wilson JM (1990): Correction of the cystic fibrosis defect in vitro by retrovirus-mediated gene transfer. *Cell* 62:1227-1233

Eloit M, Gilardi-Hebenstreit P, Toma B, Perricaudet M (1990): Construction of a defective adenovirus vector expressing the pseudorabies virus glycoprotein gp50 and its use as a live vaccine. *J Gen Virol* 71:2425-2431

Engelhardt JF, Yankaskas JR, Ernst SA, Yang Y, Marino CR, Boucher RC, Cohn

360   L. D. Stratford-Perricaudet and M. Perricaudet

JA, Wilson JM (1992): Submucosal glands are the predominant site of CFTR expression in the human bronchus. *Nature Genetics* 2:240-248

Flint SJ (1981): Structure and genomic organization of adenoviruses. In: *DNA Tumor Viruses*,2nd ed., Tooze J, ed. Cold Spring Harbor: Cold Spring Harbor Laboratory

Flint SJ, Broker TR (1981): Lytic Infection by adenoviruses. In: *DNA Tumor Viruses*, 2nd ed., Tooze J, ed. Cold Spring Harbor: Cold Spring Harbor Laboratory

Ghosh- Choudhury G, Haj-Ahmad Y, Brinkley P, Rudy J, Graham F (1986): Human adenovirus cloning vectors based on infectious bacterial plasmids. *Gene* 50:161-171

Gilardi P, Courtney M, Pavirani A, Perricaudet M (1990): Expression of human α1-antitrypsin using a recombinant adenovirus vector. *FEBS Letters* 267:60-62

Gluzman Y, Reichl H, Solnick D (1982): Helper-free adenovirus type 5 vectors. In *Eukaryotic Viral Vectors*, Gluzman Y, ed. Cold Spring Harbor: Cold Spring Harbor Laboratory

Graham FL, Smiley J, Russell WC, Nairn R (1977): Characteristics of a human cell line transformed by DNA from human adenovirus type 5. *J Gen Virol* 36:59-72

Gregory RJ, Cheng SH, Rich DP, Marshall J, Paul S, Hehir K, Ostedgaard L, Klinger KW, Welsh MJ, Smith AE (1990): Expression and characterization of the cystic fibrosis transmembrane conductance regulator. *Nature* 347:382-386

Hodges PE, Rosenberg LE (1989): The spf-ash mouse: a missense mutation in the ornithine transcarbamylase gene also causes aberrant mRNA splicing. *PNAS* 86:4142-4146

Horwitz MS (1990): Adenoviruses. In *Virology* 2nd ed., Fields BN, Knipe DM, eds. New York: Raven Press

Johnson LG, Olsen JC, Sarkadi B, Moore KL, Swanstrom R, Boucher RC (1992): Efficiency of gene transfer for restoration of normal airway epithelial function in cystic fibrosis. *Nature Genetics* 2:21-25

Le Gal La Salle G, Robert J-J, Berrard S, Ridoux V, Stratford-Perricaudet LD, Perricaudet M, Mallet J (1993): An adenovirus vector for gene transfer into neurons and glia in the brain. *Science* 259:988-990

Levrero M, Ballay A, Skellekens H, Tiollais P, Perricaudet M (1988): Hepatitis B adenovirus recombinant as a potential live vaccine. In: *Proceedings of the 8th International Biotechnology Symposium, Paris*, Saint-Just-la-Pendue, France: Imp Chirat

Levrero M, Barbant V, Ballay A, Balsamo C, Avantaggiati ML, Natoli G, Skellekens H, Tiollais P, Perricaudet M (1991): Defective and non-defective adenovirus vectors to express foreign genes in vitro and in vivo. *Gene* 101:195-202

Lubeck MD, Davis AR, Chengalvala M, Natuk RJ, Morin JE, Molnar-Kimber K, Mason BB, Bhat BM, Mizutani S, Hung PP, Purcell RH (1989): Immunogenicity and efficacy testing in chimpanzees of an oral hepatitis B vaccine based on live recombinant adenovirus. *PNAS* 86:6763-6767

Marchioli CC, Yancey RJ, Petrovskis EA, Timmins JG, Post LE (1987): Evaluation of pseudorabies virus glycoprotein gp50 as a vaccine for Aujeszky's disease in mice and swine: expression by vaccinia virus and chinese hamster ovary cells. *J Virol* 61:3977-3982

Mastrangeli A, Danel C, Rosenfeld MA, Stratford-Perricaudet LD, Perricaudet M, Pavirani A, Lecocq J-P, Crystal RG (1993): Diversity of airway epithelial cell targets for in vivo recombinant adenovirus-mediated gene transfer. *J Clin Invest* 91:225-234

Pääbo S, Bhat BM, Wold WSM, Peterson PA (1987): A short sequence in the COOH-terminus makes an adenovirus membrane glycoprotein a resident of the endoplasmic reticulum. *Cell* 50:311-317

Perricaudet M, Stratford-Perricaudet LD (1993): Adenovirus-mediated in vivo gene therapy. In: *Human Viruses in Gene Therapy*, Vos JMH, ed. Durham, NC: Carolina Academic Press

Quantin B, Stratford-Perricaudet LD, Tajbakhsh S, Mandel J-L (1992): Adenovirus as an expression vector in muscle cells in vivo. *PNAS* 89:2581-2584

Ragot T, Eloit M, Perricaudet M (1991): Recombinant E1A-defective adenoviruses expressing pseudorabies and Epstein-Barr virus glycoproteins induce immunological responses as live vaccines in rabbits and mice. In *Human Gene Transfer* Vol. 219, Cohen-Haguenauer O, Boiron M, eds. Grenoble, France: John Libbey Eurotext

Ragot T, Finerty S, Watkins PE, Perricaudet M, Morgan AJ (1993a): Replication-defective recombinant adenovirus expressing the EpsteiBarr (EBV) envelope glycoprotein gp340/220 induces protective immunity against EBV-induced lymphomas in the cottontop tamarin. *J Gen Virol* 74:501-507

Ragot T, Vincent N, Chafey P, Vigne E, Gilgenkrantz H, Couton D, Cartaud J, Briand P, Kaplan J-C, Perricaudet M, Kahn A (1993b): Efficient adenovirus-mediated transfer of a human minidystrophin gene to skeletal muscle of mdx mice. *Nature* 361:647-650

Rich DP, Anderson MP, Gregory RJ, Cheng SH, Paul S, Jefferson DM, McCann JD, Klinger KW, Smith AE, Welsh MJ (1990): Expression of cystic fibrosis transmembrane conductance regulator corrects defective chloride cannel regulation in cystic fibrosis airway epithelial cells. *Nature* 347:358-363

Riordan JR, Rommens JM, Kerem B-S, Alon N, Rozmahel R, Grzelczak Z, Zielenski J, Lok S, Plavsic N, Chou, J-L, Drumm ML, Iannuzzi MC, Collins FS, Tsui L-C (1989): Identification of the cystic fibrosis gene: cloning and characterization of complementary DNA. *Science* 245:1066-1073

Rommens JM, Iannuzzi MC, Kerem B-S, Drumm ML, Melmer G, Dean M, Rozmahel R, Cole JL, Kennedy D, Hidaka N, Zsiga M, Buchwald M, Riordan JR, Tsui L-C, Collins FS (1989): Identification of the cystic fibrosis gene: chromosome walking and jumping. *Science* 245:1059-1065

Rosenfeld MA, Siegfried W, Yoshimura K, Yoneyama K, Fukayama M, Stier LE, Paako PK, Gilardi P, Stratford-Perricaudet LD, Perricaudet M, Jallat S, Pavirani A, Lecocq J-P, Crystal RG (1991): Adenovirus-mediated transfer of a recombinant α1-antitrypsin gene to the lung epithelium in vivo. *Science* 252:431-434

Rosenfeld MA, Yoshimura K, Trapnell B, Yoneyama K, Rosenthal E, Dalemans W, Fukayama M, Bargon J, Stier L, Stratford-Perricaudet LD, Perricaudet M, Guggino W, Pavirani A, Lecocq J-P, Crystal RG (1992): In vivo transfer of the human cystic fibrosis transmembrane conductance regulator gene to the airway epithelium. *Cell* 68:143-155

Rowe WP, Huebner RJ, Gilmore LK, Parrott RH, Ward TG (1953): Isolation of a cytopathogenic agent from human adenoids undergoing spontaneous degeneration in tissue culture. *Proc Soc Exp Biol Med* 84:570-573

Severinsson L, Martens I, Peterson PA (1986): Differential association between two human MHC class I antigens and an adenoviral glycoprotein. *J Immunol* 137:1003-1009

Stratford-Perricaudet LD, Levrero M, Chasse J-F, Perricaudet M, Briand P (1990): Evaluation of the transfer and expression in mice of an enzyme-encoding gene using a human adenovirus vector. *Hum Gene Ther* 1:241-256

Stratford-Perricaudet LD, Perricaudet M (1991): Gene transfer into animals : The promise of adenovirus. In *Human Gene Transfer* Vol. 219, Cohen-Haguenauer O, Boiron M, eds. Grenoble, France: John Libbey Eurotext

Stratford-Perricaudet LD, Briand P, Perricaudet M (1992b): Feasibility of adenovirus-mediated gene transfer in vivo. *Bone Marrow Transplan* 9, S1, 151-152

Stratford-Perricaudet LD, Makeh I, Perricaudet M, Briand P (1992a): Widespread long-term gene transfer to mouse skeletal muscles and heart. *J Clin Invest* 90:626-630

Straus SE (1984): Adenovirus infections in humans. In *The Adenoviruses*, Ginsberg HS, ed. New York and London: Plenum Press

Top Jr FH, Grossman RA, Bartelloni PJ, Segal HE, Dudding BA, Russell PK, Buescher EL (1971a): Immunization with live types 7 and 4 adenovirus vaccines. I: Safety, infectivity, antigenicity, and potency of adenovirus type 7 vaccines in humans. *J Infect Dis* 124:148-155

Top Jr FH, Buescher EL, Bencroft WH, Russell PK (1971b): Immunization with live types 7 and 4 adenovirus vaccines. II: Antibody response and protective effect against acute respiratory disease due to adenovirus type 7. *J Infect Dis* 124:155-160

Williams JF (1986): Adenovirus genetics. In *Adenovirus DNA: The Viral Genome and its Expression*, Doerfler W, ed. La Hague: Martinus Nijhoff

Wold WSM, Gooding LR (1989): Adenovirus region E3 proteins that prevent cytolysis by cytotoxic T cells and tumor necrosis factor. *Mol Biol Med* 6:433-452

Wold WSM, Gooding LR (1991): Region E3 of adenovirus: A cassette of genes involved in host immunosurveillance and virus-cell interactions. *Virology* 184:1-8

Wolff JA, Malone RW, Williams P, Chong W, Acsadi G, Jani A, Felgner PL (1990): Direct gene transfer into mouse muscle in vivo. *Science* 247:1456-1468

IN VIVO GENE TRANSFER INTO THE HEART

Jeffrey M. Leiden and Eliav Barr

INTRODUCTION

The expression of recombinant genes in the human coronary arteries and myocardium holds promise for the treatment of a number of inherited and acquired cardiovascular diseases. These include the cardiomyopathy associated with Duchenne Muscular Dystrophy (DMD) (For review, Perloff, 1992), the problem of restenosis following balloon angioplasty of the coronary arteries (For review, Safian et al., 1992) and syndromes of chronic myocardial ischemia (For review, Rutherford and Braunwald, 1992). Current approaches to somatic gene therapy can be divided into two general categories: Ex vivo gene transfer involves the removal of cells from an organism followed by gene transduction in vitro and reimplantation of the genetically modified cells into the appropriate tissue in vivo. In contrast, in vivo gene transfer involves the introduction of a recombinant gene into the appropriate cell type in vivo without the need to remove and culture cells from the recipient organism.

The development of ex vivo gene transfer approaches in the heart has been limited by the unique biological properties of coronary arterial cells and cardiac myocytes. Neonatal and adult cardiac myocytes are terminally differentiated cells with a limited life span in tissue culture and little or no potential for cell replication in vitro or in vivo (Zak, 1974; Watanabe et al., 1986). Thus, it has not been possible to remove and manipulate these cells in vitro, nor to reintroduce such cells back into the heart in vivo. Similarly, although it is possible to culture arterial smooth muscle cells in vitro (Chamley et al., 1977), the technical difficulties involved in removing these cells from human coronary arteries and, in particular, of reimplanting such cells following genetic manipulation have severely limited ex vivo gene transfer approaches into the coronary vessels. Given these limitations, recent efforts have focused on devising methods for in vivo gene transfer into both the myocardium and coronary arteries. This review summarizes the current state of the art of in vivo gene transfer into the heart with particular emphasis on (i) the use of direct DNA injection into myocardium, and (ii) percutaneous transluminal gene transfer (PTGT) into the coronary vasculature and myocardium using replication-defective adenoviruses. Two additional methods of in vivo gene transfer into the coronary arteries, retroviral gene transfer and liposome-mediated gene

Gene Therapeutics: Methods and Applications of Direct Gene Transfer
Jon A. Wolff, Editor • ©1994 *Birkhäuser Boston*

transfer are described in detail in an accompanying chapter (see Plautz et al., this volume) and are therefore not discussed in this review. For additional information, the reader is also referred to several recent reviews of somatic gene therapy in the cardiovascular system (Swain, 1989; Nabel et al., 1991; Leiden and Leinwand, 1991).

IN VIVO GENE TRANSFER BY INJECTION OF PLASMID DNA INTO THE MYOCARDIUM

The capacity of skeletal muscle to express recombinant genes following direct intra-muscular injection of purified plasmid DNA was first demonstrated by Wolff and Felgner (Wolff et al., 1990) who showed that following IM injection, plasmid DNA is taken up and expressed for at least two months by a small percentage of skeletal myocytes surrounding the area of DNA injection. Three laboratories subsequently used similar techniques to demonstrate that cardiac myocytes can also take up and express recombinant genes introduced by the direct injection of purified plasmid DNA into the myocardium in vivo (Lin et al., 1990; Acsadi et al., 1991a; Kitsis et al., 1991). Interestingly, the ability to take up and express plasmid DNA in vivo appears to be limited to striated muscle as direct injection of plasmid vectors into other organs including brain, liver, spleen, uterus, stomach, lung, and kidney has failed to yield significant levels of recombinant gene expression (Acsadi et al., 1991a). As discussed below, this finding suggests that unique properties of striated muscle cells account for the as yet poorly understood mechanism of DNA uptake and expression following IM injection.

The technique of direct DNA injection into myocardium

In vivo gene transfer by direct injection of plasmid DNA into myocardium is most remarkable for its technical simplicity. Closed circular DNA is prepared from bacterial cultures by standard alkaline lysis followed by cesium chloride density centrifugation. Although plasmid DNA prepared by polyethylene glycol precipitation has been used to successfully program recombinant gene expression in cardiac myocytes, injection of this DNA appeared to result in more substantial scarring as compared to hearts injected with plasmid DNA prepared using alkaline lysis (Gal et al., 1993). Injection of linear plasmid DNA produces less efficient gene expression than closed circular DNA (Buttrick et al., 1992). Purified DNA is typically injected into the myocardium using a narrow (27-30 gauge) needle. Multiple injection vehicles including Opti-MEM, normal saline, and 5-20% sucrose in either phosphate buffered saline (PBS) or water have been used to successfully program recombinant gene expression following direct DNA injection. However, different vehicles appear to yield distinct efficiencies of recombinant gene expression and different levels of inflammation. Thus, for example, normal saline has been reported to increase the efficiency of gene transfer as compared to sucrose-containing PBS in skeletal muscle (Wolff et al., 1991). Additionally, EDTA should not be included in the injection solution as it appears to cause an increased inflammatory response. Inflammation may also be decreased by preparing endotoxin-free DNA, and by carefully removing both ethidium bromide and cesium chloride (and accompanying heavy metal ions) from the DNA solution. Finally, it should be emphasized that as compared to the injection of naked plasmid DNA, the injection of liposome/DNA complexes or Ca^{++}-PO_4/DNA precipitates results in significantly decreased efficiencies of gene transduction into both skeletal and cardiac myocytes in vivo.

The level of recombinant gene expression following DNA injection into the myocardium appears to be proportional to the amount of DNA injected over a range of approximately 10-100 μg per injection (Gal et al., 1993). Thus, most studies have utilized 25-100 μg of DNA per injection. The volume of DNA solution injected also appears to be important, with the efficiency of gene expression increasing with increasing volumes of injectate (Gal et al., 1993) between approximately 10 and 200 μl in a rodent heart. In addition, multiple injections into different regions of the myocardium increase the total level of recombinant gene expression in an additive fashion. The injected DNA is usually introduced into the left ventricular apex either through a sub-xiphoid approach or a left lateral thoracotomy. It appears that the success of the injection technique is independent of the type of anesthesia used and the method of ventilation. Finally, gene transfer into cardiac myocytes using direct injection of plasmid DNA has been demonstrated in a variety of species, including rats (Lin et al., 1990; Acsadi et al, 1991a; Kitsis et al., 1991), rabbits (Gal et al., 1993), and pigs (Gal et al., 1993).

Previous experiments have utilized several different reporter genes, including β-galactosidase (β-gal), chloramphenicol acetyltransferase (CAT), and luciferase to demonstrate myocardial gene transfer. These genes were chosen because none of them are normally expressed in the heart, and because each can be easily assayed in vitro. Each offers unique advantages in addressing basic questions regarding the specificity, efficiency, and stability of gene transfer into myocardium. The CAT and luciferase reporter genes have been used in comparisons of the efficiencies and stabilities of gene expression produced by different injection conditions because they each allow precise quantitation of the total level of recombinant gene expression following DNA injection. Luciferase has the advantage of being more sensitive than CAT so that lower levels of expression can be detected. The β-gal protein has the unique advantage of being detectable by routine histochemical techniques (Fig. 1). Thus, this reporter gene is useful in allowing the identification of individual cells that take up and express recombinant gene products in vivo. The ability to identify β-gal expression histochemically was particularly important in the heart, as cardiac myocytes comprise less than 50% of the cells in the heart.

Both viral and eukaryotic transcriptional regulatory elements have been used to regulate recombinant gene expression in cardiac muscle. The Rous sarcoma

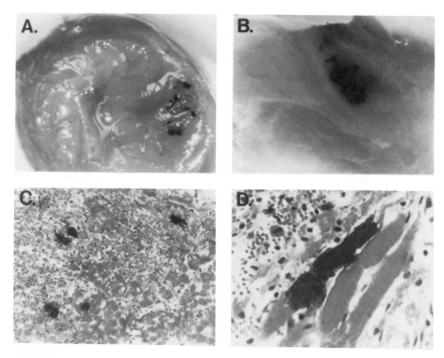

FIGURE 1. Expression of a recombinant β-galactosidase gene in cardiac myocytes in vivo after direct injection of pRSVβgal DNA into the left ventricular wall. One hundred micrograms of pRSVβgal DNA was injected into the beating apical wall of the left ventricle of Sprague-Dawley rats using a 30-g needle. Hearts were harvested 3-5 days or 3-4 weeks after injection and stained for β-galactosidase activity. Panel A: 10X view of a 3-mm section of a heart 3 days after pRSVβgal injection. Panel B: 18X view of a 3-mm section from a heart 27 days after pRSVβgal injection. Panels C and D: 125X and 250X views, respectively, of 4-μm sections from a heart 3 days after pRSVβgal injection. β-Galactosidase activity (dark-blue staining) is seen only within cardiac myocytes that can be identified by their myofibrillar architecture.

virus long terminal repeat (RSV LTR), which contains both promoter and enhancer elements, has been used extensively in these studies because previous reports have demonstrated that it programs high level recombinant gene expression in cardiac muscle both in vitro (Gustafson et al., 1987) and in vivo (Overbeek et al., 1986). The CMV promoter/enhancer has also been used successfully. However, previous studies have demonstrated that this viral element is transcriptionally down-regulated in several tissues in vivo (Dai et al., 1992). Additional studies have used the Moloney murine leukemia virus long terminal repeat (Gal et al., 1993) or cellular transcriptional regulatory elements such as the phosphoglycerol kinase promoter (Acsadi et al., 1991a), the cardiac troponin C (cTnC) promoter/enhancer (Parmacek et al., 1992), and the α-cardiac myosin heavy chain (α-MHC) promoter (Kitsis et al., 1991). Both the cTnC and α-MHC promoter/enhancers have been shown to program cardiac-specific transcription in in vitro transfection experiments (Parmacek et al., 1992; Gustafson et al., 1987; Tsika et al., 1990). The phosphoglycerol kinase and the α-cardiac myosin heavy chain promoters, but not the cardiac troponin C minimal promoter/enhancer, appear to be transcriptionally less active than the RSV LTR in cardiac myocytes following in vivo injection (Kitsis et al., 1991; Acsadi et al., 1991; Parmacek et al., 1992). Of note, the α-cardiac myosin heavy chain promoter has been shown to be responsive to thyroid hormone in vitro and has therefore been useful in studies of the hormonal regulation of recombinant genes in cardiac myocytes in vivo (Izumo et al., 1986; Lompre et al., 1984).

The specificity, efficiency and stability of recombinant gene expression following DNA injection into myocardium

The major limitation of the use of direct DNA injection to program recombinant gene expression in the myocardium revolves around the relatively low efficiency of gene transfer in vivo. Using β-galactosidase reporter plasmids both Lin et al. (1990) and Acsadi et al. (1991a) demonstrated recombinant gene expression in less than 1% of the cells in the area of DNA injection (Fig. 1). Thus, although a large area of the heart can be *effected* with multiple injections of DNA solution, the total number of cardiac myocytes that can be programmed to express a recombinant gene product remains quite limited. Ongoing studies are focused on better understanding the molecular mechanisms underlying direct DNA uptake by cardiac myocytes and on systematically altering the injection conditions in an attempt to increase the efficiency of gene transduction.

Several studies have examined the stability of recombinant gene expression following direct injection of plasmid DNA into both skeletal and cardiac muscle in vivo. Recombinant gene expression can be detected as early as 12 hours following DNA injection (Buttrick et al., 1992) and is still detectable for at least 8 months after plasmid injection into myocardium (E. Barr and J. Leiden, unpublished observations) and at least 19 months after plasmid DNA injection into skeletal muscle (Jiao et al., 1992). In most studies, the total level of recombinant gene expression appears to reach maximal levels approximately 2-4 weeks after injection and to then decline gradually. Histological studies have demonstrated that recombinant gene expression is observed only in cardiac myocytes and is never seen in connective tissue or vascular cells in the heart (Lin et al., 1990). Thus, the delivery system itself provides tissue-specificity of gene expression, an important safety consideration. Whereas most previous reports have demonstrated long-lived recombinant gene expression after a single intra-myocardial injection of plasmid DNA, a single study (Acsadi et al., 1991a) reported that recombinant gene expression was no longer detectable 28 days after DNA injection in normal rats, but could be stabilized by the use of nude rats. These results suggested an immune-mediated destruction of cells expressing recombinant gene products in the heart. The reason that this phenomenon has not been observed by other investigators in either cardiac or skeletal muscle remains unclear. However, it is possible that a more mild immune response is responsible for the gradual decay in recombinant gene expression observed in several studies between 1 and 6 months after DNA injection.

Several previous reports (Wolff et al., 1990; Acsadi et al., 1991a) have examined the physical state of the DNA in myocytes following direct DNA injections in vivo. The bulk of the DNA appears to be retained as circular and linear episomes with maintenance of the bacterial methylation pattern, suggesting a lack of DNA replication or integration in vivo. Although such studies cannot rule out rare integration events, these results are important from a safety perspective because they suggest that insertional mutagenesis may not be a significant problem following DNA injections into myocardium.

The relative efficiencies of gene transduction in skeletal versus cardiac and smooth muscle remain controversial. However, most studies have suggested that both cardiac and skeletal muscle are significantly more efficient than smooth muscle (Acsadi et al., 1991a) and that cardiac muscle can be transduced 10-100-times more efficiently than skeletal muscle (Lin et al., 1990; Kitsis et al., 1991). As discussed below, these differences may provide insights into the mechanism underlying DNA uptake and expression by myocytes.

Intra-myocardial DNA injections for studies of cardiac transcription

In addition to its potential usefulness as an approach for somatic gene therapy in the heart, the direct injection of CAT and luciferase reporter plasmids has proven to be a powerful technique for studying cardiac gene transcripition in vivo. The method is simpler, more economical, and less time-consuming than the generation of transgenic animals, and in some cases, may be more physiologically relevant than transient transfections of cultured fetal or neonatal cardiac myocytes which are known to lose their differentiated phenotype in vitro. Direct DNA injection may be particularly useful for studying the effects of specific pathophysiological states (e.g., hypertension, pressure or volume overload, or thyrotoxicosis) on cardiac transcription.

In an initial set of studies, Leinwand and co-workers demonstrated that transcriptional regulatory elements introduced into the heart using the direct injection technique are regulated in a tissue-specific fashion, and respond appropriately to thyroid hormone in vivo (Kitsis et al., 1991). Parmacek and co-workers (Parmacek et al., 1992) used the direct injection technique to define the *cis*-acting sequences regulating the cardiac-specific expression of the slow/cardiac troponin C (cTnC) gene (Fig. 2). These studies allowed the identification and characterization of a 156 bp cardiac-specific transcriptional promoter/enhancer located immediately 5' of the transcriptional start site in the cTnC gene. Taken together, these two studies demonstrated that direct DNA injection is a convenient and reproducible in vivo assay system for studies of cardiac-specific transcriptional regulatory elements.

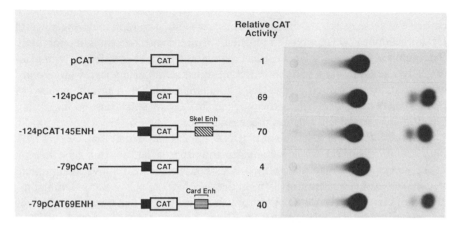

FIGURE 2. Evidence that a cardiac-specific promoter/enhancer in the 5' flanking region of the murine cTnC gene functions *in vivo* in cardiac myocytes. One hundred micrograms of cTnC/CAT reporter plasmid (schematically represented at the left) and 25 μg of the luciferase referecne plasmid pRSVL were injected directly into the left ventricular free wall of anesthetized 6-week-old Sprague-Dawley rats. Five days post-injection, the animals were sacrificed, and CAT and luciferase activities were determined from cardiac homogenates. CAT activities, corrected for differences in transfection efficiencies, are expressed relative to the CAT activity obtained following injection of the promoterless plasmid pCAT-Basic which produced 0.2% acetylation. A representative CAT assay is presented at the right.

Summary and future directions of intra-myocardial DNA injections

The studies described above have demonstrated that the direct injection of plasmid DNA into the left ventricular wall of adult animals from multiple species results in recombinant gene expression which is restricted to cardiac myocytes surrounding the area of DNA injection. These findings can be summarized as follows: (a) directly injected plasmid DNA is taken up and expressed by a small proportion of cardiac myocytes in the area immediately surrounding the injection site, (b) expression of recombinant genes introduced using direct DNA injection is significantly more efficient in the heart as compared to skeletal muscle, and (c) transcriptional regulatory elements introduced using this technique are regulated normally by both *tissueospecitic* and humoral signals. The stability of recombinant gene expression in myocardium following DNA injection remains controversial, and may be limited in some cases by an immune response against the recombinant gene products.

Most interestingly, the ability to take up and express recombinant genes following direct injection of plasmid DNA appears to be limited to skeletal and cardiac muscle. The mechanism of DNA uptake and transport to the nucleus in non-dividing striated muscle cells remains obscure. Current hypotheses include a role for muscle-specific transport systems such as the T-tubule system or a unique capacity of these cells to survive transient sarcolemmal disruption during plasmid DNA injection. This latter type of physical disruption mechanism is supported by the finding that freshly isolated cardiac myocytes cannot be transfected with plasmid DNA alone in vitro, and that efficient transduction of myocytes in vivo appears to require injection of the DNA containing solution. Current studies are focused on better understanding the mechanism of DNA uptake and on improving the efficiency of the transduction process in vivo.

Regardless of the mechanism of DNA uptake and expression, direct DNA injection offers several unique advantages as an approach to somatic gene therapy in the myocardium. First, the method does not require the removal and genetic manipulation of cardiac myoctyes from the recipient organism. Second, direct injection of plasmid DNA does not utilize infectious vectors that may carry a risk of persistent infection of the host. Third, plasmid DNA introduced by this method does not appear to integrate into the genome, thus minimizing the risk of mutagenesis of recipient cells. Finally, this method confers muscle-specific gene expression, thereby minimizing the risks of inappropriate recombinant gene expression in non-cardiac cells.

Several therapeutic applications for direct intramyocardial DNA injection are currently being explored. First, Acsadi et al. (1991b) have demonstrated that plasmids encoding both the full-length human dystrophin cDNA and the Becker-like dystrophin minigene are taken up and expressed after direct intra-muscular injection into dystrophin-deficient *mdx* mice. Dystrophin was detected in the cytoplasm of approximately 1% of the skeletal myofibers following injection. Thus, when coupled with improvements in the efficiency of gene transduction this may represent a potential therapeutic approach to both the skeletal and cardiac myopathies associated with DMD.

In a second series of experiments, Leiden and co-workers have recently started to explore the feasibility of using direct DNA injection to program angiogenesis in areas of ischemic myocardium. It is clear from previous clinical studies that patients with coronary artery disease who spontaneously develop collateral vessels in the myocardium have a better prognosis than patients lacking a collateral circulation (Sabia et al., 1992). Thus, the expression of recombinant angiogenesis factors in discreet regions of the myocardium in order to stimulate collateral blood vessel growth might represent a therapeutically important genetic approach towards revascularization. In initial studies, plasmids encoding fibroblast growth factor-5 (FGF-5) a secreted angiogenesis factor that is not normally expressed in the heart have been injected into the apical wall of the LV in 6 week old Sprague Dawley rats. We reasoned that the production of a secreted and potent cytokine like FGF-5 might circumvent the problem of inefficient gene transduction following DNA injection, and thereby stimulate neovascularization in a significant area of myocardium surrounding the injection site. Preliminary results from these experiments suggested that FGF-5 expression following direct DNA injection does increase local capillary density 3 weeks after injection in normal rat hearts (E. Barr, G. Engelman, and J. Leiden, unpublished observations). These experiments are currently being repeated in large animal models in which it is possible to determine directly the effects of neovascularization on regional blood flow, and to quantitate the protective effects of neovascularization against ischemic insults. Finally, several groups are attempting to develop both intracavitary and transcoronary artery catheter systems for localized intramyocardial DNA injection.

GENE TRANSFER MEDIATED BY REPLICATION-DEFECTIVE ADENOVIRUSES

In an attempt to develop more efficient catheter-mediated methods of gene transduction into both the coronary arteries and myocardium, several groups have recently started to explore the use of replication-defective adenoviruses delivered by intravenous or intra-arterial infusion. There were several reasons to think that adenoviruses might be useful for gene transfer in the heart. First, these vectors are capable of infecting a variety of replicating and non-replicating cell types when introduced intravenously (Stratford-Perricaudet et al., 1992; Rosenfeld et al., 1991), intra-arterially (Barr et al., in submission), intra-muscularly (Quantin et al., 1992), by inhalation (Rosenfeld et al., 1992), or directly into a target organ such as the brain (Le Gal La Salle et al., 1993). Secondly, adenovirus vectors can accommodate large cDNA inserts (up to 7.5 kb) (Haj-Ahmad and Graham, 1986; Berkner, 1988). Third, high titer (up to 10^{11} pfu/ml) stocks of these vectors can be prepared and frozen, thus potentially allowing for high efficiency gene transfer following the infusion of minimal volumes of virus in vivo. Finally, from a safety perspective, adenoviruses are common human pathogens that cause relatively low level morbidity and have not been associated with human malignancies. Adenoviruses have been previously used safely for human vaccination (Chanock et al., 1966).

Recently, two groups have demonstrated efficient gene transfer into the myocardium following intravenous or intra-arterial infusions of replication-defective adenoviruses (Stratford-Perricaudet et al., 1992; Barr et al., in submission). Additionally, Leiden and co-workers have shown that the intra-arterial infusion of replication-defective adenoviruses results in highly efficient gene transfer into coronary arterial endothelium and smooth muscle. This work is summarized below.

Replication-defective adenovirus vectors

The characteristics and the derivation of recombinant, replication-defective adenovirus vectors used in gene therapy are described in an accompanying chapter (see Stratford-Perricaudet and Perricaudet, this volume). Briefly, two serotypes of adenoviruses, serotype 2 (Ad 2) and serotype 5 (Ad 5) have been used to generate the majority of the vectors used for in vivo gene transfer experiments. These particular serotypes were chosen because they are minimally pathogenic and can be grown to high titer in vitro (Horwitz, 1990). Both viruses were made replication-

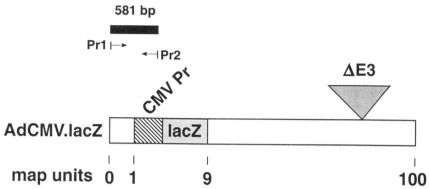

FIGURE 3. Schematic illustration of the replication-defective AdCMV.*lacZ* adenovirus. The CMV promoter/enhancer is shown by the crosshatched box and the bacterial *lacZ* gene by the shaded box. The position of the E3 deletion is noted (ΔE3). The positions of the PCR primers (Pr1 and Pr2) used to detect adenovirus DNA in infected tissues are shown above the map as is the expected 581 bp PCR product (solid black bar). Adenovirus map units are shown below the map.

defective by the deletion of two regions of the viral genome; the E1 region (map units 1-9) which encodes two early transcriptional regulatory factors that are required for both the induction of the viral lytic cycle and for the capacity of adenoviruses to transform cells in vitro, and the E3 region (map units 78.5 to 84.7) which encodes a protein that interacts with the major histocompatibility complex class I heavy chain and prevents its transport to the cell surface. The E3 protein is not required for adenovirus gene expression or growth in culture (Horwitz, 1990). However, the deletion of this region of the genome allows for the insertion of larger cDNA inserts into the recombinant viruses promoter/cDNA cassettes as large as 7.5 kb may be inserted into the E1 region of the doubly-deleted virus (Berkner, 1988). Because they lack the capacity to induce a viral lytic cycle after infection, the recombinant replication-defective adenoviruses can only be propagated by infection of a permissive cell line such as 293 human embryonic kidney cells which stably express the adenovirus E1 proteins.

Two related, but distinct recombinant, replication-defective adenoviruses have been used to examine the feasibility of adenovirus-mediated gene transfer into the heart. Both vectors are derived from Ad 5 and carry the bacterial *lacZ* reporter gene in the E1 region of the genome. The two vectors differ in the transcriptional regulatory elements controlling lacZ gene expression: Leiden and co-workers (Barr et al., in submission) have used the CMV promoter/enhancer (AdCMV.*lacZ*) (Fig. 3) while Perricaudet and co-workers (Stratford-Perricaudet et al., 1992) have used the RSV LTR (AdRSVβgal). Stocks of replication-defective adenoviruses have been prepared by infection of 293 cells at a multiplicity of infection of 2-5 pfu/cell. Prior to cell lysis, which occurs approximately 30-36 hours after initial infection, the cells are harvested, and the adenovirus particles released by repeated cycles of freezing and thawing. Virus is purified by discontinuous cesium chloride gradient centrifugation followed by dialysis against normal saline (Graham and van der Eb, 1973). These purified adenovirus stocks, which generally have titers of 10^{10}-10^{11} pfu/ml, can then be used directly for in vivo gene transfer experiments.

Specificity, efficiency, and stability of gene expression following intra-vascular adenovirus infusions

Both Perricaudet and co-workers and Leiden and co-workers have assessed the specificity, efficiency, and stability of gene expression in myocardium following intra-vascular administration of purified high-titer stocks of replication-defective recombinant adenovirus. Perricaudet and co-workers (Stratford-Perricaudet et al., 1992) injected 10^9 pfu of AdRSVβgal into the tail veins of neonatal mice and assessed the extent of gene transfer as measured by recombinant β-gal activity in the heart 15 days to one year after injection. β-gal activity was seen in a variety of organs, including the lung, liver, intestine, heart, and skeletal muscle. Histochemical staining of the heart revealed that approximately 0.2% of cardiac cells were expressing the β-gal reporter gene 15 days after injection. Expression of the transferred gene was detected as late as one year after injection, although the number of cardiac cells exhibiting β-galactosidase activity was reduced. When these same experiments were repeated in adult animals, less efficient gene transfer was noted, with a decrease in β-gal activity observed as early as 21 days after injection. Southern blot analysis was used to determine whether the adenovirus DNA had integrated into the genome. This analysis revealed that the adenovirus DNA remained extra-chromosomal in all of the organs detected. Although the sensitivity of Southern blotting does not allow for the detection of rare integration events, these results are significant, in that the potential for mutagenesis resulting from the introduction of adenovirus DNA into the myocardium would appear to be low.

Leiden and co-workers examined the pattern and stability of recombinant gene expression in the heart and coronary vasculature following percutaneous, transluminal infusion of replication-defective adenovirus directly into the coronary arteries (Barr et al., in submission). In these studies, 2 X 10^9 pfu of recombinant, replication-defective AdCMV.*lacZ* were infused via catheter into both the right and left coronary arteries of adult rabbits. Animals were sacrificed 5 days to 2 months following virus infusion, and hearts were assayed histochemically for β-gal gene expression, and by PCR for persistence of adenovirus DNA. A PCR assay also was used to determine the extent of adenovirus infection of other organs after the intra-arterial infusion of the AdCMV.*lacZ*. Intense β-gal activity was observed throughout the myocardium and the coronary arterial tree in all rabbits 5 days following adenovirus infusion (Figs 4 and 5). *LacZ* expression was observed in a large proportion of cardiac myocytes in both the atrial and ventricular myocardium and was also seen in a large number of non-myocytic connective tissue cells (Fig. 4). β-gal activity was also detected throughout the coronary arterial tree in

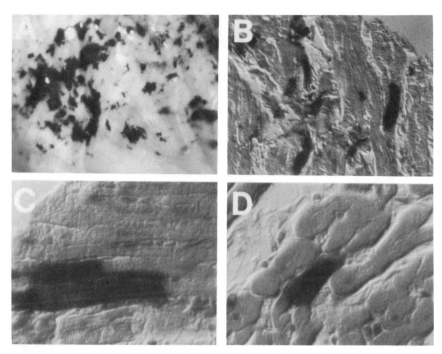

FIGURE 4. Histological detection of β-galactosidase activity in myocardium 5 days after intracoronary infusion of AdCMV.*lacZ*. A. Photomicrograph of the surface of an AdCMV.*lacZ* -infected heart (magnification = 25X). B-D. Photomicrographs of histological sections through two hearts 5 days following intracoronary infusion of AdCMV.*lacZ* (magnification = 200-400X). In each panel, blue staining represents β-galactosidase activity.

both endothelial and smooth muscle cells (Fig. 5). β-gal expression was particularly extensive in cells lining terminal capillaries in the area of distribution of the injected coronary artery. Somewhat remarkably, no inflammatory response or myocardial necrosis was observed in any of the hearts following percutaneous, transluminal infusion of the replication-defective adenoviruses. In marked contrast to the high levels of recombinant gene expression observed 5 days after intracoronary adenovirus infusions, no *lacZ* gene expression was detected in either the coronary arteries or myocardium 1 or 2 months after intrarterial infusion. Thus, recombinant gene expression in this species with this particular virus appears to be efficient but relatively short-lived.

There are several non-mutually exclusive possibilities that could explain the transient nature of recombinant gene expression observed in this system. First, the viral DNA might be lost or degraded over time. Second, the CMV promoter might be shut down in vivo, a phenomenon that has been previously reported in murine systems (Dai et al., 1992). Finally, the infected cells might die, either as a direct result of viral infection or as a result of an immune response against viral antigens.

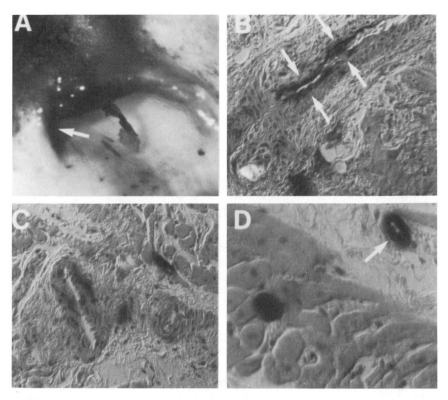

FIGURE 5. Histological detection of β-galactosidase activity in the coronary vasculature 5 days after intracoronary infusion of AdCMV.*lacZ*. A. Photomicrograph of the ascending aorta and a coronary ostium (arrow)(magnification = 40X). B. Photomicrograph of a transverse section through a large epicardial coronary artery (arrows) showing β-galactosidase activity in endothelial cells (magnification = 200X). C. Photomicrograph of a medium sized coronary artery showing β-galactosidase activity in cells in both the endothelial and medial layers (magnification = 200X). D. Photomicrograph of an intramyocardial capillary (arrow) showing β-galactosidase activity in the capillary wall (magnfication = 400X).

To determine whether the loss of recombinant gene expression demonstrated at the 1 and 2 month timepoints was due to loss of the adenovirus genome, a sensitive PCR-based assay was used to detect the presence of the adenovirus genome in cardiac lysates at various times after intra-coronary AdCMV.*lacZ* infusions. As expected, AdCMV.*lacZ* genome was present in all of the hearts examined 5 days after adenovirus infusion. However 4/7 hearts lacked detectable adenovirus DNA at 1 and 2 months after intra-arterial adenovirus infusion. These results suggested that loss of the viral genome represents at least one mechanism underlying the observed loss of viral gene expression in these animals. Whether this reflects degradation of the viral DNA, and whether this phenomenon is species- or virus-specific remains unclear. A direct lytic effect of viral infection or a potent cellular immune response against the infected cells seem less likely given the absence of a histologically detectable inflammatory response or significant myocardial necrosis.

The relatively short time course of recombinant gene expression observed by Leiden and co-workers in adult rabbit hearts contrasts significantly with the results obtained by Perricaudet and co-workers in neonatal mice. The reasons for this difference remain unclear, but may reflect differences either in the species and ages of the animals used or in the viruses used in the two studies, or both. Thus, for example, it is possible that the neonatal animals can become persistently infected by the replication-defective adenovirus and/or that their immune response to the virus differs from that of adult animals, thereby allowing long-term gene expression in the neonates. In this regard, it is of interest that Perricaudet and co-workers (Quantin et al., 1992) reported that intra-muscular injection of adenovirus results in long-term recombinant gene expression in the skeletal myocytes of neonatal mice, but in only transient expression in the muscle of similarly injected adult animals. Finally, the replication defective adenoviruses used in the two studies employed distinct transcriptional regulatory elements to control expression of the *lacZ* gene: Perricaudet and co-workers used the RSV LTR, whereas Leiden and co-workers used the CMV promoter/enhancer.

The risk of generating a systemic infection following virally mediated gene transfer in vivo remains an important safety consideration that must be addressed for all RNA and DNA viral vectors. To assess the extent of infection of non-cardiac tissues following intra-coronary infusion of AdCMV.*lacZ* in rabbits, Leiden and co-workers used a sensitive PCR assay to detect viral DNA in a variety of organs from animals 5 days after intra-coronary adenovirus infusions. Using this assay which can detect 1 copy of the adenovirus genome per 10,000 cells, AdCMV.*lacZ*-specific sequences were detected in liver, spleen, kidney, heart, lung, brain, and testis, but not in skeletal muscle or spleen. These data are important because (1) they demonstrate the wide range of cell types that can be infected with replication-defective adenoviruses in vivo and (2) the presence of adenovirus DNA in the brain and testis raises important safety concerns regarding the use intra-arterial infusions of recombinant, replication-defective adenoviruses for in vivo gene transfer.

Summary and potential applications of Adenovirus-mediated gene transfer in vivo

The two studies described above convincingly demonstrated the feasibility of using intra-vascular infusions of replication-defective adenoviruses to program high-level recombinant gene expression in both the myocardium and the coronary vasculature. The results of these studies are most remarkable because no attempt was made to ensure prolonged contact of the virus with the coronary vasculature or the myocardium. The longevity of recombinant gene expression in the heart following intra-vascular viral infusions remains unclear and to a large extent will determine the usefulness of this system for the treatment of a variety of cardiovascular diseases.

Percutaneous transluminal gene transfer into the heart using replication-defective adenoviruses has several advantages as compared to the direct injection of plasmid DNA described above. First, adenoviruses provide significantly higher efficiencies of gene transfer into both myocardium and coronary vasculature as compared to all previously described techniques. Second, in contrast to direct DNA injections, there is no evidence of an inflammatory response or myocardial necrosis and scarring at least during the first two months after intra-coronary infusions of adenovirus. Third, intra-coronary infusions of adenovirus are minimally invasive and can be carried out percutaneously using standard techniques of cardiac catheterization. Like the directly injected plasmid DNA, replication-defective adenoviruses do not appear to integrate into the genome, thereby decreasing the risk of mutagenesis of the host cell. Finally, the broad host range of the adenoviruses allows for gene transfer into multiple cardiac cell types, including cardiac myocytes and fibroblasts, and coronary artery endothelial and smooth muscle cells. On the other hand, even replication-defective adenoviruses may have a limited potential for recombination which could result in the generation of replication-competent virus and persistent infection of the host. Additionally, the capacity of adenoviruses to infect a wide variety of noncardiac tissues following intra-coronary arterial infusions represents an important safety concern. Finally, the issue of the stability of recombinant gene expression particularly in adult humans, following intra-vascular adenovirus infusions remains unclear.

Despite these possible limitations, there are several potential therapeutic applications for percutaneous transluminal gene transfer using replication- defective adenoviruses. For example, this may represent a useful approach for the prevention of restenosis following percutaneous transluminal coronary angioplasty (PTCA). Such restenosis is a significant clinical problem occurring within 6 months in 30-40% of initially successful PTCAs (Muller et al., 1992). Histological studies have demonstrated that the restenotic lesion is characterized by a reactive hyperplasia of smooth muscle cells with the concomitant production of abundant extracellular matrix in the area of plaque fracture induced by the angioplasty balloon. Recent work from Rosenberg and co-workers (Simons et al., 1992) has suggested that even short-term changes in vascular smooth muscle cell gene expression, such as those observed following the extra-vascular introduction of antisense *c-myb* oligonucleotides are sufficient to effectively prevent restenosis following PTCA. Thus, an appropriate replication-defective adenovirus that efficiently programs recombinant gene expression in vascular smooth muscle cells for a short period of time might be ideally suited to the treatment of this disorder.

Replication-defective adenovirus mediated gene transfer may also be useful in the treatment of inherited cardiovascular diseases such as the cardiomyopathy associated with Duchenne Muscular Dystrophy (DMD). Thus, for example, Perricaudet and co-workers (Le Gal La Salle et al., 1993) recently demonstrated efficient adenovirus-mediated transfer of the Becker-like dystrophin minigene into the biceps femoris muscle of neonatal *mdx* mice. Injection of approximately 2.5 $X10^9$ pfu of a recombinant, replication-defective adenovirus containing the dystrophin minigene under the control of the RSV LTR resulted in recombinant dystrophin gene expression in 6-50% of skeletal myocytes in the area of injection for periods of up to 3 months. A similar approach utilizing intra-coronary arterial infusions of a replication-defective adenovirus containing the Becker-like dystrophin minigene under the control of a cardiac myocyte-specific transcriptional regulatory element such as the cTnC promoter/enhancer might be useful for the treatment of the cardiomyopathy associated with DMD.

Despite the promise of adenovirus-mediated gene transfer into the heart, several important questions must be addressed before it is possible to accurately assess the utility and safety of this approach for human therapy. First, the stability of adenovirus-mediated gene transfer in adult animals from a number of species must be determined. These studies should employ several viruses that express different reporter genes under the control of distinct viral and cellular promoters and enhancers. Second, the finding of adenovirus DNA in several noncardiac tissues including brain and testis must be carefully addressed from a safety perspective. In particular, it will be important to determine the longevity and level of ectopic adenovirus gene expression in these organs and to attempt to minimize or abolish ectopic viral gene expression using tissue-specific transcriptional regulatory elements in conjunction with catheter-based local delivery systems and decreased amounts of virus. Finally, further work will be needed to determine if prior adenovirus infection (whether naturally occurring or as a result of an initial course of gene therapy) renders patients resistant to further infection with the replication defective adenovirus vectors.

SUMMARY

In vivo gene transfer into the heart offers unique opportunities to treat both inherited and acquired cardiovascular diseases and to study the molecular mechanisms that regulate cardiac gene expression. The development of gene transfer techniques for the heart has been complicated by technical limitations and by the unique biological properties of cardiac myocytes and coronary vascular cells. Nevertheless, novel in vivo gene transfer approaches utilizing either the direct injection of plasmid DNA or the intra-vascular administration of replication-defective, recombinant adenoviruses have recently been developed. Although each of these approaches has unique advantages and disadvantages, it seems likely that by better understanding the molecular bases of direct DNA and adenovirus gene transfer it may be possible to develop hybrid technologies that combine the efficiency of adenovirus vectors with the safety and longevity of direct DNA injection. It is likely that such hybrid gene transfer technologies will lead to the development of novel therapeutic approaches for cardiovascular disease.

REFERENCES

Acsadi G, Dickson G, Love DR, Jani A, Walsh FS, Gurusinghe A, Wolff JA, Davies KE (1991): Human dystrophin expression in *mdx* mice after intra-muscular injection of DNA constructs. *Nature* 352:815-818

Acsadi G, Jiao S, Jani A, Duke D, Williams P, Chong W, Wolff JA (1991): Direct gene transfer and expression into rat heart in vivo. *New Biol* 3:71-81

Barr E, Carroll J, Tripathy S, Kozarsky K, Wilson JM, Leiden JM (1993): Percutaneous transluminal gene transfer into the heart using replication-defective recombinant adenovirus. (Submitted.)

Berkner KL (1988): Development of adenovirus vectors for the expression of heterologous genes. *Biotechniques* 6:616-629

Buttrick PM, Kass A, Kitsis RN, Kaplan ML, Leinwand LA (1992): Behavior of genes directly injected into the rat heart in vivo. *Circ Res* 70:193-198

Chamley JH, Campbell GR, McConnell, JD, Gröschel-Stewart U (1977): Comparison of vascular smooth muscle cells from adult human, monkey, and rabbit in primary culture and in subculture. *Cell Tiss Res* 177: 503-522

Chanock RM, Ludwig W, Heubner RJ, Cate TR, Chu LW (1966): Immunization by selective infection with type 4 adenovirus grown in human diploid tissue cultures. I. Safety and lack of oncogenicity and tests for potency in volunteers. *JAMA* 195:445-452

Dai Y, Roman M, Naviaux RK, Verma I (1992): Gene therapy via primary myoblasts: Long-term expression of factor IX protein following transplantation in vivo. *Proc Natl Acad Sci USA* 89:10892-10895

Flugelman MY, Jaklitsch MT, Newman KD, Casscells W, Bratthauer GL, Dichek DA (1992): Low level in vivo gene transfer into the arterial wall thromgh a perforated balloon catheter. *Circulation* 85:1110-1117

Gal D, Weir L, LeClerc G, Pickering JG, Hogan J, Isner JM (1993): Direct myocardial transfection in two animal models. Evaluation of parameters affecting gene expression and percutaneous gene delivery. *Lab Invest* 68:18-25

Graham FL, Eb AJ-van-der (1973): Transformation of rat cells by DNA of human adenovirus 5. *Virology* 54:536-539

Graham FL, Smiley J, Russell WC, Nairn R (1977): Characteristics of a human cell line transformed by DNA from adenovirus type 5. *J Gen Virol* 36:59-74

Gustafson T, Markham B, Bahl JJ, Morkin E (1987): Thyroid hormone regulates expression of a transfected a myosin heavy chain fusion gene in fetal heart cells. *Proc Natl Acad Sci USA* 84:3122-3126

Haj-Ahmad Y, Graham FL (1986): Development of a helper-independent human adenovirus vector and its use in the transfer of the herpes simplex virus thymidine kinase gene. *J Virol* 57:267-274

Horwitz MS (1990): The Adenoviruses. In *Virology*, Fields BN, Knipe DM, eds. New York: Raven Press

Izumo S, Nadal-Ginard B, Mahdavi V (1986): All members of the MHC multigene family respond to thyroid hormone in a highly tissue-specific manner. *Science*

231:597-600

Jiao S, Williams P, Berg RK, Hodgeman BA, Liu L, Repetto G, Wolff JA (1992): Direct gene transfer into nonhuman primate myofibers in vivo. *Hum Gene Ther* 3:21-33

Kitsis R, Buttrick P, McNally E, Kaplan M, Leinwand LA (1991): Hormonal modulation of a gene injected into rat heart in vivo. *Proc Natl Acad Sci USA* 88:4138-4142

Le Gal La Salle G, Robert JJ, Berrard RS, Ridoux V, Stratford-Perricaudet LD, Perricaudet M, Mallet J (1993): An adenovirus vector for gene transfer into neurons and glia in the brain. *Science* 259:988-990

Leinwand LA, Leiden JM (1991): Gene transfer into cardiac myocytes in vivo. *Trends Card Med* 1: 271-276

Lin H, Parmacek MS, Morle G, Bolling S, Leiden JM (1990): Expression of recombinant genes in myocardium in vivo after direct injection of DNA. *Circulation* 82:2217-2221

Lompre A-M, Nadal-Ginard B, Mahdavi V (1984): Expression of the cardiac ventricular a- and b-myosin heavy chain genes is developmentally and hormonally regulated. *J Biol Chem* 259:6437-6446

Muller DW, Ellis SG, Topol EJ (1992): Experimental models of coronary artery restenosis. *J Am Coll Cardiol* 19:418-432

Nabel EG, Plautz G, Boyce FM, Stanley JC, Nabel GJ (1989): Recombinant gene expression in vivo within endothelial cells of the arterial wall. *Science* 244:1342-1344

Nabel EG, Plautz G, Nabel GJ (1990): Site-specific gene expression in vivo by direct gene transfer into the arterial wall. *Science* 249:1285-1288

Nabel EG, Plautz G, Nabel GJ (1991): Gene transfer into vascular cells. *J Am Coll Cardiol* 17:189B-194B

Overbeek PA, Lai S-P, Van Quill KR, Westphal H (1986): Tissue-specific expression in transgenic mice of a fused gene containing RSV terminal sequences. *Science* 231:1574-1577

Parmacek MS, Vora AJ, Shen T, Barr E, Jung F, Leiden JM (1992): Identification and characterization of a cardiac-specific transcriptional regultory element in the slow/cardiac troponin C gene. *Mol Cell Biol* 12:1967-1976

Perloff JK (1992): Congenital heart disease in adults. In: *Heart Disease*, Braunwald E, ed. Philadelphia: Saunders Press

Quantin B, Perricaudet LD, Tajbakhsh S, Mandel J-L (1992): Adenovirus as an expression vector in muscle cells in vivo. *Proc Natl Acad Sci USA* 89:2581-2584

Ragot T, Vincent N, Chafey P, Vigne E, Gilgenkrantz H, et al. (1993): Efficient adenovirus-mediated transfer of a human minidystrophin gene to skeletal muscle of *mdx* mice. *Nature* 361:647-650

Rosenfeld MA, Siegfried W, Yoshimura K, Yoneyama K, et al. (1991): Adenovirus-mediated transfer of a recombinant a1-antitrypsin gene to the lung epithelium in vivo. *Science* 252:431-434

Rosenfeld MA, Yoshimura K, Trapnell BC, Yonyama K, et al. (1992): In vivo transfer of the human cystic fibrosis transmembrane conductance regulator gene to the airway epithelium. *Cell* 68:143-155

Rutherford JD, Braunwald E (1992): Chronic ischemic heart disease. In: *Heart Disease*, Braunwald E, ed. Philadelphia: Saunders Press

Sabia PJ, Powers ER, Ragosta M, Sarembock IJ, Burwell LR, Kaul S (1992): An association between collateral blood flow and myocardial viability in patients with recent myocardial infarction. *N Eng J Med* 327:1825-1831

Safian RD, Gelbfish JS, Erny RE, Schnitt SJ, Schmidt DA, Baim DS (1990): Coronary atherectomy. Clinical, angiographic, and histological findings and observations regarding potential mechanims. *Circulation* 82:69-79

Simons M, Edelman ER, DeKeyser J-LL, Langer R, Rosenberg RD (1992): Antisense *c-myb* oligonucleotides inhibit intimal arterial smooth muscle cell accumulation in vivo. *Nature* 359:67-70

Simons M, Rosenberg RD (1992): Antisense nonmuscle myosin heaavy chain and *c-myb* oligonucleotides suppress smooth muscle cell proliferation in vitro. *Circ Res* 70:835-843

Steinhelper ME, Lanson NA, Dresdner KP, et al. (1990): Proliferation in vivo and in culture of differentiated adult atrial cardiomyocytes from transgenic mice. *Am J Physiol* 259:H1826-H1834

Stratford-Pericaudet LD, Makeh I, Perricaudet M, Briand P (1992): Widespread long-term gene transfer to mouse skeletal muscles and heart. *J Clin Invest* 90:626-630

Swain JL (1989): Gene therapy: a new approach to the treatment of cardiovascular disease. *Circulation* 80:1495-1496

Tsika R, Bahl J, Leinwand L, Morkin E (1990): Thyroid hormone regulates expression of a transfected human a-myosin heavy chain fusion gene in fetal rat heart cells. *Proc Natl Acad Sci USA* 87:379-383

Watanabe AM, Green FJ, Farmer BB (1986): Preparation and use of cardiac myocytes in experimental cardiology. In:*The Heart and Cardiovascular System*. Fozzard HA, Haber E, Jennings RB, Katz AM, Morgan, HE, eds. New York: Raven Press

Wolff JA, Malone RW, Williams P, et al. (1990): Direct gene transfer into mouse muscle in vivo. *Science* 247:1465-1468

Wolff JA, Williams P, Acsadi G, Jiao S, Jani A, Chong W (1991): Conditions affecting direct gene transfer into rodent muscle in vivo. *BioTechniques* 11:474-485

Wu CH, Wilson JM, Wu GY (1989): Targeting genes: delivery and persistent expression of a foreign gene driven by mammalian regulatory elements in vivo. *J Biol Chem* 264:16985-16987

Zak R (1974): Development and proliferation capacity of cardiac muscle cells. *Circ Res* 34-35 (suppl II):II-17

RECEPTOR-MEDIATED TARGETED GENE DELIVERY USING ASIALOGLYCOPROTEIN-POLYLYSINE CONJUGATES

Stephen Furs and George Y. Wu

Delivery of exogenous DNA into cells has been in the forefront of genetic research, both in basic and clinical sciences. Many techniques have been developed to introduce foreign genes into mammalian cells in vitro (Gopal, 1985; Harland and Weintraub, 1985; Potter et al., 1984; Williams et al., 1984; Nicolau and Sene, 1982; Zhou et al., 1991; Graham and Van der Eb, 1973). For example, one of the oldest and most popular methods involves a co-precipitation of DNA with calcium phosphate. These insoluble particles are internalized within the host cells (Loyter et al., 1982). A portion of the DNA containing a gene of interest can be expressed in vitro. Indeed, calcium phosphate precipitates have also been used successfully in vivo by direct injection into organs resulting in transfection of cells in animals and subsequent expression (Dubensky et al., 1984a; Benvenisty and Reshef, 1986a). For example, Benvenisty and Reshef detected expression of chloramphenicol acetyltransferase (CAT), in mainly liver and spleen, after intraperitoneal injection of calcium phosphate precipitated plasmids which contained CAT marker gene (Benvenisty and Reshef, 1986b). Similarly, Dubensky and associates were able to demonstrate viral replication and acute infection after polyoma viral DNA was directly introduced into the liver or spleens of mice (Dubensky et al., 1984b).

Other applications of foreign gene transfection using viral vectors have been investigated because of the efficiency of transfection of some viruses. Retroviruses are efficient at gene transfer in replicating cells, and integrate the transferred genes into cellular DNA (Miller, 1992). One disadvantage of retroviral vectors is an inability to infect nondividing cells (Miller et al., 1990). Adenovirus vectors do not have this limitation (Svensson and Persson, 1984; Tibetts and Giam, 1979). For example, Rosenfeld et al. used adenovirus to demonstrate expression of human cystic transmembrane conductance regulator gene in tracheal epithelium in cotton rats (Rosenfeld et al., 1992).

Liposomes are also an attractive vehicle for gene transfer. In this technique, DNA is trapped on or within a membrane vesicle which can be delivered to living cells. For example, Nicolau et al. utilized liposomes to incorporate rat proinsulin gene into liver via intravenous injection; however, there was also significant uptake in the spleen (Nicolau et al., 1983). Zhou and colleagues demonstrated target specificity and efficient transfection activity of a liposome model by using a lipophilic moiety to synthesize a polylysine-phospholipid conjugate (i.e. a lipopolylysine) (Zhou et al., 1991).

Most of the aforementioned methods of gene delivery were developed with in vitro models; however, when applied in vivo, their potential for gene delivery is limited by their lack of cell specificity. This lack of cell specificity can result in non-targeted genetic delivery in possibly undesirable locations. Also, many of these techniques developed for transfection of mammalian cells in vivo are technically difficult.

Liver cells have highly specific cell-surface receptors that recognize galactose-terminal glycoproteins or asialoglycoproteins (ASGP) (Ashwell and Morell, 1974). By taking advantage of this receptor, substances could be targeted specifically to liver cells. Once the asialoglycoprotein receptor is recognized, endocytosis occurs and the glycoprotein is internalized by membrane-bound endosomal vesicles which eventually fuse with lysosomes. Usually proteolytic breakdown of the glycoprotein occurs, subsequently (Wall et al., 1980; Dunn et al., 1980; Stockert and Morrell, 1982). Several investigators have demonstrated ligand specificity for hepatocytes by covalently linking various agents to asialoglycoproteins (Molema et al., 1991; Fiume et al., 1987). Specificity to hepatocytes was demonstrated in an in vivo model where a targetable carrier antagonist conjugate was developed to protect normal hepatocytes from damage by a highly specific hepatotoxin, galactosamine. Intravenous injection of the antagonist conjugate resulted in selective uptake by the liver (Keegan-Rogers and Wu, 1990). Based on these studies, experiments were undertaken to determine whether foreign genetic material could be targeted to hepatocytes in a similar fashion.

To prepare a targetable DNA carrier, an ASGP was covalently coupled to a polycation. Taking advantage of the inherent negative charge of DNA (from its exposed phosphate moieties) DNA was then bound to a polycation, polylysine, by electrostatic interactions resulting in *non-covalent* bonds. Such linkages could occur without irreversibly changing or damaging the DNA (Wu and Wu, 1992).

To test this system, an experiment was designed to deliver a piece of DNA in the form of a bacterial plasmid, pSV2 CAT which contains the gene for chloramphenicol acetyltransferase (CAT). The marker for gene transformation was CAT enzyme expression in the target cells (Wu and Wu, 1987).

An asialoglycoprotein was created, asialoorosomucoid (ASOR), by isolating orosomucoid from pooled human sera and desialylating it to expose galactose residues using neuraminidase (Whitehead and Sammons, 1966); Kawasaki and Ashwell, 1977). The ASOR was purified and iodinated with carrier-free $Na^{125}I$ (Greenwood et al., 1963) using a solid phase lactoperoxidase system. A targetable DNA carrier system was prepared by coupling ASOR to poly-L-lysine in a 5:1 molar ratio using N-succinimidyl 3-(2-pyridyldithio) propionate (Jung et al., 1981). The conjugate was separated from non-coupled ASOR and polylysine on a Bio-Gel A-1.5m molecular sieve column (Laemmli, 1970).

In order to determine the proportion of ASOR-polylysine conjugate that should be mixed with plasmid DNA for formation of targetable complexes, increasing amounts of ^{125}I-labeled conjugate were added to tubes containing equal amounts of DNA. Samples were incubated, dialyzed and filtered, and the filtrate electrophoresed on a agarose gel (Maniatis et al., 1982). After staining with ethidium bromide to visualize DNA, an autoradiograph was also obtained to detect the location of the ^{125}I-ASOR-PL conjugate. Progressively increasing amounts of DNA appeared to be retained by the ASOR-PL conjugate as the proportion of conjugate to DNA was increased in the samples. To confirm that DNA was indeed being retarded at the top of the gels, pSV2 CAT plasmid was labeled with ^{32}P by nick-translation (Maniatis et al., 1975a). Samples with increasing ratios of conjugate to DNA were prepared as described before. However, after filtration, the filters were also washed and counted. The gel showed that increasing the proportion of ASOR-PL to DNA did bind progressively greater amounts of DNA. In addition, counting of the filters showed that conjugate to DNA ratios >3.27:1 resulted in progressive increases in amounts of retained insoluble DNA on the filters (Wu and Wu, 1988).

An in vitro model was designed to assay for foreign gene expression using four cell lines: human hepatoma cell line HepG2 (ASGP receptor +); hepatoma cell line SK-Hep 1 (ASGP receptor -); human lung fibroblast IMR-90 (ASGP receptor -); and uterine smooth muscle (ASGP receptor -). Samples were filtered, then incubated with each cell line for 48 hours at 37°C under 5% CO_2. Equal numbers of cells were assayed for CAT activity by incubation with ^{14}C-chloramphenicol. Standard CAT enzyme incubated with ^{14}C-chloramphenicol was spotted onto each plate for quantification of CAT activity in the cell samples and enzyme activity was detected by the presence of 1- and 3-acetylchloramphenicol derivatives on the plates.

The SK-Hep 1 cell line demonstrated no gene transformation with either the ASOR-PL-DNA conjugate, ASOR-DNA, PL-DNA, or DNA alone. The HepG2 cell line *did* demonstrate gene transformation, but with only the ASOR-PL-DNA complex and not with any of the controls. Of note, competition by an excess of ASOR inhibited transformation and expression of the CAT gene in the cells, indicating that the HepG2 cells recognized the ASOR-PL-DNA complex by the asialoglycoprotein portion of the complex.

To investigate the efficiency of the transformation, pSV2 CAT DNA was also introduced into the HepG2 cell line by a calcium phosphate method. The transformation efficiency of the complex was found to be approximately double that of the calcium phosphate method (Wu and Wu, 1987b).

The specificity and relative efficiency of the targeted gene delivery to cell lines with the ASGP receptor was further demonstrated by incubation of the ASOR-PL-DNA complex with human lung fibroblast IMR-90 cells, and uterine smooth muscle cells, both of which do not possess ASGP receptors as found with SK-Hep 1, receptor (-) hepatoma cells. No detectable CAT activity was found in any of these cells.

The targeted gene expression in HepG2 hepatoma cells was found to be transient; CAT activity maximized at 0.028 unit/10^6 cells measured immediately after the transformation. A decline was noted to 0.003 unit/10^6 cells by the third passage (sixth-post transformation day), and no CAT activity detected by the fourth passage (Wu and Wu, 1988).

In summary, these series of experiments showed that soluble asialoglycoprotein-polylysine conjugates could be used to target genes with specific delivery to hepatocytes via receptor mediated endocytosis. This resulted in transient expression of foreign genes by these cells.

To test whether hepatic asialoglycoprotein receptors would recognize this DNA carrier in vivo, the DNA carrier was prepared (as described previously) and complexed to pSV2 CAT, a plasmid which contains the CAT gene driven by an SV40 promoter. For in vivo uptake and hybridization studies, the plasmid was labeled with ^{32}P by nick-translation (Maniatis et al., 1975b). The conjugate was complexed in a 2:1 molar ratio (based on ASOR content of the complex) to the plasmid.

To determine whether the DNA-conjugate complex retained its ability to be recognized by hepatic ASGP receptors in vivo, groups of male Sprague-Dawley rats, 200-250 grams, were injected intravenously with ^{125}I-ASOR, ASOR-PL-^{32}P-DNA, or ^{32}P-DNA, all in sterile saline. Ten minutes later, the animals were sacrificed and samples of various organs (liver, spleen, lung, kidney and blood) were taken and portions counted for radioactivity. After injection of DNA alone, most of the residual ^{32}P-radioactivity remained circulating in the blood, 46%; while 24% was found in kidney. Injection of labeled DNA complexed with the carrier conjugate targeted to liver with 85% of the injected counts taken up by that organ after 10 minutes, compared to 17% of the counts when the same amount of labeled DNA alone was injected under the same conditions. Only 5% of the injected counts remained in the blood, and 5% taken up by the spleen. When ^{125}I-ASOR was injected into rats, the organ distribution, determined by radioactivity 10 minutes after injection, was similar to that found for the complex.

To assess the integrity of the pSV2-CAT plasmid DNA beyond the 10 minute post-injection period, a group of rats was intravenously injected with pSV2-CAT DNA as a complex in saline. The animals were sacrificed after 24 hours, the livers removed and homogenized; the DNA was extracted and assayed by dot-blot hybridization with a ^{32}P-DNA probe to detect pSV2 CAT DNA sequences. Targeted pSV2 CAT DNA was detected in the samples from rats injected with complex, but not from control saline-treated rats indicating that the hybridization was due to delivered foreign gene and not host gene sequences.

Homogenates of livers taken 24 hours after injection of the complex showed functional CAT gene activity. When the dose of the complexed DNA was increased from 250 micrograms to 750 micrograms/200 gram rat, CAT activity increased from 2.5 to 6.0 units/gram liver. No significant difference in increase of CAT activity was found when more than 750 microgram/200 gr rat was used (Wu and Wu, 1992b). Injection of components of the complex (DNA alone, DNA-PL, ASOR-PL) and saline alone showed no detectable CAT activity under any of these conditions. Also, no detectable CAT activity in other organs, lungs, kidneys, and spleen, was found. A molar excess of ASOR injected along with ASOR-PL-DNA complex, resulted in no detectable CAT activity (Wu and Wu, 1988b).

A plasmid, palb-CAT, containing the gene for chloramphenicol acetyltransferase driven by a mouse albumin regulatory elements (natural mammalian regulatory sequences) was prepared by replacement of the SV40 promoter sequences by mouse albumin promoter and enhancer sequences in the MTBV.JT. (Pinkert et al., 1987). The plasmid was complexed to the carrier ASOR-PL. Targeted gene expression was assessed by intravenously injecting Sprague-Dawley rats with saline containing palb-CAT DNA in the form of a complex, or controls. At 24 hour intervals, animals were sacrificed. Liver samples were removed, homogenized, and samples assayed for protein content and CAT activity. The results showed that CAT gene expression was transient, reaching maximum activity at 24 hours with a decline to no detectable activity by 96 hours (Wu et al., 1989).

To examine the possibility of prolonging targeted gene expression, 66% partial hepatectomies were performed on groups of rats shortly after injection of DNA complex. The idea was to initiate cellular division and hepatocyte regeneration in order to increase the probability of integration of the transfected gene into the host genome. Over an 8 week period, rats were sacrificed at various intervals and CAT activity assays were performed at each time point. The results showed that CAT activity was first detected at 48 hours after 66% hepatectomy and persisted at each time point. Maximum activity occurred by the 8th week and remained with significant levels even at the final time point (11th week) (Wu et al., 1989b).

The state of the targeted DNA in livers with persistent CAT gene expression was investigated. DNA was extracted from liver homogenates from ASOR-PL-palb-CAT plasmid treated livers 11 weeks after partial hepatectomy. Samples of DNA were digested with *Bste* II which does not cut the palb-CAT plasmid, *Xba*I which cuts the plasmid at a single site, and *Bam* HI which excises the CAT insert from the plasmid. All digestions were carried out at 37°C. The DNA was then transferred to nitrocellulose and CAT sequences detected by hybridization with a ^{32}P-labeled CAT cDNA probe (Southern, 1975). Hybridization was seen in liver samples from rats treated with targetable DNA complex. Distinct bands were detected rather than a smear of high molecular weight material that would be expected if integration had occurred. High levels of transgene DNA (100-10,000 copies/cell) were found. Additional series of Southern blot analyses demonstrated that the predominant form of the transgene DNA was that of an episome. It was also demonstrated that the episome persisted as a stabilized, nonreplicating plasmid based on patterns of DNA methylation (Wilson et al., 1992).

Experiments were performed to determine whether the targetable soluble DNA delivery system could target a normal gene to correct a metabolic abnormality caused by a defect in a corresponding endogenous gene. For initial studies, Nagase analbuminemic rats were selected (Nagase et al., 1979). These rats have a splicing defect in serum albumin mRNA resulting in virtually undetectable levels of circulating albumin. A vector that expresses human serum albumin, the plasmid palb[3] driven by the rat albumin promoter and mouse enhancer regions was constructed.

The carrier was complexed to the palb³ plasmid. Nagase analbuminemic rats were injected intravenously with either controls or the DNA complex, followed by a 66% partial hepatectomy to stimulate liver cell replication. At various time intervals, blood was drawn, the rats sacrificed and livers removed and homogenized. A cDNA probe for human albumin sequences using Southern blot assay, detected hybridizable sequences in the rats treated with the complex (ASOR-PL-palb³), but not in the controls. No significant rearrangements involving the albumin structural gene were found. The targeted DNA was found to exist mainly in plasmid form. Most importantly, circulating human albumin *was* detected in the serum of ASOR-PL-palb³ treated rats. Albumin first became detectable within 48 hours after injection, reaching a maximum by 2 weeks postinjection, and expression remained detectable through 4 weeks postinjection. Of note, the maximum amount of albumin detected in the treated Nagase analbuminemic rats was 0.1% of normal levels. Control rats failed to express the gene (Wu et al., 1991).

The Watanabe heritable hyperlipidemic (WHHL) rabbit was selected as a model of an inheritable disease caused by a deficiency in the receptor for LDL (Watanabe, 1980). An asialoglycoprotein-polylysine conjugate was complexed to DNA containing a LDL receptor gene. WHHL rabbits were injected intravenously with the complexed DNA. The cellular and organ distribution of the DNA-complexes was found primarily in liver (85%), but there was rapid clearing of the complexes after 10 minutes. The hepatocyte was the target cell with evidence of >90% cell specificity noted. Small amounts of the DNA-complex was taken up by non-parenchymal liver cells (Kupffer cells).

Total cellular DNA analyses of the liver samples taken at various time intervals after injection showed that treated animals had high levels of the intact DNA fragments along with some partially degraded plasmid DNA when compared to control groups. There was progressive degradation and decline in the amount of intact plasmid over 48 hours after injection. Using a quantitative RNase protection assay (Wilson et al., 1990), recombinant human LDL receptor transcripts in the liver samples was assayed. LDL receptor RNA was detected at 4 hours, maximal at 24 hours, but declined to undetectable levels by 72 hours after injection of the complexes. The levels of LDL receptor RNA was 2-4% of endogenous levels at 24 hours, the maximum time interval (Wilson et al., 1992).

Metabolically, it was demonstrated that a transient decrease in the total serum cholesterol (approximately 25-30% of the pretreatment values) occurred in rabbits that received the complexed DNA containing the LDL receptor gene (Wilson et al., 1992b).

In a very different approach, one designed to inhibit rather than initiate gene expression, an antisense oligonucleotide complex was targeted via asialoglycoprotein receptors to a cell line permanently transfected with hepatitis B virus. This resulted in specific inhibition of hepatitis B viral gene expression and replication (Wu and Wu, 1992).

In conclusion, targeted gene delivery can be accomplished utilizing a simple, soluble DNA delivery system that takes advantage of a highly specific receptor on hepatocytes. Gene expression could be made to persist when hepatocytes were stimulated to replicate. This novel approach may allow for a noninvasive, clinically practical means for somatic gene therapy to treat inherited metabolic disorders and other disease states.

ACKNOWLEDGMENTS

We thank Ms. Mary Simons and Mrs. Rosemary Pavlick for kindly providing assistance with the preparation of this manuscript.

REFERENCES

Ashwell G, Morell A (1974): The role of surface carbohydrates in the hepatic recognition and transport of circulating glycoproteins. *Adv Enzymol* 41:99-128

Benvenisty N, Reshef L (1986): Direct introduction of genes into rats and expression of the genes. *Proc Natl Acad Sci USA* 83:9551-9555

Dubensky T, Campbell B, Villarreal L (1984): Direct transfection of viral and plasmid DNA into liver or spleen of mice. *Proc Natl Acad Sci USA* 81:7529-7533

Dunn W, Hubbard A, Aronson N (1980): Low temperature selectively inhibits fusion of pinocytic vesicles and lysosomes during heterophagy of ^{125}I-asialofetuin by the perfused rat liver. *J Biol Chem* 255:5971-5978

Fiume L, Mattioli A, Spinoza G (1987): Distribution of a conjugate of 9-beta-D-arabino furanosyladenine monophosphate (ara-AMP) with lactosaminated albumin in parenchymal and sinusoidal cells of rat liver. *Cancer Drug Delivery* 4:11-16

Gopal T (1985): Gene transfer method for transient gene expression, stable transformation, and co-transformation of suspension cell cultures. *Mol Cell Biol* 5:1188-1193

Graham F, Van der Eb A (1973): A new technique for the assay of infectivity of human adenovirus 5 DNA. *Virology* 52:456-467

Greenwood F, Hunter W, Glover J (1963): The preparation of ^{131}I labeled human growth hormone of high specific radioactivity. *Biochemistry* 10:114-119

Harland R, Weintraub H (1985): Translation of mRNA injected into *Xenopus* oocytes is specifically inhibited by antisense RNA. *J Cell Biol* 101:1094-1099

Jung G, et al. (1981): Biological activity of the antitumor protein neocarzinostatin coupled in a monoclonal antibody by N-succinidyl 3-(2-pyridylthio-)-propionate. *Biochem Biophys Res Commun* 101:599-606

Kawasaki T, Ashwell G (1977): Isolation and characterization of an avian hepatic binding protein specific for N-acetylglucosamine-terminated glycoproteins. *J Biol Chem* 252:6536-6543

Keegan-Rogers V, Wu G (1990): Targeted protection of hepatocytes from galactosamine toxicity in vivo. *Cancer Chemother and Pharmacol* 26(2):93-96

Laemmli U (1970): Cleavage of structural proteins during the assembly of the head of bacteriophage T4. *Nature* 277:680-685

Loyter A, Scangos G, Ruddle F (1982): Mechnisms of DNA uptake by mammalian cells: Fate of exogenously added DNA monitored by use of fluorescent dyes. *Proc Natl Acad Sci USA* 79:422-426

Maniatis T, Fritsch E, Sambrook G (1982): Technique for isolation of molecular clones. In *Molecular Cloning, A laboratory manual,* Cold Spring Harbor Laboratory, Cold Spring Harbor, NY

Maniatis T, Jeffrey A, Klein D (1975): Nucleotide sequence of the rightward operator of phage T. *Proc Natl Acad Sci USA* 72:1184-1188

Miller AD (1992): Human gene therapy comes of age. *Nature* 357:455-460

Miller D, Adam M, Miller AD (1990): Gene transfer by retrovirus vectors occurs only in cells that are actively replicating at the time of infection. *Mol Cell Biol* 10:4239-4242

Molema G, Jansen RW, Visser J, Herdewijn P, Moolnaar F, Meijer DKF (1991): Neoglycoproteins as carriers for antiviral drugs: Synthesis and analysis of protein-drug conjugates. *J Med Chem* 34:1137-1141

Nagase S, Shimamune S, Shumiya S (1979): Albumin deficient rat mutant. *Science* 205:590-591

Nicolau C, et al. (1983): In vivo expression of rat insulin after intravenous administration of the liposome entrapped gene for rat insulin I. *Proc Natl Acad Sci USA* 80:1068-1072

Nicolau C, Sene C (1982): Liposome-mediated DNA transfer in eukaryotic cells. *Biochim Biophys Acta* 721:185-190

Pinkert C, Ornitz D, Brinster R, Palmiter R (1987): An albumin enhancer located 101 cb upstream functions along with its promoter to direct efficient, liver-specific expression in transgenic mice. *Genes and Dev* 1:268-276

Potter H, et al. (1984): Enhancer dependent expression of human B immunoglobulin genes introduced into mouse pre-B lymphocytes by electroporation. *Proc Natl Acad Sci USA* 81:7161-7165

Rosenfeld MA, et al. (1992): In Vivo transfer of the human cystic fibrosis transmembrane conductance regulator gene to the airway epithelium. *Cell* 68:143-155

Southern E (1975): Detection of specific sequences among DNA fragments separated by gel electrophoresis. *J Mol Biol* 98:503-517

Stockert R, Morell A (1982): Endocytosis of glycoproteins. *The Liver: Biology and Pathobiologyy,* IM Arias, H Popper, D Shafritz, D Schachter, W Jakoby, eds. Raven Press. pp. 205-217

Svensson U, Persson R (1984): Entry of adenovirus 2 into HeLa cells. *J Virology* 51(3):687-694

Tibbetts C, Giam C (1979): In Vitro association of empty adenovirus capsids with double stranded DNA. *J Virology* 32(3):995-1005

Wall D, Wilson G, Hubbard A (1980): The galactose specific recognition system of mammalian liver: receptor distribution on the hepatocyte surface. *Cell* 21:79-93

Watanabe Y (1980): Serial inbreeding of rabbits with hyperlipidemia. *Atherosclerosis* 36:261-268

Whitehead D, Sammons H (1966): A simple technique for the isolation of orosomucoid from normal and pathological sera. *Biochim Biophys Acta* 124:209-211

Williams DA, et al. (1984): Introduction of new genetic material into pleuripotent hematopoietic stem cells of the mouse. *Nature* 310:476-480

Wilson J, et al. (1992): A novel mechanism for achieving transgene persistence in vivo after somatic gene transfer into hepatocytes. *J Biol Chem* 267:11483-11489

Wilson J, et al. (1992): Hepatocyte directed gene transfer in vivo leads to transient improvement of hypercholesterolemia in low density lipoprotein receptor deficient rabbits. *J Biol Chem* 267:963-967

Wilson J, et al. (1990): Temporary amelioration of hyperlipidemia on low density lipoprotein receptor-deficient rabbits transplanted with genetically modified hepatocytes. *Proc Natl Acad Sci USA* 87:8437-8441

Wu C, Wilson J, Wu G (1989): Targeting genes: delivery and persistent expression of a foreign gene driven by mammalian regulatory elements in vivo. *J Biol Chem* 264:16985-16987

Wu G, et al. (1991): Receptor-mediated gene delivery in vivo, partial correction of genetic analbuminemia in Nagase rats. *J Biol Chem* 266:14338-14342

Wu G, Wu C (1988): Evidence for targeted gene delivery to HepG2 hepatoma cells in vitro. *Biochemistry* 27:887-892

Wu G, Wu C (1987): Receptor mediated in vitro gene transformation by a soluble DNA carrier system. *J Biol Chem* 262:4429-4432

Wu G, Wu C (1992): Targeted delivery and expression of foreign genes in hepatocytes. *Liver Diseases*, G Wu, C Wu, eds. Marcel Dekker, NY. pp. 127-149

Wu G, Wu C (1992): Specific inhibition of hepatitis B viral gene expression in vitro by targeted antisense oligonucleotides. *J Biol Chem* 267:12436-12439

Zhou X, Klibanov A, Huang L (1991): Lipophilic polylysines mediate effecient DNA transfection in mammalian cells. *Biochim Biophys Acta* 1065:8-14

RETROVIRAL-MEDIATED GENE TRANSFER AND DUCHENNE MUSCULAR DYSTROPHY

Matthew G. Dunckley and George Dickson

THE SUITABILITY OF DUCHENNE MUSCULAR DYSTROPHY FOR GENE THERAPY

Over 70 human diseases have been named as potential beneficiaries of somatic cell gene therapy, ranging from inherited disorders, such as cystic fibrosis and forms of severe combined immune deficiency, to cancer and AIDS (Scarpa and Caskey, 1989). Intervention by 'designer genes' incorporated into patients' own cells could replace absent or defective molecules, synthesize metabolic enzymes or drugs, or manipulate the body's immune responses (Ledley, 1990; Miller, 1990a). The realisation that recombinant DNA technology, now familiar in a diagnostic context, can be applied to the correction of diagnosed diseases is leading to a renewed optimism in the clinic for treating conditions that have so far persistently defeated more conventional therapeutic strategies.

One such disease is the most common inherited disorder of skeletal muscle, affecting over 1 in 3500 of the male population (Wessel, 1990). First described in 1868 by a French physician, Guillaume Duchenne, the X-linked myopathy now called Duchenne's muscular dystrophy (DMD) continues to defy attempts to alleviate or control the relentless degenerative course of the disease, which confines sufferers to a wheelchair by the age of 12 and ultimately proves fatal within their third decade. The major characteristic of DMD pathology is the progressive degeneration of skeletal muscle leading to diminishing strength and secondary deformities of the underlying skeleton, such as scoliosis, due to a lack of muscular support (Emery, 1988). Attempts to repair damaged myofibers are unable to compensate for recurrent phases of degeneration and are further hindered by a gradual deposition of fibrotic connective tissue at severely myopathic sites (Nonaka, 1991).

Duchenne muscular dystrophy is a highly suitable target for gene therapy for a number of reasons. Firstly, it is an exceptionally severe condition with a high morbidity and for which no effective alternative therapy exists. Moreover, a high proportion of cases occur with no previous family history due to an unusually high spontaneous mutation rate in the DMD gene (Roses, 1988). Thus, any improvements that can be brought about in the condition will be significant and those risks associated with novel therapeutic approaches are likely to be far outweighed by potential benefits. Secondly, as the primary cause of DMD lies with defects in a single, recessively inherited gene, now identified and cloned (Koenig et al., 1987; see below), introduction of just one normal copy of the dystrophin gene per dystrophic nucleus could theoretically prevent the disease phenotype. In practice, normal physiological levels of dystrophin may not be necessary as there appears to be a threshold of expression below which the amount of dystrophin present is insufficient to prevent the myopathic pathology. Examination of a number of Duchenne and Becker muscular dystrophy patients synthesizing normal, full-length dystrophin molecules but at variable levels suggests that if dystrophin is produced in less than 30-40% of normal quantities, the patient will develop a Duchenne phenotype (Hoffman et al., 1988). Hence, this should represent a minimal therapeutic target for dystrophin gene expression.

Many of the distinctive properties of skeletal muscle are also favorable for stable gene transfer. Indeed, for these reasons many groups worldwide are using this tissue for the stable expression of a number of heterologous genes not normally specifically associated with muscle, such as Factor IX and human growth hormone (Barr and Leiden, 1991; Dhawan et al., 1991). Firstly, the fusion of differentiating embryonic myoblasts during development forms a syncytium in which the component nuclei migrate to the periphery of the 'sarcolemma' plasma membrane and contribute to the molecular composition of the whole 'myofiber' (Bischoff, 1978; Grounds and McGeachie, 1987). These myofibers fuse together to build larger fibers which make up the various muscle groups and, unless injured, form a highly stable tissue. This suggests that transfer of recombinant dystrophin genes into even a proportion of myofiber nuclei may significantly contribute to the function of the whole myofiber. Secondly, a proportion of the myoblast precursors remain as mononucleate cells and lie at intervals along the outside surface of each myofiber in a dormant state, where they are termed 'satellite cells.' These cells form an important resource available for the repair and regeneration of locally damaged areas of muscle (Grounds et al., 1992). If these cells are the targets of gene transfer, they may act as long-term depositories of transgene for expression in regenerated muscle in the future.

The remarkable capacity of skeletal muscle to regenerate after injury has been well documented and is an early feature of the myopathic phenotype of DMD (Emery, 1988; Nonaka, 1991). If this regeneration was able to replace dystrophin-deficient muscle with functional muscle fibers, subsequent rounds of degeneration may be avoided, preventing progressive muscular weakness. Efficient retroviral-mediated gene transfer could exploit this situation to the full, whereby recombinant retroviral vectors carrying a biologically active dystrophin gene could be injected into myopathic muscle undergoing active regeneration in order to transduce a large proportion of the activated satellite cell population. Fusion of these cells to regenerate destroyed muscle fibers could then lead to the constitutive expression of recombinant dystrophin along their length. In addition, some transduced cells may reconstitute the satellite cell pool, ready to regenerate sites of myopathic damage with myonuclei expressing recombinant dystrophin.

Inevitably, many limitations of the available systems provide problems to overcome. In the case of DMD, however, the most significant difficulty lies with the enormous size of the gene itself.

DYSTROPHIN AND THE DMD GENE

The modern strategy of molecular genetics known as 'positional cloning' or 'reverse genetics' led to the identification and sequencing of the gene affected in DMD by Koenig et al. in 1987. The DMD gene is the largest known in the entire human genome, covering some 2.3 megabases (Mb) along the short arm of the X chromosome and comprising 79 exons (DenDunnen et al., 1989). Transcription of the gene in skeletal muscle produces an mRNA of approximately 14 kb including an open reading frame of almost 12kb encoding the protein 'dystrophin' (Hoffman et al., 1987)(Fig.1a). More recently, an array of alternatively spliced isoforms have been identified transcribed from at least three distinct promoters in tissues ranging from CNS neurones to hepatocytes (Feener et al., 1989; Barnea et al., 1990; Bar et al., 1990; Blake et al., 1992). As the most debilitating pathological features of DMD involve skeletal muscle, the major isoform of dystrophin found here has naturally received most attention. However, when considering ultimate clinical gene transfer applications on a broader spectrum, it may be necessary to take account of other tissue-specific isoforms. At present, therapeutic targets are likely to be limited to selected groups of skeletal muscles in order to restrain the most disabling consequences of dystrophin deficiency.

The discovery of the gene enabled the isolation of dystrophin, a 427 kDa rod-shaped protein absent from the muscles of DMD patients and the corresponding animal models of the disease (Hoffman et al., 1987; Koenig et al., 1988). Further information derived from sequence similarities with other proteins and immunological analyses indicate that dystrophin forms part of the muscle peripheral cytoskeleton where it comprises up to 5% of the total protein (Ohlendieck and Campbell, 1991).

Structurally (Fig.1b), dystrophin has α-actinin-like actin-binding domains at the amino-terminus followed by a series of 24 spectrin-like α-helical repeats that form the largest section of the molecule, the so-called 'rod domain.' Towards the 3' end, a cysteine-rich region (again with sequence similarities to α-actinin) is adjacent to the unique carboxy-terminus which is especially subject to alternative splicing (Feener et al., 1989). Recently, a complex of membrane-associated glycoproteins has been described (Ervasti and Campbell, 1991), of which at least one binds the cysteine-rich or 5' C-terminal domains of dystrophin (Suzuki et al., 1992) and which are observed at much reduced levels in dystrophin-deficient muscle tissues (Ervasti et al., 1990). Furthermore, immunolocalisation studies and immunoprecipitation of these molecules with homogenates of excised skeletal muscles have further demonstrated a close association with laminin, a major component of the extracellular matrix or basal lamina (Ibraghimov-Beskrovnaya et al., 1992; Dickson et al., 1992). These data strongly suggest that dystrophin is an important

A

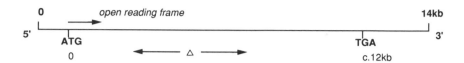

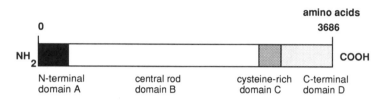

B

FIGURE 1. (A) Linear representation of the 14 kb human dystrophin cDNA showing the extent of the coding sequence (open reading frame). A 6.3 kb dystrophin cDNA bearing a large (5.1 kb) central in-frame deletion (indicated Δ) was derived from a mildly affected Becker muscular dystrophy patient and shown to be compatible with the packaging limits of retroviral vectors. (B) Schematic diagram of human dystrophin indicating the four major polypeptide domains. The truncated dystrophin molecule encoded by the Becker gene described above apparently retains a high level of functional activity despite lacking over 40% of the central rod domain.

structural element of the muscle membrane, perhaps contributing to force transduction or stabilization of the sarcolemma. On this basis, the scenario has been proposed whereby an absence of dystrophin, as in DMD, weakens the molecular connections across the sarcolemma between the muscle cytoskeleton and the basal lamina. Consequently, unrestrained stresses during muscle contraction rupture the membrane leading to an excessive influx of ions such as Ca^{2+}, then hypercontraction, proteolysis and degeneration of the muscle fiber (Duncan, 1989).

Such a hypothesis suggests that reconstitution of dystrophic skeletal muscle with functional dystrophin molecules could prevent the effects of dystrophin deficiency. Delivery of intact dystrophin protein to the muscles is not feasible and would be highly transient. Instead, the most effective and stable way to constitutively supply dystrophin to muscle fibers is by transfer of functional copies of the gene itself to muscle nuclei. This has been attempted by three distinct approaches: (i) direct injection of expression plasmids bearing dystrophin cDNAs into skeletal muscle (Acsadi et al., 1991); (ii) transplantation of normal myoblasts into dystrophin-deficient muscle (Partridge et al., 1989), and (iii) delivery of recombinant dystrophin genes to dystrophic muscle by viral vector systems (Dunckley et al., 1992). The first of these is reviewed in detail by Dr. Jon Wolff in this volume and myoblast transfer has been extensively discussed elsewhere (e.g. Partridge, 1991a), so we shall focus on the third and, in particular, on retroviral vectors and how they may be applied to dystrophin gene transfer into muscle.

RETROVIRAL VECTORS

Retroviruses have many biological properties that make them highly suitable vehicles for the transport of foreign DNA into mammalian cells. The most obvious of these is their ability to infect a wide variety of cell types, although the species infectable by a given 'pseudotype' of retrovirus may be restricted to certain groups of animals (Chatis et al., 1983). Once their genomic 'proviral' sequences have entered the host cell, retroviruses integrate permanently into the host genome and remain, unlike adenoviruses and herpesviruses, as permanent nonlytic occupants - the guests who never leave! (Weiss et al., 1984). By way of introduction, we shall briefly outline the essential features of retrovirus biology that enable them to be manipulated as highly efficient gene transfer vectors before considering how they can be applied to potential gene therapeutic approaches to alleviate the pathology of Duchenne muscular dystrophy.

The retrovirus virion

The 'wild-type' retrovirus most studied and most commonly adapted as a gene transfer vector is the Moloney murine leukemia virus (Mo-MuLV). Most aspects of its biology are common to all retroviruses, so we shall consider it as a typical example.

In essence, there are two components to an infectious retroviral particle: (i) the double-stranded RNA genome and (ii) its associated structural and functional elements - the viral envelope containing the enzymes required for successful entry and integration into the host cell genome. The basic features of the retroviral genome are illustrated in Fig. 2. The most distinctive elements are the two flanking regions called the Long Terminal Repeats (LTRs) containing regulatory sequences such as the retroviral promoter and enhancer. The LTRs define the 'provirus' which is reverse transcribed into DNA after entry into a target cell and is subsequently integrated into an apparently random site in the host chromosome. In addition, a sequence within the 3' LTR encodes the terminal polyadenylation signal. The remainder of the provirus is taken up by sequences essential for successful packaging of transcribed proviral RNA into virions (the ψ site and packaging signal), primer start sites for synthesis of + and - strands, and the genes *gag*, *pol* and *env* encoding the ribonucleoprotein core, the retroviral reverse transcriptase and integrase enzymes and the envelope glycoproteins respectively (Varmus, 1982). Since these components can be simply grouped into those which act in cis and those able to be supplied in trans (Table 1), the retrovirus can be easily manipulated into a replication-defective gene transfer vehicle by replacement of those

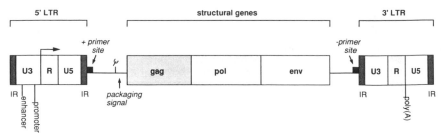

FIGURE 2. Components of a retroviral genome (based on MoMuLV). Long terminal repeats (LTRs) at each end contain promoter and enhancer sequences for constitutive gene expression (5' LTR), a polyadenylation signal (3' LTR) and inverted repeat sequences (IR) necessary for integration into the host cell genome. The genes *gag*, *pol* and *env* encode essential viral enzymes and structural proteins necessary for infection and replication. Sequences around the ψ site ensure packaging into virions and primer sites enable synthesis of + and - strands.

genes normally required for ongoing cycles of viral reproduction with foreign DNA (Eglitis and Anderson, 1988).

Replication-defective retroviruses

Virologists had previously reported unusual retrovirus mutants that were incapable of self-replication. Only when 'wild-type' replication-competent 'helper virus' infected the cells in which they were present could these mutants form successful infectious virions (Goldfarb and Weinberg, 1981). Further studies revealed that the replication-incompetent mutants had defective *gag*, *pol* and *env* genes, the products of which could only be supplied in trans by a concurrent infection of

TABLE 1. The retroviral genome can be divided into *cis*- and *trans*-acting elements. *Trans*-acting sequences can be replaced by foreign DNA to create retroviral vectors able to be packaged into replication-defective virions by 'producer cells' expressing *gag*, *pol* and *env* genes.

cis-acting	*trans*-acting
promoter	*gag*: encodes core proteins
enhancer	*pol*: encodes reverse transcriptase
polyadenylation site	*env*: encodes envelope glycoproteins
+/- primer sites	
packaging signal	

TABLE 2. The surface glycoprotein encoded by the retroviral *env* gene interacts with cell surface ligands on target cells. Retroviruses can therefore be grouped into pseudotypes according to the infectable host range allowed by their *env* gene.

Pseudotype	Host Range
Ecotropic	mouse and rat only
Amphotropic	most mammalian cells
Xenotropic	most species except mouse
Polytropic	most mammalian cells

wild-type virus. As a result of these observations, *gag*, *pol* and *env* genes from MoMuLV were cloned into expression vectors and transfected into NIH-3T3 cells to create cell lines with 'helper' function (Mann et al., 1983; Miller, 1990b). Proviral DNA in which the *gag*, *pol* and *env* genes had been replaced by a heterologous recombinant gene was cloned into a separate vector bearing an intact packaging signal. Transfection of such a retroviral vector into 'helper' or packaging cell lines results in the production of recombinant virions able to transport the foreign gene into target cells but unable to produce progeny retroviral particles. Such combinations of transfected retroviral vector and packaging cell are called producer cell lines and are able to package retroviral RNA up to approximately 12 kb in size, including up to about 8 kb of foreign DNA (Morgenstern and Land, 1991).

Retroviral transduction

The cycle of retroviral infection, like the retrovirus itself, can also be considered in two parts: adsorption/integration and gene expression. An infectious virion bears on its surface specific glycoproteins which act as ligands for noncovalent interactions with molecules on the surface membrane of a variety of cells, i.e. retroviral 'receptors' (Yoshimoto et al., 1992). The specific glycoprotein encoded by the *env* gene within the virus or producer cell line can be allocated to four categories depending on the range of host species bearing its corresponding receptor molecule on the cell surface (Weiss et al., 1984; Battini et al., 1992)(Table 2). For instance, the ecotropic glycoprotein of MoMuLV (gp70 or SU protein) binds a molecule found only on the cells of rats and mice, recently identified as a cationic amino acid transporter (Kim et al., 1991). The ligand-receptor interaction allows adsorption of the retrovirus onto the surface of the target cell which is followed by fusion of the retroviral envelope with the plasma membrane, releasing the contents of the virion into the cytoplasm (Andersen and Nexo, 1983; Gilbert et al., 1992). The retroviral reverse transcriptase (RT) initially transcribes one of the RNA strands into DNA to form an RNA-DNA hybrid molecule which is then subject to digestion by this enzyme's RNase H activity followed by further DNA synthesis via the retroviral polymerase to form the complementary DNA strand. Once completed, a retroviral integrase (IN) permanently incorporates the whole DNA provirus into an accessible site within the host chromatin (Goodrich and Duesberg, 1990; Kulkosky et al., 1992). The retroviral promoter and enhancer elements in the 5' LTR (and any additional internal promoters cloned into the recombinant vector) may now lie in a suitable context from which to drive expression of the introduced genes.

The increasing knowledge of retroviral biology has produced a series of refinements to the first retroviral vectors and packaging cells, with the aim of both increasing the titers of retrovirus released by each producer cell and reducing to a minimum the risk of accidentally producing wild-type helper virus that could lead to uncontrolled viremia with subsequent unpredictable effects on the patient's health. Current 'third generation' packaging cell lines and various complex retroviral vectors have led to a position now where the risk of such helper virus generation has been effectively eliminated (Danos and Mulligan, 1988; Markowitz et al., 1988). In addition, the discovery that the sequences necessary for efficient packaging of the retroviral RNA extend into the *gag* gene (Bender et al., 1987) have resulted in greatly increased titers using vectors incorporating these developments (e.g. Armentano et al., 1987).

DYSTROPHIN GENE TRANSFER

Current gene therapy proposals are limited to the transformation of somatic (i.e. nongermline) cells (Anderson, 1992). This means that disease phenotypes may be corrected in affected individuals but, however successful, the genetic constitution of the patients' offspring will be unaffected. Quite apart from the technical difficulties of germ-line genetic manipulation in man and the unknown long-term consequences of manipulating the human genome in this way, germline gene therapy raises considerably greater ethical hurdles than treatments affecting somatic tissues. Many of these latter questions have been met and evaluated already in the field of organ transplantation - itself a somewhat crude form of somatic gene therapy. Nevertheless, germ cell gene transfer continues to be a valuable technique in the laboratory in the development of transgenic animals both as models of human disease and as in vivo test systems for novel gene constructs.

Animal models of DMD

The murine model for DMD, called the '*mdx* mouse' (for X-linked muscular dystrophy), was first described before the gene had been identified (Bulfield et al., 1984) based upon the skeletal muscle histology, elevated creatine kinase levels and X-linked inheritance of this phenotype in mice from a colony of normal C57Bl/ 10 animals. Following the publication of the DMD gene sequence and the discovery that the muscle of *mdx* mice did not contain detectable levels of dystrophin,

Sicinski et al. (1989) analysed the corresponding dystrophin gene sequence in the *mdx* mouse genome and found that dystrophin translation was curtailed in these animals by a point mutation towards the 5' end of the gene. Interestingly, the consequences of dystrophin deficiency in the *mdx* mouse are remarkably milder relative to DMD patients and especially differ in the lack of progression of the myopathy in these animals. Instead, phases of muscle degeneration, especially in 3-6 week old animals, are followed by regeneration which is sufficiently effective to prevent the development of muscular weakness (Carnwath and Shotton, 1987; Anderson et al., 1988). More recently, however, the diaphragm and intercostal muscles of older (> 6 months) *mdx* mice have been shown to exhibit a progressively severe and fibrotic myopathy and fibrosis similar to the human disease (Stedman et al., 1991). Furthermore, as the biochemical abnormality is similar to the human DMD patient, the *mdx* mouse is highly suitable for testing dystrophin gene transfer approaches both in vitro and in the whole animal.

In recent years, a larger animal model - a family of Golden Retriever dogs (the *xmd* dog) -has also been described (Cooper et al., 1988). Unlike the *mdx* mouse, X-linked muscular dystrophy in these animals follows a highly comparable course to DMD in man, exhibiting progressive muscular weakness, hypertrophy of defined muscle groups and premature death due to respiratory insufficiency (although *xmd* dogs are euthanised on development of distress prior to the terminal stage of the disease) (Valentine et al., 1990). The disadvantage of this model relative to the *mdx* mouse is primarily, in common with other large animal models of disease, the much slower generation time resulting in a very limited supply of experimental animals. In addition, the breeding success of dogs suffering from this disease is somewhat lower than healthy animals. Nevertheless, these animals are proving to be highly beneficial in the understanding of DMD pathology and cells derived from *xmd* dogs are currently being used for gene transfer studies. Such a large animal model should be useful for evaluating clinical approaches to the gene therapy of DMD immediately prior to clinical trials in man (Partridge, 1991b).

Physical gene transfer methods

Recently, it has been possible to incorporate the entire native dystrophin gene within a yeast artificial chromosome (YAC) construct (DenDunnen et al., 1992). Nevertheless, while microinjection and lipid-mediated transfer of YACs into mammalian cells has been achieved (Gnirke and Huxley, 1991; Strauss and Jaenisch, 1992), the incorporation of such large recombinant DNA molecules in mammalian cells is unlikely to represent a clinically useful technique in the near future. To date most gene transfer experiments have utilized plasmid expression vectors containing recombinant cDNA constructs. Such vectors can accommodate foreign genes at least as large as the 12 kb coding region of dystrophin. The full-length sequences corresponding to both human (Dickson et al., 1991) and mouse (Lee et al., 1991) dystrophin skeletal muscle mRNAs have been cloned as cDNA genes and transferred to cultured cells by standard physical transfection methods. In addition, concentrated plasmid preparations containing human dystrophin cDNAs have been injected directly into the dystrophin-deficient muscle tissue of *mdx* mice in vivo and shown to produce intact dystrophin molecules correctly localised to the sarcolemma (Acsadi et al., 1991). Physical transfection methods such as these, however, are far from efficient normally achieving gene transfer in considerably less than 2% of target cells (Wolff et al., 1990; Acsadi et al., 1991). While this may be adequate for the analysis of novel gene constructs, it is highly unlikely to lead to any detectable functional change in a muscle as a whole.

Retroviral-mediated gene transfer

Viral vectors, on the other hand, consistently achieve widespread gene transfer both in vitro and also in vivo (Hwang and Gilboa, 1984; Miller and Rosman, 1989). Their main limitation, which is unimportant for most genes, is their physical capacity to package genetic material within an infectious protein particle (virion). Current adeno- and retroviral vectors, at least, are unable to accommodate more than 8 kb of foreign DNA in addition to the sequences necessary for essential viral functions (approx. 3 kb). Hence, the 12 kb full-length dystrophin cDNA is excluded from packaging in these vectors and has thus far been restricted to the existing low efficiency physical gene transfer techniques.

A potential solution to this problem came with the discovery of a group of patients with a very mild form of the allelic disorder of DMD Becker muscular dystrophy (BMD) (Love et al., 1991). On analysis of their particular dystrophin gene mutation, it was found that over 40% of the coding region had been deleted. The resulting dystrophin molecule was severely reduced in size, bearing a deletion of about 46% of the central rod domain, yet retained intact amino- and carboxy-terminal domains (England et al., 1990). Despite such a dramatic modification of normal dystrophin in these patients, the truncated molecule was clearly able to function adequately in skeletal muscle. Moreover, as the mRNA from these patients was merely 6.3 kb in size, a cDNA corresponding to such a minigene could offer an alternative for gene transfer which was compatible with packaging by viral vectors.

Once such a cDNA was constructed (Acsadi et al., 1991), we incorporated it within a retroviral vector based on MoMuLV (Fig.3a) and isolated a high titre producer cell line manufacturing replication-deficient yet infectious recombinant dystrophin retrovirus (Dunckley et al., 1992). Primary myoblasts isolated from *mdx* mice were co-cultured with these producer cells in the presence of polybrene and allowed to differentiate into myotubes. Subsequent immunostaining of the cultures revealed significant numbers (>10%) of myotubes labelled at the sarcolemma by anti-dystrophin antibodies against the C-terminus of the molecule. Simultaneous immunostaining with an antibody against the central rod domain, deleted from the Becker molecule, did not label these cells. Comparisons of C-terminal labelling between normal mouse myotubes and *mdx* myotubes transduced

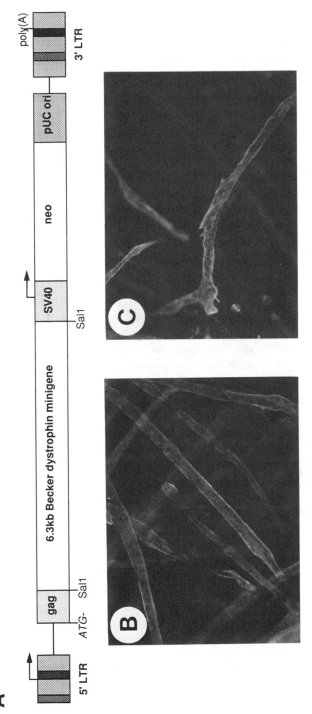

FIGURE 3. (A) Diagram of the retroviral vector pBabeNeo incorporating a 6.3 kb human dystrophin cDNA (Dunckley et al., 1992). The dystrophin minigene is transcribed from the MoMuLV retroviral promoter and an internal SV40 promoter drives expression of the selectable marker gene *neo*. (B) Differentiated normal C57BJ/10 mouse myotubes in culture labelled with an antibody to the C-terminal domain of dystrophin. (C) Myotubes grown from primary myoblasts of the dystrophin-deficient *mdx* mouse co-cultured with a cell line manufacturing the Becker dystrophin recombinant retrovirus. Immunostaining with the dystrophin C-terminal antibody labelled some 10% of these myotubes in a pattern indistinguishable from normal myotubes as in (B) but they were not labelled by antibodies to epitopes in the rod domain deleted from the Becker construct clearly demonstrating retroviral transfer of the minigene.

by recombinant retrovirus showed that the pattern of immunostaining was identical (Fig.3b and c).

Meanwhile, the Becker dystrophin retroviral construct was linearized and injected into fertilised normal (C57Bl/10 x CBA-J) mouse ova to produce transgenic mice (Wells et al., 1992). 'Founder' male offspring were bred with homozygous *mdx* females and second generation male animals analyzed for gene transmission. Transgenic *mdx* mice expressing the Becker dystrophin molecule revealed that a number of the characteristic pathological features of the *mdx* dystrophic mouse had been considerably reduced in severity. Most importantly, the degree of central nucleation of muscle fibers in the transgenic animals (an indicator of previous phases of degeneration and regeneration) was reduced to near-normal levels in 4 week old animals and dramatically lower than non-transgenic littermates.

These results inspired us to move to the in vivo situation to attempt direct retroviral-mediated transduction of *mdx* skeletal muscle in the intact animal (Dunckley et al., 1993). Initial pilot experiments involved a simple injection of filtered producer cell line culture media with added polybrene into the quadriceps muscle of *mdx* mice at the peak of their myopathic phase (i.e. 4-6 weeks after birth). Retroviruses can only infect and successfully integrate into actively dividing cells (Miller et al., 1990c), so it was hoped that the satellite myoblasts proliferating to repair myopathic muscle would be targeted by injected recombinant retrovirus and subsequently fuse to form myofibers expressing the Becker dystrophin. Two weeks after these injections, quadriceps muscles were excised, frozen and cryostat sections immunostained with antibodies against the C-terminus and rod domain of dystrophin. Large groups of positively labelled myofibers were observed at the sarcolemma using a C-terminal dystrophin antibody, just like normal dystrophin-positive fibers (Fig.4a and b). In addition, the dystrophin rod domain antibody (against a region of dystrophin absent from the recombinant Becker molecule) did not label these muscle fibers suggesting that they derived from the fusion of transduced satellite cells.

In order to further prove that gene transfer was being achieved via satellite cells and to attempt to improve transduction efficiency, the active satellite cell pool was increased by inducing acute muscle damage using an injection of bupivacaine. Bupivacaine (BPVC / Marcain[R]) is a local anaesthetic which is also specifically myotoxic to differentiated skeletal muscle (Benoit and Belt, 1970). Following a single injection into the tibialis anterior muscle, the myofibers lose their normal morphology within 24 hours and the muscle is rapidly invaded by macrophages. However, over the next 14-21 days the muscle regenerates until myofibers are fully restored (Hall-Craggs, 1974). This remarkable recovery is achieved by the proliferation of satellite cells. Once activated, they rapidly divide and fuse to one another and into neighboring fibers, regenerating the muscle architecture (McGeachie and Grounds, 1987).

Recombinant stocks of retrovirus were concentrated by centrifugation (Cepko, 1989) and small volumes of resuspended virus injected into regenerating *mdx* tibialis anterior muscles 48-60 hours after they had received a bupivacaine injection. At

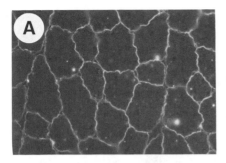 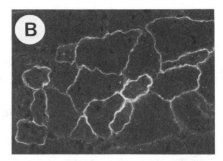

FIGURE 4. Immunolabelling of cryostat sections of mouse muscle with dystrophin antisera. (A) Normal C57Bl/10 mouse muscle labelled at the sarcolemma with a dystrophin C-terminal antibody. (B) Quadriceps muscle of an *mdx* mouse previously injected with recombinant dystrophin retrovirus and labelled with a dystrophin C-terminal antibody. A group of myofibers expressed the recombinant dystrophin correctly localized to the sarcolemma. Simultaneous incubation with an antibody to a dystrophin rod domain epitope deleted from the recombinant molecule did not label these fibers.

various time intervals after regeneration, muscles were removed and immunostained for dystrophin immunoreactivity. Analysis of transduced myofibers demonstrated that preinjection of the muscle with bupivacaine significantly enhanced the efficiency of in vivo gene transfer into skeletal muscle with up to 12% of myofibers labelled by dystrophin antisera. This confirmed that retroviruses were indeed transducing activated satellite cells in regenerating muscle and also indicated that refinement of such a protocol could conceivably lead to highly efficient gene transfer into skeletal muscle in vivo. Immunostaining of injected muscle with an antibody to one of the dystrophin-associated glycoproteins (normally undetectable in *mdx* mouse muscle) showed a restoration of apparently normal levels of this protein in transduced myofibers expressing the recombinant human dystrophin molecule. If these membrane glycoproteins are indeed mediators of membrane stability via dystrophin and laminin linkages across the sarcolemma, this would suggest that membrane integrity had been restored.

The limiting factor of transduction in this system is likely to be the number of infectious recombinant viral particles rather than the number of active satellite cells in the regenerating muscle, as a large proportion of the muscle is degenerated by the bupivacaine injection. Therefore, it is imperative to develop higher titer retrovirus preparations in order to achieve close to saturation with gene transfer vehicles. Currently, this is generally achieved by screening clones of producer cells for viral titer. Variability between cell lines may be due to the chromosomal location of the integrated provirus and is probably largely influenced by the nature of the retroviral vector. In the case of the recombinant dystrophin retrovirus, packaging efficiency may be reduced due to the large size of the construct. Novel vectors and other functional minigenes of reduced size (e.g. lacking selectable marker genes) may help to raise titers still further.

In addition to these measures, recombinant retroviruses may be concentrated from the tissue culture supernatants of these cells by ultrafiltration or high speed centrifugation, followed by resuspension in small volumes of serum or media (Mathes et al., 1977; Cepko, 1989). Alternative strategies have attempted to increase the number of copies of proviral DNA within each producer cell, such as the so-called "ping-pong" technique (Kozak and Kabat, 1990; Lynch and Miller, 1991). Co-cultures of ecotropic and amphotropic producer cells lead to multiple cross-infections and a gradual amplification of provirus copy number. However, in practice this invariably leads to the rapid generation of replication-competent retroviruses due to an increased chance of recombination events taking place. Careful modification of this method (e.g. selection of producer cells and vectors with minimal homologous sequences) may nevertheless increase retroviral titers without helper virus production.

Safety issues

Risk factors associated with retroviral-mediated gene transfer have been extensively addressed, especially prior to the commencement of clinical human gene therapy programs in 1990 (reviewed Cornetta et al., 1991a). Most concerns focussed on the possibility of integrated proviruses causing the activation of cellular oncogenes and the chances of spontaneous generation of replication-competent retroviruses. Data from primates used in preclinical gene therapy studies have strongly indicated the safety of murine retroviral vectors even if the initial preparation is contaminated with helper virus (Cornetta et al., 1991b). Moreover, modern retroviral vectors and packaging cell lines incorporate numerous safety features which reduce these risks to negligible levels, especially when considered in relation to the seriousness of such target diseases as DMD.

CONCLUSIONS AND FUTURE PROSPECTS

Retroviral vectors currently offer the only truly permanent gene transfer system whereby foreign genes can be stably incorporated into the genome of somatic cells. For this reason and the high efficiency of gene transfer that can be achieved, virtually all clinical gene therapy protocols have adopted retroviral gene transfer for a wide variety of genes and diseases.

While cell proliferation (required for retroviral integration) is not normally associated with differentiated muscle, the activity of muscle stem cells in regenerating muscle is a major characteristic of DMD pathology. Recently, the feasibility of transfer of functional recombinant dystrophin genes by retroviral vectors has been clearly demonstrated, leading to the correct localization and apparent functional complementation of dystrophin deficiency in the *mdx* mouse model of the disease. Retroviral gene transfer of other genes into primary myoblasts in culture has been followed by replacement of these cells into the syngeneic recipient animals (Barr and Leiden, 1991; Dhawan et al., 1991). This avoids the complications of immune rejection encountered in heterogeneic myoblast transfer therapy, yet the technical difficulties of growing the vast numbers of cells required remains. While this is a promising strategy for treating diseases, such as haemophilia B, which may not require full reconstitution of normal gene expression for therapeutic effect, a more direct gene transfer approach is probably necessary to correct primary defects of muscle, such as in DMD. Hence, strategies for increasing retroviral titers and gene transfer efficiency using dystrophin minigenes are a high priority. An alternative approach may be to implant producer cells within regenerating muscle to provide a steady supply of recombinant retrovirus to the muscle. These cells could be contained within some form of 'caged' environment or be created from myogenic cell lines for incorporation within the muscle fibers themselves. Ongoing studies of retrovirus molecular biology may also lead to the development of tissue-specific retroviral vectors, either by modifying surface glycoproteins via the *env* gene for interactions with muscle-specific cell surface ligands and/or by incorporating muscle-specific promoters within the retroviral vector (Petropoulos et al., 1992).

In conclusion, Duchenne muscular dystrophy remains a challenge to both clinicians and scientists alike, but prospects for an effective gene therapy are continually increasing. The remarkable attributes of a common pathogen—the retrovirus—have already proved highly adaptable for the treatment of human disease by gene transfer and it may well be the recombinant retrovirus which finally leads to the defeat of this debilitating disease.

REFERENCES

Acsadi G, Dickson G, Love DR, Jani A, Walsh FS, Gurusinghe A, Wolff JA, Davies KE (1991): Human dystrophin expression in *mdx* mice after intramuscular injection of DNA constructs. *Nature* 352:815-818

Andersen KB, Nexo BA (1983): Entry of murine retrovirus into mouse fibroblasts. *Virology* 125:85-98

Anderson JE, Bressler BH, Ovalle WK (1988): Functional regeneration in the hindlimb skeletal muscle of the *mdx* mouse. *J Musc Res Cell Motil* 9:499-515

Anderson WF (1992): Human gene therapy. *Science* 256:808-813

Armentano D, Yu S-F, Kantoff PW, von Ruden T, Anderson WF, Gilboa E (1987): Effect of internal viral sequences on the utility of retroviral vectors. *J Virol* 61:1647-1650

Bar S, Barnea E, Levy Z, Neuman S, Yaffe D, Nudel U (1990): A novel product of the Duchenne muscular dystrophy gene which greatly differs from the known isoforms in its structure and tissue distribution. *Biochem J* 272:557-560

Barnea E, Zuk D, Simantov R, Nudel U, Yaffe D (1990): Specificity of expression of the muscle and brain dystrophin gene promoters in muscle and brain cells. *Neuron* 5:881-888

Barr E, Leiden JM (1991): Systemic delivery of recombinant proteins by genetically modified myoblasts. *Science* 254:1507-1509

Battini J-L, Heard JM, Danos O (1992): Receptor choice determinants in the envelope glycoproteins of amphotropic, xenotropic and polytropic murine leukemia viruses. *J Virol* 66:1468-1475

Bender MA, Palmer TD, Gelinas RE, Miller AD (1987): Evidence that the packaging signal of Moloney murine leukemia virus exiends into the *gag* region. *J Virol* 61:1639-1646

Benoit PW, Belt WD (1970): Destruction and regeneration of skeletal muscle after treatment with a local anaesthetic, bupivacaine (Marcain[R]). *J Anat* 107:547-556

Bischoff R (1978): Myoblast fusion. In: *Membrane Fusion.* Cell Surface Reviews, Vol.5:127-179. Poste G, Nicolson GL, eds.

Blake DJ, Love DR, Tinsley J, Morris GE, Turley H, Gatter K, Dickson G, Edwards YH, Davies KE (1992): Characterisation of a 4.8 kb transcript from the Duchenne muscular dystrophy locus expressed in Schwannoma cells. *Hum Mol Genet* 1:103-109

Bulfield G, Siller WG, Wight PAL, Moore KJ (1984): X chromosome-linked muscular dystrophy (*mdx*) in the mouse. *Proc Natl Acad Sci USA* 81:1189-1192

Carnwath JW, Shotton DW (1987): Muscular dystrophy in the *mdx* mouse: histopathology of the soleus and extensor digitorum longus muscles. *J Neurol Sci* 80:39-54

Cepko C (1989): Lineage analysis in the vertebrate nervous system by retrovirus-mediated gene transfer. In: *Cell Culture.* Methods in Neurosciences, Vol.1:367-392. Conn PM, ed. San Diego, CA: Academic Press

Chatis PA, Holland CA, Hartley JW, Rowe WP, Hopkins N (1983): Role for the 3' end of the genome in determining disease specificity of Friend and Moloney murine leukemia viruses. *Proc Natl Acad Sci USA* 80:4408-4411

Cooper BJ, Winand NJ, Stedman H, Valentine BA, Hoffman EP, Kunkel LM, Scott M-O, Fischbeck KH, Kornegay JN, Avery RJ, Williams JR, Schmickel RD, Sylvester JE (1988): The homologue of the Duchenne locus is defective in X-linked muscular dystrophy of dogs. *Nature* 334:154-156

Cornetta K, Morgan RA, Anderson WF (1991a): Safety issues related to retroviral-mediated gene transfer in humans. *Hum Gene Ther* 2:5-14

Cornetta K, Morgan RA, Gillio A, Sturm S, Baltrucki L, O'Reilly R, Anderson WF (1991b): No retroviremia or pathology in long-term follow-up of monkeys exposed to a murine amphotropic retrovirus. *Hum Gene Ther* 2:215-219

Danos O, Mulligan RC (1988): Safe and efficient generation of recombinant retroviruses with amphotropic and ecotropic host ranges. *Proc Natl Acad Sci USA* 85:6460-6464

DenDunnen JT, Backer E, VanOmmen GJB, Pearson PL (1989): The DMD gene analysed by field inversion gel electrophoresis. *Br Med Bull* 45:644-658

DenDunnen JT, Grootscholten PM, Dauwerse JG, Walker AP, Monaco AP, Butler R, Anand R, Coffey AJ, Bentley DR, Steensma HY, VanOmmen GJB (1992): Reconstruction of the 2.4 Mb human DMD-gene by homologous YAC recombination. *Hum Mol Genet* 1:19-28

Dhawan J, Pan LC, Pavlath GK, Travis MA, Lanctot AM, Blau HM (1991): Systemic delivery of human growth hormone by injection of genetically engineered myoblasts. *Science* 254:1509-1512

Dickson G, Love DR, Davies KE, Wells KE, Piper TA, Walsh FS (1991): Human dystrophin gene transfer: production and expression of a functional recombinant DNA-based gene. *Human Genetics* 88:53-58

Dickson G, Azad A, Morris GE, Simon H, Noursadeghi M, Walsh FS (1992): Co-localisation and molecular association of dystrophin with laminin at the surface of mouse and human myotubes. *J Cell Sci* 103:1223-1233

Duchenne GBA (1868): Recherches sur la paralysie musculaire pseudohypertrophique ou paralysie myo-sclérosique. *Arch Gén Méd* 11:5-25; 179-209; 305-321; 421-443; 552-588

Duncan CJ (1989): Dystrophin and the integrity of the sarcolemma in Duchenne muscular dystrophy. *Experientia* 45:175-177

Dunckley MG, Love DR, Davies KE, Walsh FS, Morris GE, Dickson, G (1992): Retroviral-mediated transfer of a dystrophin minigene into *mdx* myoblasts in vitro. *FEBS Lett* 296:128-134

Dunckley MG, Wells DJ, Walsh FS, Dickson G (1993): Direct retroviral-mediated transfer of a dystrophin minigene into *mdx* mouse muscle in vivo. *Hum Mol Genet* 2:717-723

Eglitis MA, Anderson WF (1988): Retroviral vectors for introduction of genes into mammalian cells. *Biotechniques* 6:608-614

Emery AEH (1988): *Duchenne Muscular Dystrophy.* (2nd edn.). Oxford: Oxford University Press

England SB, Nicholson LVB, Johnson MA, Forrest SM, Love DR, Zubrzycka-Gaarn EE, Bulman DE, Harris JB, Davies KE (1990): Very mild muscular dystrophy associated with deletion of 46% of dystrophin. *Nature* 343:180-182

Ervasti JM, Ohlendieck K, Kahl SD, Gaver MG, Campbell KP (1990): Deficiency of a glycoprotein component of the dystrophin complex in dystrophic muscle. *Nature* 345:315-319

Ervasti JM, Campbell KP (1991): Membrane-organisation of the dystrophin-glycoprotein complex. *Cell* 66:1121-1131

Feener CA, Koenig M, Kunkel LM (1989): Alternative splicing of human dystrophin mRNA generates isoforms at the carboxy terminus. *Nature* 338:509-511

Gilbert MA, Charreau B, Vicart P, Paulin D, Nandi PK (1992): Mechanism of entry of a xenotropic MMuLV-derived recombinant retrovirus into porcine cells using the expression of the reporter *nlslacZ* gene. *Arch Virol* 124:57-67

Gnirke A, Huxley C (1991): Transfer of the human HPRT and GART genes from yeast to mammalian cells by microinjection of YAC DNA. *Som Cell Mol Genet* 17:573-580

Goldfarb MP, Weinberg RA (1981): Generation of novel, biologically active Harvey sarcoma viruses via apparent illegitimate recombination. *J Virol* 38:136-150

Goodrich DW, Duesberg PH (1990): Evidence that retroviral transduction is mediated by DNA, not by RNA. *Proc Natl Acad Sci USA* 87:3604-3608

Grounds MD, McGeachie JK (1987): A model of myogenesis in vivo, derived from detailed autoradiographic studies of regenerating skeletal muscle, challenges the concept of quantal mitosis. *Cell Tissue Res* 250:563-569

Grounds MD, Garrett KL, Lai MC, Wright W, Beilharz MW (1992): Identification of skeletal muscle precursor cells in vivo by use of MyoD1 and myogenin probes. *Cell Tissue Res* 267:99-104

Hall-Craggs ECB (1974): Rapid degeneration and regeneration of a whole skeletal muscle following treatment with bupivacaine (Marcain). *Exp Neurol* 43:349-358

Hoffman EP, Brown RH, Kunkel LM (1987): Dystrophin: the protein product of the Duchenne muscular dystrophy locus. *Cell* 51:919-928

Hoffman EP, Fischbeck KH, Brown RH, Johnson M, Medori R, Loike JD, Harris JB, Waterston R, Brooke M, Specht L, et al. (1988): Characterisation of dystrophin in muscle-biopsy specimens from patients with Duchenne's and Becker's muscular dystrophy. *N Engl J Med* 318:1363-1368

Hwang SLH, Gilboa E (1984): Expression of genes introduced into cells by retroviral infection is more efficient than that of genes introduced into cells by DNA transfection. *J Virol* 50:417-424

Ibraghimov-Beskrovnaya O, Ervasti JM, Leveille CJ, Slaughter CA, Sernett SW, Campbell KP (1992): Primary structure of dystrophin-associated glycoproteins linking dystrophin to the extracellular matrix. *Nature* 355:696-702

Kim JW, Closs EI, Albritton LM, Cunningham JM (1991): Transport of cationic amino acids by the mouse ecotropic retrovirus receptor. *Nature* 352:725-728

Koenig M, Hoffman EP, Bertelson CJ, Monaco AP, Feener C, Kunkel LM (1987): Complete cloning of the Duchenne muscular dystrophy (DMD) cDNA and preliminary genomic organisation of the DMD gene in normal and affected individuals. *Cell* 50:509-517

Koenig M, Monaco AP, Kunkel LM (1988): The complete sequence of dystrophin predicts a rod-shaped cytoskeletal protein. *Cell* 53:219-228

Kozak SL, Kabat D (1990): Ping-pong amplification of a retroviral vector achieves high-level gene expression: human growth hormone production. *J Virol* 64:3500-3508

Kulkosky J, Jones KS, Katz RA, Mack JPG, Skalka AM (1992): Residues critical for retroviral integrative recombination in a region that is highly conserved among retroviral/retrotransposon integrases and bacterial insertion sequence transposases. *Mol Cell Biol* 12:2331-2338

Ledley, FD (1990): Clinical application of somatic gene therapy in inborn errors of metabolism. *J Inher Metab Dis* 13:597-616

Lee CC, Pearlman JA, Chamberlain JS, Caskey CT (1991): Expression of recombinant dystrophin and its localisation to the cell membrane. *Nature* 349:334-336

Love DR, Flint TJ, Genet SA, Middleton-Price HR, Davies KE (1991): Becker muscular dystrophy patient with large intragenic dystrophin deletion: implications for functional minigenes and gene therapy. *J Med Genet* 28:860-864

Lynch CM, Miller AD (1991): Production of high-titer helper virus-free retroviral vectors by cocultivation of packaging cells with different host ranges. *J Virol*

65:3887-3890

Mann R, Mulligan RC, Baltimore D (1983): Construction of a retrovirus packaging mutant and its use to produce helper free defective retrovirus. *Cell* 33:153-159

Markowitz D, Goff S, Bank A (1988): A safe packaging cell line for gene transfer: separating viral genes on two different plasmids. *J Virol* 62:1120-1124

Mathes LE, Yohn DS, Olsen RG (1977): Purification of infectious feline leukemia virus from large volumes of tissue culture fluids. *J Clin Micro* 5:372-374

McGeachie JK, Grounds MD (1987): Initiation and duration of muscle precursor replication after mild and severe injury to skeletal muscle of mice: an autoradiographic study. *Cell Tissue Res* 248:125-130

Miller AD, Rosman GJ (1989): Improved retroviral vectors for gene transfer and expression. *Biotechniques* 7:980-990

Miller AD (1990a): Progress toward human gene therapy. *Blood* 76:271-278

Miller AD (1990b): Retrovirus packaging cells. *Hum Gene Ther* 1:5-14

Miller DG, Adam MA, Miller AD (1990c): Gene transfer by retrovirus vectors occurs only in cells that are actively replicating at the time of infection. *Mol Cell Biol* 10:4239-4242

Morgenstern JP, Land H (1991): Choice and Manipulation of Retroviral Vectors. In: *Gene Transfer and Expression Protocols*. Methods in Molecular Biology, Vol.7:181-205. Murray EJ, ed. Clifton, NJ: Humana Press

Nonaka I (1991): Progressive muscular dystrophy with particular reference to muscle regeneration. *Acta Paediatr Jpn* 33:222-227

Ohlendieck K, Campbell KP (1991): Dystrophin constitutes 5% of membrane cytoskeleton in skeletal muscle. *FEBS Lett* 283:230-234

Partridge TA, Morgan JE, Coulton GR, Hoffman EP, Kunkel LM (1989): Conversion of *mdx* myofibers from dystrophin-negative to -positive by injection of normal myoblasts. *Nature* 337:176-179

Partridge TA (1991a): Myoblast transfer: a possible therapy for inherited myopathies? *Muscle Nerve* 14:197-212

Partridge TA (1991b): Animal models of muscular dystrophy - what can they teach us? *Neuropath Appl Neurobiol* 17:353-363

Petropoulos CJ, Payne W, Salter DW, Hughes SH (1992): Appropriate in vivo expression of a muscle-specific promoter by using avian retroviral vectors for gene transfer. *J Virol* 66:3391-3397

Roses AD (1988): Mutants in Duchenne muscular dystrophy. Implications for prevention. *Arch Neurol* 45:84-85

Scarpa M, Caskey CT (1989): The use of retroviral vectors in human disorders. In: *Experimental Hematology Today* - 1988, 81-91. Baum SJ, Dicke KA, Lotzova E, Pluznik DH, eds. New York: Springer-Verlag

Sicinski P, Geng Y, Ryder-Cook AS, Barnard EA, Darlison MG, Barnard PJ (1989): The molecular basis of muscular dystrophy in the *mdx* mouse: a point mutation. *Science* 244:1578-1580

Stedman HH, Sweeney HL, Shrager JB, Maguire HC, Panettieri RA, Petrof B, Narusawa M, Leferovich JM, Sladky JT, Kelly AM (1991): The *mdx* mouse diaphragm reproduces the degenerative changes of Duchenne muscular dystrophy. *Nature* 352:536-539

Strauss WM, Jaenisch R (1992): Molecular complementation of a collagen mutation in mammalian cells using yeast artificial chromosomes. *EMBO J* 11:417-421

Suzuki A, Yoshida M, Yamamoto H, Ozawa E (1992): Glycoprotein-binding site of dystrophin is confined to the cysteine-rich domain and the first half of the carboxy-terminal domain. *FEBS Lett* 308:154-160

Valentine BA, Cooper BJ, Cummings JF, DeLahunta A (1990): Canine X-linked muscular dystrophy: morphologic lesions. *J Neurol Sci* 97:1-23

Varmus HE (1982): Form and function of retroviral proviruses. *Science* 216:812-820

Wells DJ, Wells KE, Walsh FS, Davies KE, Goldspink G, Love DR, Chan-Thomas P, Dunckley MG, Piper T, Dickson G (1992): Human dystrophin expression corrects the myopathic phenotype in transgenic *mdx* mice. *Hum Mol Genet* 1:35-40

Weiss R, Teich N, Varmus H, Coffin J (1984): *RNA Tumor Viruses*. Cold Spring Harbor: Cold Spring Harbor Laboratory

Wessel HB (1990): Dystrophin: a clinical perspective. *Ped Neurol* 6:3-12

Wolff JA, Malone RW, Williams P, Chong W, Acsadi G, Jani A, Felgner PL (1990): Direct gene transfer into mouse muscle in vivo. *Science* 247:1465-1468

Yoshimoto T, Yoshimoto E, Meruelo D (1992): Enhanced gene expression of the murine ecotropic retroviral receptor and its human homolog in proliferating cells. *J Virol* 66:4377-4381

Keyword Index

This index was established according to the keywords supplied by the editor. Page numbers refer to the beginning of the chapter.

RELATED TITLES

Steroid Hormone Receptors
Basic and Clinical Aspects
V. K. Moudgil, Editor
1993   536 Pages   Hardcover   ISBN 0-8176-3694-3

The Polymerase Chain Reaction
Kary B. Mullis, François Ferré, and Richard A. Gibbs, Editors
1994   432 Pages
Hardcover   ISBN 0-8176-3607-2
Softcover   ISBN 0-8176-3750-8

Gene Expression
General and Cell-Type-Specific
Michael Karin, Editior
1993   320 Pages   Hardcover   ISBN 0-8176-3605-6

The Search for Antiviral Drugs
Case Histories from Concept to Clinic
Julian Adams and Vincent J. Merluzzi, Editors
1993   256 Pages   Hardcover   ISBN 0-8176-3606-4

Cytotoxic Cells
Recognition, Effector Function, Generation, and Methods
M. V. Sitkovsky and P. A. Henkart, Editors
1993   544 Pages   Hardcover   ISBN 0-8176-3608-0

RELATED TITLES

Angiogenesis
Key Principles • Science • Technology • Medicine
R. Steiner, P. B. Weisz, and R. Langer, Editors
1992   494 Pages   Hardcover   ISBN 0-8176-2674-3

DNA Methylation
Molecular Biology and Biological Significance
J.-P. Jost and H. P. Saluz, Editors
1993   572 Pages   Hardcover   ISBN 0-8176-2778-2

Tissue Engineering
Current Perspectives
Eugene Bell, Editor
1993   256 Pages   Hardcover   ISBN 0-8176-3687-0

Peptides
Design, Synthesis, and Biological Activity
Channa Basava and G. M. Anantharamaiah, Editors
1994   320 Pages   Hardcover   ISBN 0-8176-3703-6

Tissue Culture Techniques
An Introduction
By Bernice M. Martin
1994
Hardcover   ISBN 0-8176-3718-4
Softcover   ISBN 0-8176-3643-9